D1287543

Clinical
Reproductive
Medicine

CLINICAL REPRODUCTIVE MEDICINE

Edited by

Bryan D. Cowan, M.D.
Professor and Director
Division of Reproductive Endocrinology
Department of Obstetrics and Gynecology
University of Mississippi Medical Center
Jackson, Mississippi

David B. Seifer, M.D.
Director, Division of Reproductive
Endocrinology and Infertility
Associate Professor, Department of
Obstetrics and Gynecology
The Ohio State University Medical Center
Columbus, Ohio

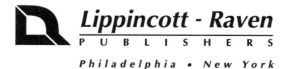

Lippincott - Raven
P U B L I S H E R S

Philadelphia • New York

Acquisitions Editor: Lisa McAllister
Developmental Editor: Rebecca Irwin Diehl
Manufacturing Manager: Dennis Teston
Production Manager: Lawrence Bernstein
Production Editor: Bob Berkel
Cover Designer: Ede Dreikurs
Indexer: Victoria Boyle
Compositor: Lippincott–Raven Electronic Production
Printer: Maple-Vail Press

Printed in the United States of America

9 8 7 6 5 4 3 2 1

Library of Congress Cataloging-in-Publication Data

Clinical reproductive medicine / Bryan D. Cowan, David B. Seifer,
    editors.
        p. cm.
    Includes bibliographical references and index.
    ISBN 0-397-51186-8
    1. Female infertility—Treatment.   2. Human reproduction—Endocrine aspects.
3. Human reproductive technology.   I. Cowan, Bryan D., 1949–   . II. Seifer, David B., 1955–
    [DNLM: 1. Reproduction—physiology.   2. Endocrine Diseases—physiopathology.
3. Infertility—therapy.   4. Reproduction Techniques.   5. Reproductive Medicine.
WQ 205 C64056 1997]
RG201.C57   1997
618.1'78—dc20
DNLM/DLC
For Library of Congress   96-28717
                                                                        CIP

To our parents for a legacy of intellectual curiosity and love and to
Harriette (bdc)
and
Cindy, Ben and Charlie (dbs)
who remain our most valued partners in this great adventure.

Contents

Contributors ix

Preface xi

Section I: Endocrinology

1. Neuroregulation of the HPO Axis 3
Victoria M. Sopelak

2. Steroid Biosynthesis 11
Bryan D. Cowan

3. Reproductive Peptide Hormones 21
Bryan D. Cowan

4. Ovarian Phylogeny 29
Halina P. Wiczyk

5. Normal and Abnormal Sexual Development 37
Patricia E. Bailey

6. Disorders of Puberty 49
Cynthia H. Meyers-Seifer and David B. Seifer

7. Regulation of the Ovarian-Menstrual Cycle 61
Victoria M. Sopelak

8. Dysfunctional Uterine Bleeding 69
Bryan D. Cowan

9. Amenorrhea 75
Bryan D. Cowan

10. Hyperprolactinemia 85
Vivian Lewis

11. Androgen Excess Disorders 95
Stephen R. Lincoln

12. Menopause 103
Delbert L. Booher

13. Dynamic Testing of Glandular Reserve 115
Lisa Barrie Schwartz and David B. Seifer

14. Oral Contraceptives 131
Michael D. Fox

Section Two: Reproduction

15. Gametogenesis 143
Victoria M. Sopelak

16. Implantation Biology 159
Bryan D. Cowan

17. Infertility Evaluation 167
Bryan D. Cowan

18. Endometriosis 175
Steve N. London

19. Mullerian Anomalies 181
Harriette L. Hampton

20. Ectopic Pregnancy 191
Bryan D. Cowan

21. Reproductive Surgery 201
Michael S. Opsahl and Edwin D. Robins

22. Gamete Technologies 213
Alan S. Penzias

23. Gonadotropin-Releasing Hormone Analogs 225
John D. Isaacs, Jr.

24. Ovulation Induction: Clomiphene Citrate and Menotropins 231
John D. Isaacs, Jr.

25. Recurrent Pregnancy Loss 239
Michael J. Gast

26. Reproductive Immunology 247
William A. Bennett

27. Molecular Technologies in Reproductive Medicine 267
Cecil A. Long

Appendix 281

Index 283

Contributors

Patricia E. Bailey, M.D. (5) Normal and Abnormal Sexual Development. *Director, Pediatric and Adolescent Gynecology Services, Department of Obstetrics and Gynecology, Bay State Medical Center, Springfield, Massachusetts.*

William A. Bennett, Ph.D. (26) Reproductive Immunology. *Assistant Professor, Division of Reproductive Endocrinology, Department of Obstetrics and Gynecology, University of Mississippi Medical Center, Jackson, Mississippi.*

Delbert L. Booher, M.D. (12) Menopause. *Assistant Professor, Department of Obstetrics and Gynecology, The Cleveland Clinic Foundation, Health Sciences Center for the Ohio State University; Associate Clinical Professor, Department of Reproductive Biology, Case Western Reserve University; Director, Program for Mature Women, Department of Gynecology and Obstetrics, Cleveland Clinic Foundation, Cleveland, Ohio.*

Bryan D. Cowan, M.D. (2) Steroid Biosynthesis; (3) Reproductive Peptide Hormones; (8) Dysfunctional Uterine Bleeding; (9) Amenorrhea; (16) Implantation Biology; (17) Infertility Evaluation; (20) Ectopic Pregnancy. *Professor and Director, Division of Reproductive Endocrinology, Department of Obstetrics and Gynecology, University of Mississippi Medical Center, Jackson, Mississippi.*

Michael D. Fox, M.D. (14) Oral Contraceptives. *Reproductive Endocrinology, Saint Vincent's Hospital and Memorial Hospital, Jacksonville, Florida.*

Michael J. Gast, M.D., Ph.D. (25) Recurrent Pregnancy Loss. *Associate Professor, Clinical Obstetrics and Gynecology, Washington University School of Medicine, St. Louis, Missouri; Vice President, Women's Healthcare, Research and Development, Wyeth-Ayerst Research, Radnor, Pennsylvania.*

Harriette L. Hampton, M.D. (19) Müllerian Anomalies. *Division of Reproductive Endocrinology, Department of Obstetrics and Gynecology, University of Mississippi Medical Center, Jackson, Mississippi.*

John D. Isaacs, Jr., M.D. (23) Gonadotropin-Releasing Hormone Analogs; (24) Ovulation Induction: Clomiphene Citrate and Menotropins. *Assistant Professor, Division of Reproductive Endocrinology, Department of Obstetrics and Gynecology, University of Mississippi Medical Center, Jackson, Mississippi.*

Vivian Lewis, M.D. (10) Hyperprolactinemia. *Division of Reproductive Endocrinology, Department of Obstetrics and Gynecology, University of Rochester Medical Center, Strong Memorial Hospital, Rochester, New York.*

Stephen R. Lincoln, M.D. (11) Androgen Excess Disorders. *Assistant Professor, Division of Reproductive Endocrinology and Infertility, Department of Obstetrics and Gynecology, University of Tennessee at Memphis, Memphis, Tennessee.*

Steve N. London, M.D. (18) Endometriosis. *Professor and Chair, Department of Obstetrics and Gynecology, Louisiana State University Medical Center, Shreveport, Louisiana.*

Cecil A. Long, M.D. (27) Molecular Technologies in Reproductive Medicine. *Assistant Professor, Department of Obstetrics and Gynecology, ART Program at Birmingham, Birmingham, Alabama.*

Cynthia H. Meyers-Seifer, M.D. (6) Disorders of Puberty. *Assistant Professor of Clinical Pediatrics, Department of Endocrinology, The Ohio State University, Children's Hospital, Columbus, Ohio.*

Michael S. Opsahl, M.D. (21) Reproductive Surgery. *Clinical Associate Professor of Obstetrics and Gynecology, Uniformed Services University of Health Sciences, Genetics and* In Vitro *Fertilization Institute, Fairfax, Virginia.*

Alan S. Penzias, M.D. (22) Gamete Technologies. *Assistant Professor of Obstetrics and Gynecology, Director,* In Vitro *Fertilization, Division of Reproductive Endocrinology, Tufts University School of Medicine, Boston, Massachusetts.*

Edwin D. Robins, M.D., L.C.D.R., M.C., U.S.N.R. (21) Reproductive Surgery. *Institute of Reproductive Medicine and Science, Saint Barnabas Medical Center, Livingston, New Jersey.*

Lisa Barrie Schwartz, M.D. (13) Dynamic Testing of Glandular Reserve. *Assistant Professor of Reproductive Endocrinology, Department of Obstetrics and Gynecology, New York University Medical Center, New York, New York.*

David B. Seifer, M.D. (6) Disorders of Puberty; (13) Dynamic Testing of Glandular Reserve. *Director, Division of Reproductive Endocrinology and Infertility, Associate Professor, Department of Obstetrics and Gynecology, The Ohio State University Medical Center, Columbus, Ohio.*

Victoria M. Sopelak, Ph.D. (1) Neuroregulation of the HPO Axis; (7) Regulation of the Ovarian-Menstrual Cycle; (15) Gametogenesis. *Associate Professor, Department of Obstetrics and Gynecology, Division of Reproductive Endocrinology, University of Mississippi Medical Center, Jackson, Mississippi.*

Halina P. Wiczyk, M.D. (4) Ovarian Phylogeny. *Chief and Assistant Professor, Division of Reproductive Endocrinology, Department of Obstetrics and Gynecology, Bay State Medical Center, Springfield, Massachusetts.*

Preface

Any practitioner of reproductive medicine understands the emotional difficulties that our patients confront daily. Infertile couples often suffer the intense anguish of unfulfilled hopes for a family. Many women with acquired or congenital reproductive endocrinopathies contend with life-long clinical and often psychological manifestations of their diseases. Our special responsibilities to each of them include genuine and meaningful counseling, care, and diligence. It is our intention that this textbook will guide others in those endeavors.

Clinical Reproductive Medicine presents to students and physicians contemporary clinical applications of reproductive medicine. It is intended for the general practitioner, internist, and general obstetrician-gynecologist. There are two sections: the first contains the underlying physiology and pathophysiology of reproductive endocrinopathies while the second section focuses upon the treatments of infertility. This organizational scheme comfortably compliments the clinical management of patients. Each treatment plan presents an evidence-based recommendation and discusses important clinical treatments that are both logical and common. The fundamentals that guide our present-day clinical decisions are emphasized to the end that we may forge our future considerations on evidence and knowledge.

Acknowledgments

We wish to acknowledge the teachers who developed our excitement in this practice of reproductive biology and medicine. Joseph C. Daniel, Jr., Ph.D., Dwain D. Hagerman, M.D., and Frederick Naftolin, M.D., D.Phil. showed us the discipline of reproductive science and the rigors of scientific thought. Winfred L. Wiser, M.D. and Alan H. DeCherney, M.D. helped to mature our compassionate delivery of clinical care.

SECTION I

Endocrinology

Clinical Reproductive Medicine,
Edited by Bryan D. Cowan and David B. Seifer
Lippincott-Raven Publishers, Philadelphia © 1997

CHAPTER 1

Neuroregulation of the HPO Axis

Victoria M. Sopelak

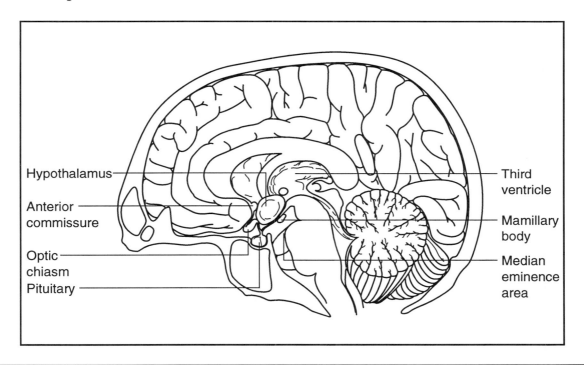

Anatomy and Secretion
  Hypothalamus
  Pituitary
  Ovary
Hypothalamic-Pituitary Function

Menstrual Cyclicity and the Hypothalamic-Pituitary Axis
Conclusion
Suggested Reading

V. M. Sopelak: Department of Obstetrics and Gynecology, Division of Reproductive Endocrinology, University of Mississippi Medical Center, Jackson MS 39216

Reproductive function in the human female is dependent on complex interactions between the central nervous system (CNS), pituitary gland, ovaries, and the accessory reproductive tract organs. The cascade of events culminating in normal menstrual cyclicity begins with events in the hypothalamus. This chapter will review the anatomy and function of the hypothalamic-pituitary complex and describe how these ultimately regulate ovarian function.

ANATOMY AND SECRETION

Hypothalamus

The hypothalamus is a portion of the diencephalon (forebrain) lying below the third ventricle between the optic chiasma, the unpaired infundibulum (median eminence), which extends by way of the infundibular stalk (hypophyseal stalk) into the posterior lobe of the hypophysis (pituitary), and the paired mamillary bodies (Fig. 1-1). It is bounded anteriorly by the lamina terminalis, anterior commissure, and optic chiasm; posteriorly by the brainstem; and dorsally by the thalamus, which is adjacent to the third ventricle. The hypothalamus is extensively connected with the brain and pituitary (anterior and posterior) via circulatory and neural pathways, to be described subsequently. The hypothalamus is composed of nerve cells grouped into a large number of bundles called nuclei (Fig. 1-2). The nuclei of the hypothalamus with important reproductive function include the supraoptic and paraventricular nuclei, the preoptic area, the mediobasal hypothalamus, the median eminence, the arcuate nuclei, and the suprachiasmatic nuclei.

The supraoptic and paraventricular nuclei have direct neural connection with the posterior pituitary (Fig. 1-3). The supraoptic nuclei secretes mainly vasopressin whereas oxytocin is secreted predominantly by the paraventricular nuclei and transported by nerve fibers to the posterior pituitary for storage and release. In contrast, other nuclei produce the releasing and inhibitory factors, such as gonadotropin-releasing hormone (GnRH), thyrotropin-releasing hormone (TRH), growth hormone release–inhibiting hormone or somatostatin, corticotropin-releasing hormone (CRH), and growth hormone–releasing hormone (GHRH), which control anterior pituitary secretion (Table 1-1). These substances are transported to the anterior pituitary via the blood portal system.

The functional connection of the hypothalamus with the anterior lobe of the pituitary is established by a system of hypothalamohypophysial blood vessels (see Fig. 1-3). The hypothalamic factors are transported along the nerve fibers to the median eminence where they permeate into the capillary walls, enter into the portal circulation, and are carried to the anterior pituitary (see Figs. 1-2 and 1-3). These factors then affect endocrine cells of the pituitary, eliciting specific hormonal responses.

The hypothalamus also has intrahypothalamic neural connections, afferent fiber connections with the midbrain and limbic systems, and efferent fiber connections with the midbrain and limbic systems as well as with the posterior lobe of the pituitary. An example of the multitude of communication pathways can be seen in the median eminence (infundibulum). Blood is supplied to the median eminence via the superior hypophyseal arteries (see Fig. 1-3). Venous drainage from the median eminence is via the portal veins to the anterior pituitary. The capillary plexus in the lower portion of the pituitary stalk is supplied by the inferior hypophyseal artery and is drained by short portal veins that enter the pituitary directly. Reverse blood flow from the pituitary to the median eminence can occur by way of the short portal vessels that drain both the anterior and posterior pituitary and may provide short-loop feedback control of the hypothalamus. In addition, the median eminence itself is divided into areas: the ependymal layer (or zona interna), subependymal layer (fibrous layer), and palisade layer composed of cells similar to those found in the region of the third ventricle

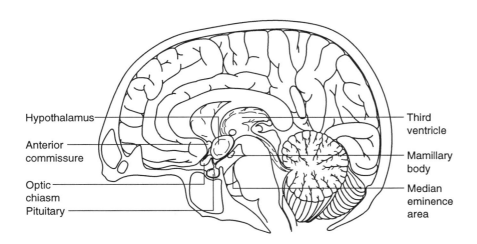

FIG. 1-1. A sagittal section of the human hypothalamic-pituitary unit showing the relationship to the optic chiasm, third ventricle, and brain.

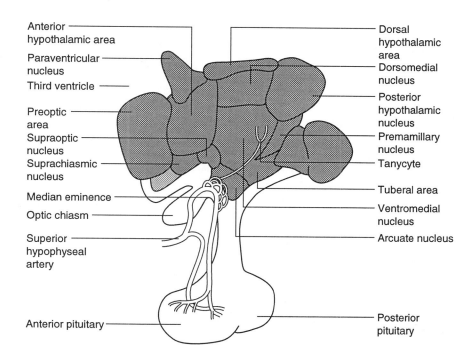

FIG. 1-2. Diagrammatic representation of the hypothalamus showing the relative positions of the major nuclei, the vascular components of the median eminence, and the attachment to the pituitary gland.

(Fig. 1-4). The ependymal cells in this area are modified and called tanycytes (see Figs. 1-2 and 1-4). Each tanycyte has numerous microvilli, can extend throughout the entire width of the median eminence, ends in the capillary plexus in the palisade layer, and may carry substances to and/or from the third ventricle or from the cerebrospinal fluid into the portal circulation. As depicted in Fig. 1-4, other neural interactions are possible.

The close proximity of aminergic and peptidergic (releasing-factor producing) neurons, glial cells, and other nerve endings of unknown origin may facilitate multifactoral hypothalamic control. A portion of the median eminence is covered by specialized glial cells known as astrocytes, which are replaced by the pericapillaries in the palisade layer, forming the portal capillaries. These capillaries are fenestrated, allowing passage of fairly large

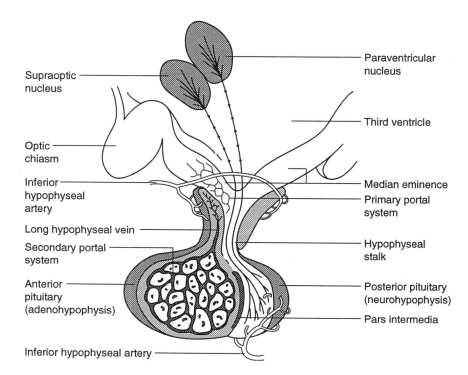

FIG. 1-3. Sagittal depiction of the pituitary and its important anatomic features. Hypothalamic hormones are delivered to the anterior lobe via the median eminence and hypothalamic-portal circulation. Cell bodies aggregated in the paraventricular and supraoptic nuclei of the hypothalamus extend into the posterior pituitary where release of vasopressin, oxytocin, and neurophysins occurs.

TABLE 1-1. *Anterior pituitary and principal hypophysiotropic factors*

Anterior pituitary hormone	Principal hypophysiotropic controlling factor
LH	GnRH = gonadotropin-releasing hormone
FSH	GnRH = gonadotropin-releasing hormone
GH	GHRH = growth hormone–releasing hormone Somatostatin or growth hormone–inhibiting hormone
TSH	TRH = thyrotropin-releasing hormone
PRL	PRF = prolactin-releasing factor & ? TRH (thyrotropin-releasing factor) & ? VIP (vasoactive intestinal polypeptide) PIH = prolactin release–inhibiting hormone (dopamine)
POMC, ACTH, β-LPH, etc.	CRH = corticotropin-releasing hormone

LH, luteinizing hormone; FSH, follicle-stimulating hormone; GH, growth hormone; TSH, thyrotropin-stimulating hormone; PRL, prolactin; POMC, proopiomelanocortin; ACTH, adrenocorticotropic hormone; β-LPH, β-lipotropin.

molecules, and are outside of the blood–brain barrier. Thus, various portions of the hypothalamus can receive and send a diversity of signals.

Pituitary

The pituitary gland lies in the sella turcica at the base of the brain. It is connected with the hypothalamus by the hypophyseal stalk (pituitary stalk). The pituitary is phys- iologically divided into the adenohypophysis (anterior) and neurohypophysis (posterior) pituitary with a small, avascular zone, the pars intermedia, dividing these two regions (see Fig. 1-3).

The anterior pituitary gland is composed of five different types of cell types, based on immunocytologic and ultrastructural findings. These cells in the anterior pituitary produce the six known anterior pituitary hormones (Tables 1-1 and 1-2). The two cell types in the acidophilic series, somatotropes and lactotropes (mammotropes), produce growth hormone (GH) and prolactin (PRL), respectively. Three other cell types—the corticotropes, thyrotropes, and gonadotropes— belong to the basophilic series. The corticotropes produce adrenocorticotropin (ACTH) and other fractions of the proopiomelanocortin molecule (POMC), such as β-lipotropin (β-LPH) and endorphins. Thyrotropes synthesize thyroid-stimulating hormone (TSH) and the gonadotropes produce luteinizing hormone (LH) and follicle-stimulating hormone (FSH). Secretion of these six hormones by the anterior pituitary is primarily controlled by the hypothalamic releasing and inhibitory factors secreted within the hypothalamus and transferred to the anterior pituitary through the hypothalamic-hypophyseal portal vessels (see Figs. 1-2 and 1-3, Tables 1-2 and 1-3). However, other substances, produced locally (such as β-endorphins) or at distant sites (such as estradiol), may influence pituitary cell production and secretion of trophic hormones (discussed subsequently).

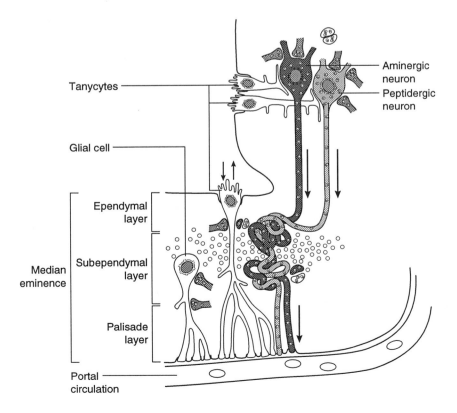

FIG. 1-4. Cellular layers of the median eminence and the probable arrangement of ependymal tanycytes, glial cells, and aminergic and peptidergic neurons. These cellular associations allow for communication and transport of substances to and from the third ventricle, cerebrospinal fluid, other hypothalamic nuclei, and the portal circulation.

Tanycytes

Glial cell

Aminergic neuron

Peptidergic neuron

Ependymal layer

Subependymal layer

Median eminence

Palisade layer

Portal circulation

TABLE 1-2. *Anterior pituitary cell types and primary hormones produced*

Pituitary cell type	Primary hormone produced
Gonadotropes	LH = luteinizing hormone
	FSH = follicle-stimulating hormone
Somatotropes	GH = growth hormone
Thyrotropes	TSH = thyroid-stimulating hormone (thyrotropin)
Lactotropes	PRL = prolactin
Corticotropes	POMC = proopiomelanocortin (precursor molecule)
	1) ACTH = adrenocorticotropic hormone
	a) α-MSH = α-melanocyte-stimulating hormone
	b) CLIP = corticotropin-like intermediate lobe peptide
	2) γ-MSH = γ-melanocyte-stimulating hormone
	3) β-LPH = β-lipotropin
	a) γ-LPH = γ-lipotropin
	b) β-endorphin

TABLE 1-3. *Hypothalamic controlling factors and their principal sites of production*

Hypothalamic controlling factor	Principal hypothalamic production site
GnRH	Arcuate nucleus
	Preoptic area
	Mediobasal hypothalamus
GnRH	Arcuate nucleus
	Median eminence
	Pituitary stalk
Somatostatin (growth hormone release-inhibiting hormone)	Paraventricular nucleus
	Ventromedial–arcuate complex
	Suprachiasmatic nucleus
	Ventral premammillary nuclei
TRH	Paraventricular nucleus
PRF	? Paraventricular nucleus
Dopamine (prolactin release–inhibiting hormone)	Arcuate nucleus
	Paraventricular nucleus

GnRH, gonadotropin-releasing hormone; TRH, thyrotropin-releasing hormone; PRF, prolactin-releasing factor.

The posterior pituitary (neurohypophysis) includes the neural (hypophyseal) stalk, the neural lobe, and the median eminence (specialized neural tissue at the base of the hypothalamus forming the crucial region for the transfer of pituitary-regulating neurosecretion to the anterior pituitary) (Fig. 1-3). The two hormones secreted by the posterior pituitary, vasopressin (AVP) and oxytocin (OT), are synthesized in the cell bodies of the supraoptic and paraventricular nuclei, packaged in granules with their respective neurophysines, transported down the axons, and stored in the terminal regions of the axons until appropriate stimulation causes their release from the posterior pituitary (Figs. 1-3 and 1-5). The neuropeptides are released from the secretory granules by exocytosis. This process involves the fusion of the neurosecretory granule membrane and a small portion of the cell membrane at the axon terminal. The granule contents are then extruded into the extracellular space where it enters the circulation. Recently, it

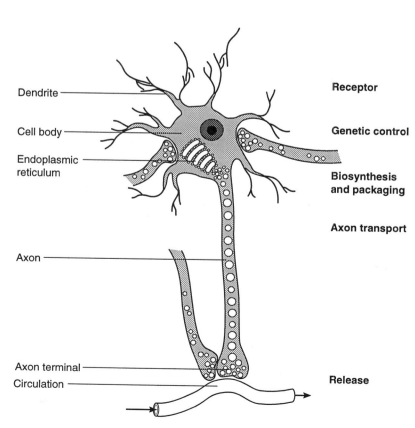

FIG. 1-5. Neurotransmitters and neurohormones are synthesized by enzymes in the cell body, packaged into secretory granules, transported down the axons, and stored in the axon terminals. Appropriate stimulation causes release (exocytosis) of the granule's contents into the circulation.

was found that oxytocin-producing neurons also contain cholecystokinin and that vasopressin-producing neurons also contain dynorphin. The importance of coexisting peptides within certain neurons is still under investigation.

Ovary

The ovary is composed of follicles containing oocytes as well as corpora luteal and stromal tissue. Each follicle in turn is composed of an outer layer of theca cells that surrounds the inner granulosa cell layer. The theca and granulosa cells are the primary steroid-secreting components within the ovary. These cells have gonadotropin receptors and respond to stimuli from the pituitary. The theca cells, in response to LH stimulation, synthesize androgens. The major products of ovarian androgen synthesis are dehydroepiandrosterone (DHEA) and androstenedione. In addition, the theca cells secrete small amounts of progesterone and testosterone. The granulosa cells, initially in response to FSH stimulation, metabolize the theca-derived androgens to estrogens by aromatization (primarily during the follicular phase) and synthesize progesterone during the luteal phase of the menstrual cycle. After ovulation, the theca and granulosa cells derived from the dominant follicle are transformed by LH into luteal cells, which primarily secrete progesterone and some estrogens. In addition to steroid secretion, the ovary also produces oocyte maturation inhibitor, growth factors, interleukins, inhibins, activins, and follistatin.

HYPOTHALAMIC-PITUITARY FUNCTION

The hypothalamus plays a critical role in the control of anterior and posterior pituitary secretion. As previously mentioned, the six known anterior pituitary hormones are under the control of one or more hypothalamic peptidergic factors. Additionally, they may be influenced by hormone feedback from steroid-producing tissues, biogenic amines, and other neurotransmitters found in the hypothalamus and at other diffuse neuroendocrine sites.

Table 1-1 lists the pituitary hormones and the principle hypophysiotropic factors that control their secretion. Many of the releasing hormones are secreted by hypothalamic cells within particular nuclei, whereas other releasing hormones are more widely distributed within the hypothalamus. The principal sites of production of the hypothalamic controlling factors is presented in Table 1-3. The axons from these nuclei traverse different routes before reaching the median eminence and discharging their releasing factors into the hypothalamic-pituitary portal circulation. The structure of prolactin-releasing hormone has not been identified; however, under experimental conditions, both thyrotropin-releasing hormone and vasoactive intestinal polypeptide (VIP) can bring about the release of prolactin.

Our understanding of hypothalamic-pituitary physiology is constantly changing. The close proximity of the various cell bodies, nerve axons, and terminals within the hypothalamus, in addition to a variety of biogenic amines and other neurotransmitters found there, may lead to discovery of other controlling mechanisms. Many cells produce both peptides and neurotransmitters such as the coexistence of neuropeptide Y and γ-aminobutyric acid (GABA) in somatostatin- producing cells. The functional significance of many of these types of relationships remains unclear.

MENSTRUAL CYCLICITY AND THE HYPOTHALAMIC-PITUITARY AXIS

The pituitary gonadotropic hormones LH and FSH are responsible for follicular development, oocyte maturation, ovulation, and luteal function during the menstrual cycle. LH and FSH consists of two subunits (α and β), which are synthesized as precursors that undergo posttranslational modifications and glycosylation (see Chapter 3). The individual subunits have little biological activity.

The hypothalamus controls pituitary secretion of LH and FSH through the decapeptide known as gonadotropin-releasing hormone (GnRH) produced in the region of the arcuate nucleus and possibly in the preoptic-anterior hypothalamic area in the human. GnRH is synthesized as part of a larger 92-amino-acid precursor molecule. This molecule is broken down into GnRH, a 56-amino-acid peptide termed gonadotropin-releasing hormone–associated peptide (GAP, with undetermined function), and other fragments. GnRH is packaged into granules within the Golgi apparatus and transported by axonal flow to terminals in the median eminence. GnRH is released in a pulsatile fashion. It is transported to the pituitary via the hypothalamic-pituitary circulation (see Fig. 1-3).

Within the anterior pituitary, GnRH binds to a plasma membrane receptor on the gonadotropes and initiates a cascade of intracellular events. GnRH binding to its receptor alters intracellular and extracellular calcium within the gonadotrope, regulates its own receptor population, and causes synthesis (via gene expression) of LH and FSH (see Chapter 3). GnRH membrane receptor concentration, maximal expression of the LH- and FSH-β subunit genes, and gonadotropin release are all determined by the amplitude and frequency of pituitary GnRH stimulation.

The importance of a pulsatile pattern of GnRH stimulation of the gonadotrope has been clearly demonstrated in monkeys that have lesions created in the arcuate region of the hypothalamus. During continuous infusion, LH and FSH secretion may be initially stimulated, but this is followed by a decline in the gonadotropins and cessation of menstrual cyclicity. Pituitary desensitization may be due to depletion of cellular LH and FSH, loss of GnRH receptors, and changes in calcium levels. It is postulated that pituitary downregulation occurs because most receptors are occupied with GnRH after continuous stimulation and are internalized. Thus, the gonadotroph is essentially "blind" to further GnRH stimulation because the occupied receptors have been removed from the membrane surface.

The reason that GnRH is secreted episodically is unknown. Presumably the GnRH pulse generator is located in the medial basal hypothalamus within the vicinity of the arcuate nucleus. There is evidence that several neurotransmitters, including norepinephrine, dopamine, β-endorphin, and possibly GABA, influence GnRH secretion. Their effects may be stimulatory or inhibitory, depending on the endocrine parameters. It appears that norepinephrine is released in the vicinity of the GnRH pulse generator and is synchronous with GnRH release from the median eminence. Because α-adrenergic blockers result in suppression of GnRH and LH pulses in the primate, norepinephrine may play a role in GnRH pulsatility. Dopamine, a suppressor of prolactin synthesis and release, also inhibits the release of LH. The endogenous opiate β-endorphin inhibits LH and FSH secretion by reducing GnRH release into the hypophyseal portal circulation. When levels of estradiol are low, during days 1–5 of the menstrual cycle, hypothalamic β-endorphin concentrations are also low. During the late follicular phase, when estradiol is high, or during the luteal phase, in the presence of both estradiol and progesterone, hypothalamic β-endorphin release increases although pituitary β-endorphin release is unaffected by these ovarian changes. Administration of naloxone, an opiate antagonist, will increase gonadotropin release by decreasing the inhibition of GnRH secretion caused by the endogenous opioid peptides. This naloxone-induced increase in gonadotropins is maximal in the presence of gonadal steroids, indicating that the inhibitory influence that endogenous opioids exert on GnRH secretion is influenced by gonadal steroids.

The pituitary capacity to secrete LH and FSH is dependent on two functionally separate pools of gonadotropin. One pool is represented as the acutely releasable forms of LH and FSH. The second pool (reserve) is released only after sustained GnRH stimulation and probably reflects new gonadotropin synthesis. During the early follicular phase, when estradiol (E_2) levels are low, the releasable and reserve pools of gonadotropins are at a minimum and the sensitivity of the gonadotrope to GnRH stimulation is at its nadir. In response to FSH, a cohort of follicles begin developing and secreting estradiol. As E_2 levels rise during the midfollicular phase, a preferential increase in the reserve pool of gonadotropins occurs. At midcycle, when E_2 concentrations are at their apex, both releasable and reserve pools of gonadotropins become maximal. During the midluteal phase, in the presence of progesterone and estrogen, gonadotrope sensitivity to GnRH is similar to that in the mid- to late follicular phase.

Each pulse of GnRH released by the hypothalamus into the hypothalamic-hypophyseal portal circulation can result in a pulse of LH and FSH. However, the secretion of LH and FSH may be divergent. Explanations for the divergence include the possibility of another FSH-releasing hormone in addition to GnRH, differences in the half-lives of LH and FSH, changes in GnRH pulse frequency and amplitude, or feedback influences of gonadal peptides, such as inhibin and activin, on gonadotropin subunit expression. FSH has a longer half-life than LH. This longer half-life often masks subsequent low-amplitude releases of FSH and makes correlating FSH response to changes in GnRH pulse frequency more difficult. Changes in the pulse frequency of GnRH can selectively regulate gonadotropin subunit gene transcription. It appears that a fast GnRH pulse frequency favors LH β-mRNA, whereas a slow frequency favors FSH β-mRNA. Nonsteroid ovarian factors may also influence FSH release. Inhibin and activin are composed of dimers (Chapter 3), are closely related members of the transforming growth factor-β (TGF-β) superfamily, and are secreted by the follicle and corpus luteum into the peripheral circulation. Inhibin has been shown to decrease FSH secretion at the level of the pituitary via long-loop feedback inhibition.

CONCLUSION

From the foregoing discussion it becomes apparent that the neuroregulation of the HPO axis is highly complex. Hypothalamic factors exert inhibitory or stimulatory influence on pituitary secretion. Inhibitory factors interact with the respective releasing factors to exert dual control over such hormones as prolactin, GH, and TSH, for instance. The actions of the hypophyseotropic hormones may not be limited to a single pituitary hormone. Examples include TRH release of TSH, as well as PRL, ACTH, and GH; GnRH release of both LH and FSH; somatostatin inhibition of GH, TSH, and other nonpituitary hormones; and dopamine inhibition of PRL, TSH, gonadotropin, and GH release. Secretion of releasing hormones is regulated by local neurotransmitters and neuropeptides, which interact with the effects of circulating hormones such as gonadal steroids. Lastly, there is additional evidence for feedback effects of hypophysiotropic factors on themselves (ultrashort-loop feedback control) and for feedback effects of anterior pituitary hormones (short-loop feedback control). Thus, the hypothalamic-pituitary unit is acted on by neurotransmitters, by feedback effects of hormones secreted by target glands, by pituitary peptide hormones, and by neuropeptide modulators.

SELECTED READING

Anatomy and Secretion

Conn PM. The molecular mechanism of gonadotropin-releasing hormone action in the pituitary. In: Knobil E, Neill JD, eds. *The Physiology of Reproduction,* 2nd ed, vol 1. New York: Raven Press, 1994;1815–1832.

Kovacs K, Horvath E. *Morphology of the Pituitary in Health and Disease.* In: Becker KL, ed. *Principles and Practice of Endocrinology and Metabolism.* Philadelphia: JB Lippincott, 1990;109–124.

Page RB. The anatomy of the hypothalamo-hypophysial complex. In: Knobil E, Neill JD, eds. *The Physiology of Reproduction,* 2nd ed, vol 1. New York: Raven Press, 1994;1527–1619.

Reichlin S. Neuroendocrinology. In: Wilson JD, Foster DW, eds. *Williams Textbook of Endocrinology,* 8th ed. Philadelphia: WB Saunders, 1992; 135–219.

Sladek JR, Sladek CD. Morphology of the endocrine brain, hypothalamus, and neurohypophysis. In: Becker KL, ed. *Principles and Practice of Endocrinology and Metabolism.* Philadelphia: JB Lippincott, 1990;92–98.

Sopelak VM. The neuroendocrine component: the hypothalamic-pituitary unit. In: Ferin M, Jewelewicz R, Warren M, eds. *The Menstrual Cycle.* New York: Oxford University Press, 1993;8–24.

Thorner MO, Vance ML, Horvath E, Kovacs K. The anterior pituitary. In: Wilson JD, Foster DW, eds. *Williams Textbook of Endocrinology,* 8th ed. Philadelphia: WB Saunders, 1992;221–310.

Speroff L, Glass RH, Kase NG, eds. Neuroendocrinology. In: *Clinical Gynecologic Endocrinology and Infertility,* 5th ed. Baltimore: Williams and Wilkins, 1994;141–181.

HPO Axis and Reproduction

Catt KJ, Pierce JG. Gonadotropic hormones of the adenohypophysis. In: Yen SSC, Jaffe RB, eds. *Reproductive Endocrinology,* 2nd ed. Philadelphia: WB Saunders, 1986;75–114.

Everett JW. Pituitary and hypothalamus: perspectives and overview. In: Knobil E, Neill JD, eds. *The Physiology of Reproduction,* 2nd ed, vol 1. New York: Raven Press, 1994;1509–1526.

Hylka VW, DiZerega GS. Reproductive hormones and their mechanism of action. In: Mishell DR, Davajan V, Lobo RA, eds. *Infertility, Contraception and Reproductive Endocrinology,* 3rd ed. Boston: Blackwell Scientific, 1991;34–52.

Kletzky OA, Lobo RA. Reproductive neuroendocrinology. In: Mishell DR, Davajan V, Lobo RA, eds. *Infertility, Contraception and Reproductive Endocrinology,* 3rd ed. Boston: Blackwell Scientific, 1991;3–33.

Rasmussen DD. The interaction between mediobasohypothalamic dopaminergic and endorphinergic neuronal systems as a key regulator of reproduction: an hypothesis. *J Endocrinol Invest* 1991;14:323–352.

Sopelak VM. Hypothalamic-pituitary-ovarian communication. In: Ferin M, Jewelewicz R, Warren M, eds. *The Menstrual Cycle.* New York: Oxford University Press, 1993;42–61.

Clinical Reproductive Medicine,
Edited by Bryan D. Cowan and David B. Seifer
Lippincott-Raven Publishers, Philadelphia © 1997

CHAPTER 2

Steroid Biosynthesis

Bryan D. Cowan

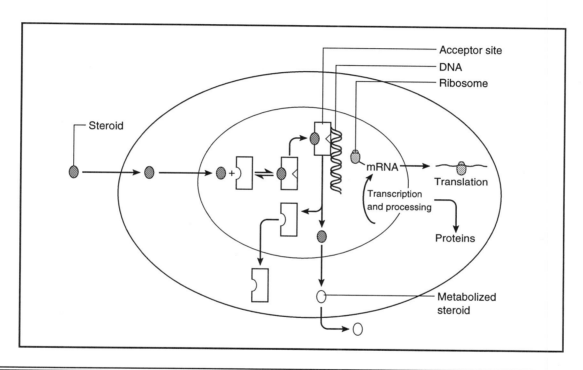

Nomenclature
Cholesterol Uptake and Utilization
Mineralocorticoid and Glucocorticoid Biosynthesis
Progesterone Biosynthesis
Androgen Biosynthesis

Estrogen Biosynthesis
Steroid Elimination
Mechanisms of Steroid Hormone Action
Suggested Reading

B. D. Cowan: Division of Reproductive Endocrinology, Department of Obstetrics and Gynecology, University of Mississippi Medical Center, Jackson MS 39216

Steroid hormones regulate several physiologic and reproductive endocrine responses. Five groups of steroid hormones (mineralocorticoid, glucocorticoid, progestin, androgen, estrogen) are recognized by the physiologic responses they induce. Mineralocorticoids and glucocorticoids regulate physiologic homeostasis during all ages of life and are produced by the adrenal glands. The mineralocorticoids promote renal tubular sodium retention, and glucocorticoids have carbohydrate-mobilizing properties as well as other peripheral effects. The reproductive hormones are principally secreted by the gonads during the reproductive times of adulthood. Progestins promote reproduction, androgens induce male secondary sexual characteristics, and estrogens induce female secondary sexual characteristics.

Steroid hormones are structurally similar to each other and arise from a common series of precursors and metabolic pathways. Adrenocortical steroid synthesis is stimulated by pituitary adrenocorticotropic hormone (ACTH). The production of sex steroids is stimulated by the tropic hormones luteinizing hormone (LH), follicle-stimulating hormone (FSH), and human chorionic gonadotropin (hCG). Steroids interact with one or more specific nuclear receptors contained in target tissues. The steroid–receptor complexes ultimately regulate tissue-specific chromatin expression and cellular activity.

NOMENCLATURE

For purposes of steroid nomenclature, the cyclopentano-phenanthrane ring represents a contrived "steroid frame" that exists on the drawing pads but does not exist naturally. This structure has four ring units attached adjacent to each other, named A, B, C, and D (Fig. 2-1). The A, B, and C rings form the familiar phenanthrane chemical structure and are joined to the additional closed 5-carbon (cyclopentano-) D ring. The carbons that constitute a 21-carbon structure are numbered as described in Fig. 2-2. Carbon 18 is added to the configuration in the "saddle" between ring C and D, and carbon 19 is added in the saddle between ring A and B. Carbons 20 and 21 are attached to the 17 position at ring D. Important steroid substitutions principally occur at carbon locations 3, 11, and 17. Additional "isomerization" reactions occur at positions 4–5, and aromatization is accomplished after enzymatic deletion of carbon 19.

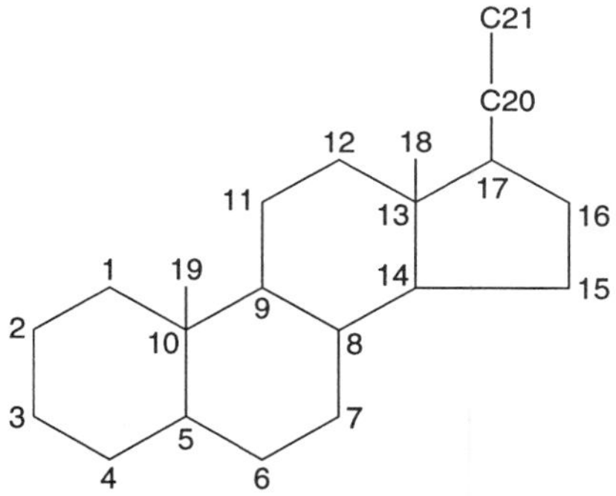

This steroid nucleus forms a geometric plane in space and as such provides steric conformation requirements for many positional substitutions. The substitutions that are oriented behind the plane of the molecule are termed α and are designated schematically as a broken or dotted line (eg, cortisol; see Fig. 2-8). The substitutions above the plane are termed β and are written with a solid line (eg, 17β-estradiol; see Fig. 2-16). Such annotation is important both chemically and biologically. For example, the naturally occurring 17β-estradiol has potent estrogen activity, but a substitution of the 17-hydroxy group renders the molecule biologically inactive.

Cholesterol is a 27-carbon steroid that undergoes side chain cleavage to yield the 21-carbon precursor compound pregnenolone. In general, mineralocorticoids, glucocorticoids, and progestins contain 21 carbons. Androgens contain 19 carbons, and estrogens lose the 19th carbon between ring A and B to form an 18-carbon structure with a completely saturated (aromatized) A ring (Table 2-1). The steroid biosynthetic pathway (Fig. 2-3) demonstrating steroid biosynthesis to aldosterone is called the mineralocorticoid pathway. Alternatively, cortisol production after 17-hydroxylation of pregnenolone is known as the glucocorticoid pathway. Removal of carbon 20 and 21 ($P450_{C17}$) transforms precursor steroids to the androgen/estrogen pathway. The pathway from cholesterol to dehydroepiandrosterone (DHEA) is referred to as the Δ5 pathway because the double bond of these precur-

FIG. 2-2. Numeric schema for steroid.

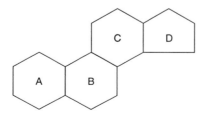

FIG. 2-1. Cyclopentanophenanthrane ring.

TABLE 2-1. *Carbon content of steroids*

Steroid	Number of carbons
Cholesterol	27
Mineralocorticoids	21
Glucocorticoids	21
Progestins	21
Androgens	19
Estrogens	18

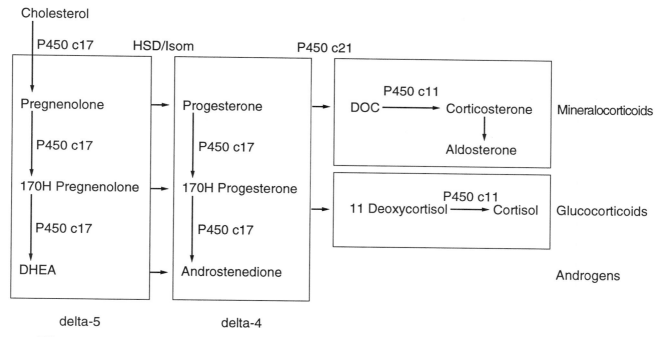

FIG. 2-3. Steroid biosynthesis in the adrenal and gonads. The principle pathways and enzymes are depicted.

sors connects the 5–6 carbons. Steroid biosynthesis on the right side of 3β-hydroxysteroid dehydrogenase/isomerase is referred to as the Δ4 pathway. In this configuration, all steroids have a double bond connecting the 4–5 carbons. In general, steroids with the Δ4 configuration have potent biologic activity, while steroids with the Δ5 structure are considered precursors and have much weaker end-organ biological activity.

CHOLESTEROL UPTAKE AND UTILIZATION

The parent compound for steroid biosynthesis is cholesterol (Fig. 2-4). Human steroidogenic cells derive most of their cholesterol from the uptake of circulating cholesterol contained in low-density lipoproteins (LDLs). Although steroidogenic tissues synthesize cholesterol de

novo, most of the cholesterol available for steroid synthesis is provided by cellular uptake of LDL cholesterol (Fig. 2-5). LDL-cholesterol esters are taken up from circulation by receptor-mediated endocytosis. The internalized LDL cholesterol ester is either stored directly in the cell or is converted to free cholesterol to be used for steroid hormone synthesis. The LDL molecule consists of an outer shell of protein with an inner core of cholesterol and free fatty acids. The protein in the outer crust is generally apolipoprotein B. When apolipoprotein B interacts with the LDL receptor on a steroid-producing cell, the lipoproteins bind with specific receptor sites on the cell membrane (Fig. 2-6). The receptor–lipoprotein complex is then transferred to a special region on the cell surface referred to as a "coated pit" where the lipoproteins are internalized by absorptive endocytosis. The intracellular vesicles formed by this process subsequently fuse with lysosomes, lipoproteins are then degraded, and cholesterol is released into the cytosol.

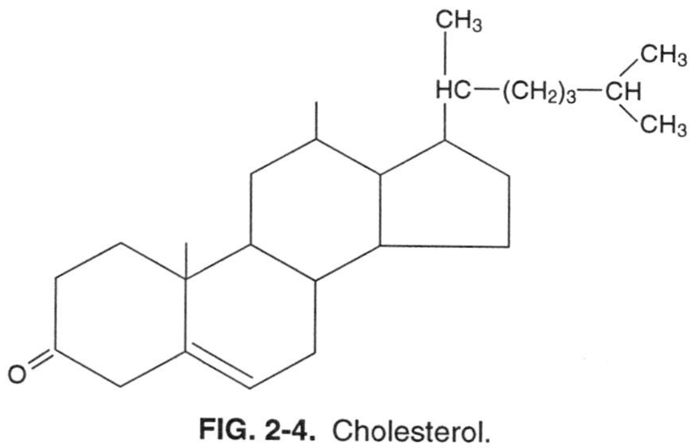

As cytosolic cholesterol accumulates, it is stored in an esterified pool. Cholesterol storage is controlled by the action of two opposing enzymes, cholesterolesterase and cholesterol ester synthetase. In general, trophic hormones (ACTH, LH) stimulate the esterase and inhibit the synthetase, thus increasing the availability of free cholesterol for steroid biosynthesis.

Before cholesterol can be converted to steroids, it must be transported to and internalized within the mitochondria. Two peptides appear to be responsible for this phenomenon. One peptide (sterol carrier protein 2) transports unesterified cholesterol to the mitochondria and a

FIG. 2-4. Cholesterol.

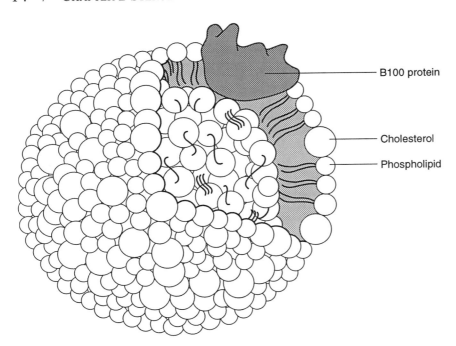

FIG. 2-5. Structure of low-density lipo-protein (LDL).

second peptide (steroidogenesis activator peptide) enhances flux of cholesterol across the mitochondrial membrane to the site of the cholesterol side chain cleavage enzyme (below).

Most steroidogenic enzymes that convert cholesterol to steroid precursors and biologically active steroids are members of the cytochrome P450 group of oxidase reactions. Cytochrome P450 is a generic term for the large number of oxidative enzymes, each of which consists of about 500 amino acids and contain iron. They are termed P450 enzymes because they exhibit a characteristic light shift under special treatment conditions. Most cytochrome P450 enzymes are found in the endoplasmic reticulum of the liver. They metabolize an array of toxins,

drugs, environmental pollutants, and other lipid-soluble substrates. Despite this huge variety of substrates, fewer than 200 types of cytochrome P450 enzymes exist. Only five distinct cytochrome P450 enzymes are involved in sex steroid biosynthesis (Table 2-2). Four are associated with adrenal steroidogenesis and one additional P450 enzyme is associated with estrogen biosynthesis. The three-dimensional structure of the cytochrome P450 enzymes is curious. The proteins appear to form a tubular or tunnel structure. The precursor steroid enters on one side of the enzyme (substrate), traverses the length of the enzyme and leaves on the other side (product), and may be sequentially modified by other longitudinally oriented cytochrome P450 enzymes.

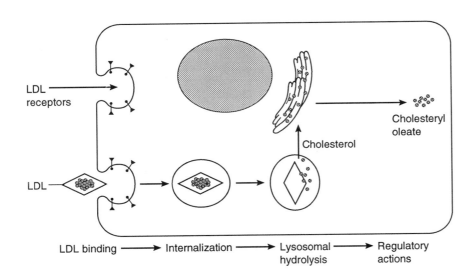

FIG. 2-6. LDL–apoprotein B receptor interaction.

TABLE 2-2. *P450 nomenclature of five enzymes involved in steroid biosynthesis*

P450 name	Old name
$P450_{scc}$	20:22-Desmolase
$P450_{c17}$	17:20-Desmolase
$P450_{c21}$	21-Hydroxylase
$P450_{c11}$	11β-Hydroxylase
$P450_{arom}$	Aromatase

Cholesterol transformation to pregnenolone in the mitochondria is the rate-limiting step of all hormonally regulated sex steroid biosynthesis. Hydroxylation occurs at carbon 22 and carbon 20, and the bond between these two carbons is divided. The enzyme responsible for these reactions is referred to as the side chain cleavage enzyme of the P450 complex, $P450_{scc}$.

MINERALOCORTICOID AND GLUCOCORTICOID BIOSYNTHESIS

Figure 2-7 shows the structure of aldosterone and cortisol is shown in Fig. 2-8. Six enzymes are required to synthesize aldosterone from cholesterol. Both aldosterone and deoxycorticosterone (DOC) possess potent mineralocorticoid activity and induce hypertension in patients who overproduce the steroids, eg, 11β-hydroxylase ($P450_{C11}$). Only one additional enzyme is required to convert mineralocorticoids to glucocorticoids. Pregnenolone is converted to 17-hydroxypregnenolone by $P450_{c17}$ (previously known as 17-hydroxylase), which performs the same action on progesterone, converting that precursor to 17-hydroxyprogesterone. Cortisol is the end product of adrenal steroid biosynthesis and regulates pituitary ACTH stimulation of the adrenal cortex. Finally, 17-hydroxypregnenolone and 17-hydroxyprogesterone are converted to DHEA and androstenedione, respectively, by $P450_{c17}$ (previously called 17:20-desmolase). This reaction is responsible for the production of adrenal androgens.

The adrenal cortex is divided into three zones: outer zona glomerulosa, zona fasciculata, and zona reticularis. The zona glomerulosa is chiefly concerned with biosynthesis of the mineralocorticoid aldosterone, which is reg-

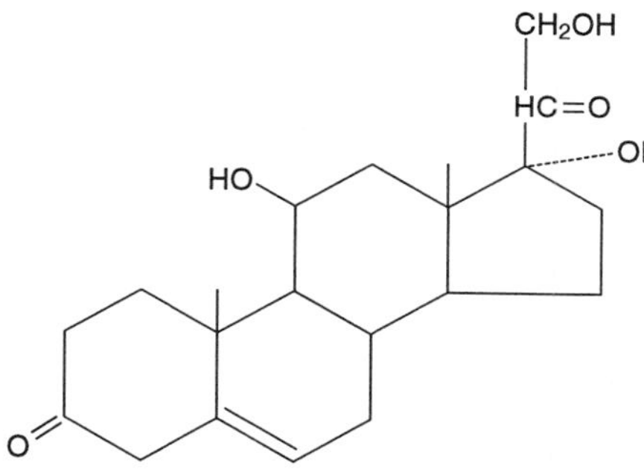

FIG. 2-8. Structure of cortisol.

ulated by serum levels of potassium and angiotensin but is only minimally influenced by ACTH. The two innermost zones are controlled primarily by pituitary ACTH secretion and produce adrenal androgens (androstenedione and DHEA) and glucocorticoids (Fig. 2-9). Cortisol biosynthesis is regulated by the interaction of four regulatory compartments. The central nervous system (CNS) regulates the diurnal secretion of ACTH and influences ACTH during stressful crises. The hypothalamus releases corticotropin-releasing hormone (CRH), a 41-amino-acid peptide synthesized principally in the paraventricular nucleus of the hypothalamus. CRH is secreted into the portal circulation of the infundibular stalk, delivered to the anterior pituitary, and stimulates ACTH release.

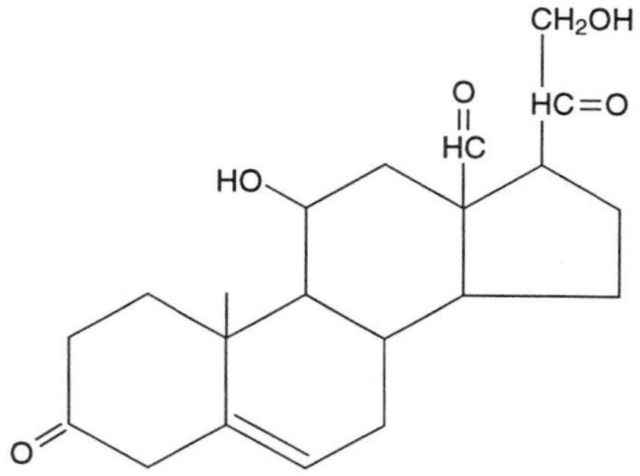

PROGESTERONE BIOSYNTHESIS

Progesterone (Fig. 2-10) is an obligatory metabolic precursor of mineralocorticoid, glucocorticoid, and androgen production. As a hormone product, it is synthesized only by the luteal cells of the ovary after ovulation and the trophoblast cells of the placenta during pregnancy. Progesterone cannot be 21-hydroxylated by the ovary or placenta because these endocrine tissues lack the enzyme $P450_{C21}$. Production of progesterone by the ovary requires gonadotropin-mediated follicular maturation, transformation of granulosa cells to luteal cells, and sustained LH or hCG stimulation.

ANDROGEN BIOSYNTHESIS

Androgen biosynthesis is performed in the adrenal gland and the gonads (ovaries and testes). DHEA, the sulfated metabolite DHEA-S, and androstenedione are the major androgens secreted by the adrenal gland (Figs. 2-11 to 2-13), whereas testosterone (Fig. 2-14) and androstenedione are the predominate androgens of the gonads. The amount of androgen production by the gonads is dependent on the sex of the individual. The testes secrete approximately five times more androgens than the ovaries (Table 2-3). The pathway for androgen biosynthe-

FIG. 2-7. Structure of aldosterone.

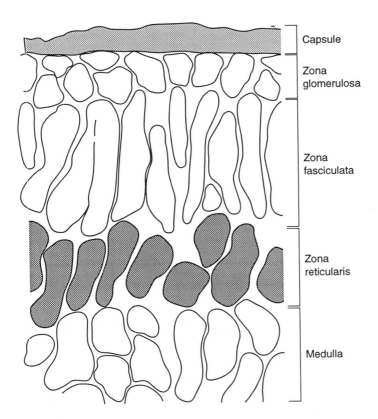

Capsule

Zona
glomerulosa

Zona
fasciculata

Zona
reticularis

Medulla

FIG. 2-9. Sites of adrenal hormone synthesis. Aldosterone is produced in the glomerulosa and androgens and cortisol are synthesized in the fasciculata and reticularis.

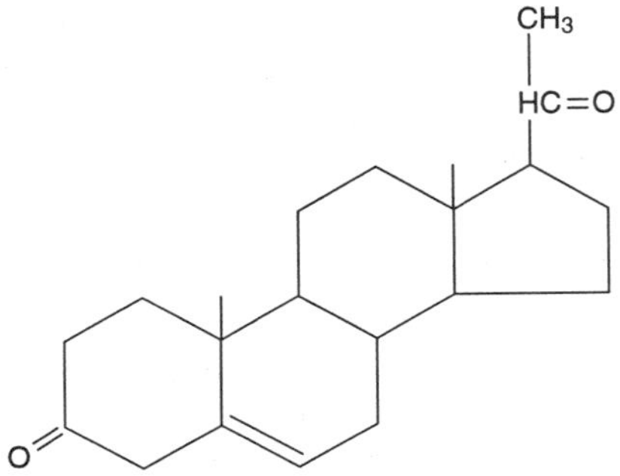

FIG. 2-10. Progesterone.

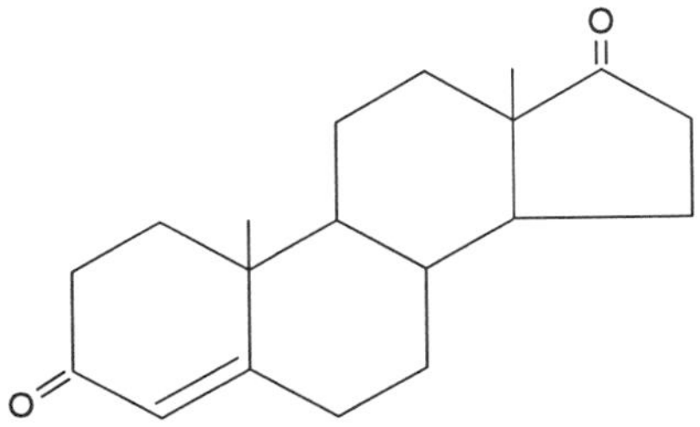

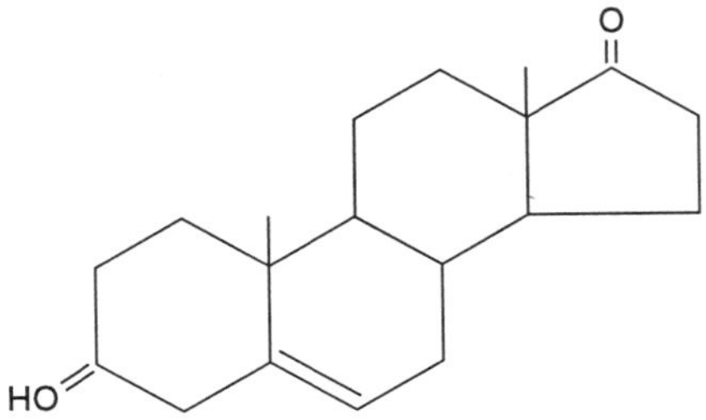

FIG. 2-11. Dehydroepiandrosterone.

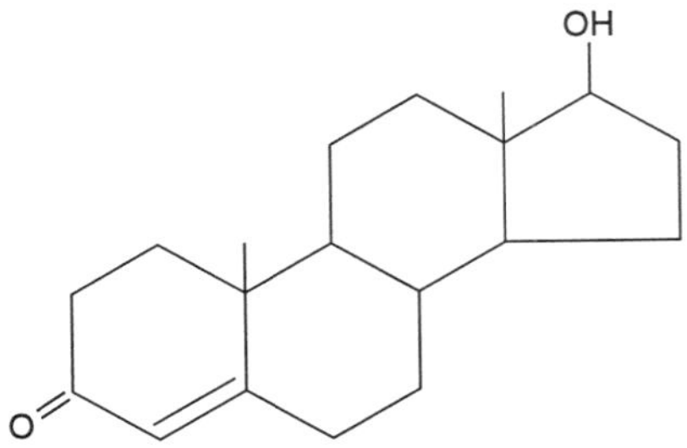

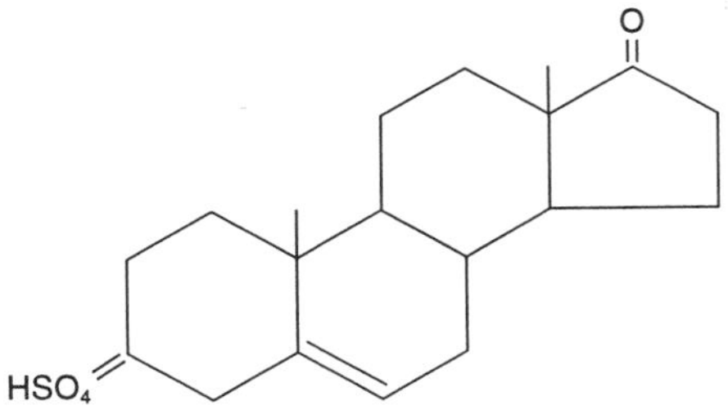

FIG. 2-12. Dehydroepiandrosterone sulfate.

FIG. 2-13. Androstenedione.

FIG. 2-14. Testosterone.

TABLE 2-3. *Androgen production rates in men and women (mg/day)*

Androgen	Men	Women
Testosterone	6	0.2
Androstenedione	3	2

sis is outlined in Fig. 2-3. In men, testosterone is the principal androgen secreted by the testes, and testosterone production is approximately twice that of androstenedione. In women, the principal ovarian androgen is androstenedione and androstenedione production is approximately 10 times that of testosterone. Men produce approximately 5 mg of testosterone per day, and women produce approximately 0.2 mg of testosterone per day.

ESTROGEN BIOSYNTHESIS

Estrogen biosynthesis is derived from previous androgen formation. A single reaction $P450_{arom}$ (aromatase) converts androstenedione to estrone (Fig. 2-15) or testosterone to 17β-estradiol (Fig. 2-16). In women the daily

production of estrogen is quite variable, depending on the reproductive maturity of the individual (premenarchial versus postmenopausal) and the phase of the ovarian menstrual cycle.

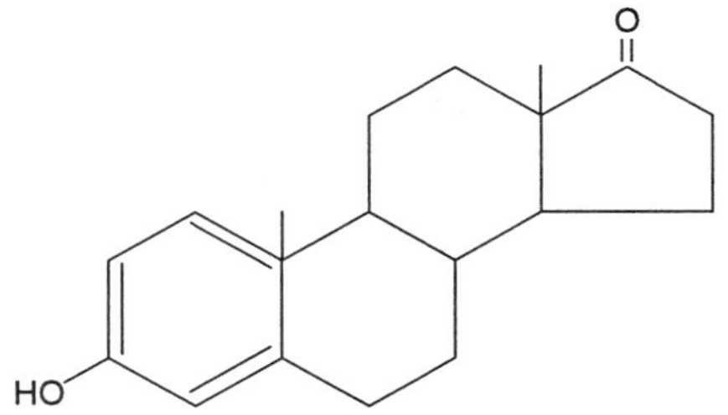

STEROID ELIMINATION

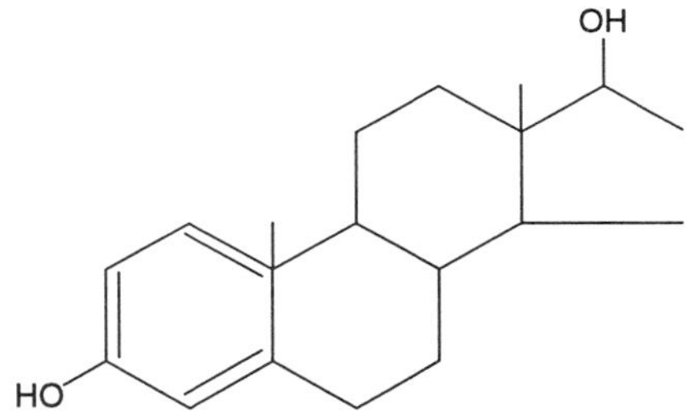

Steroid elimination is accomplished by ring A reduction, oxidation and/or reduction of oxygen containing residues, conjugation of hydroxy groups, or a combination of these processes (Table 2-4). All steroid modifications prior to elimination are designed to reduce the biological activity of the steroid and to increase its hydrophilic properties to enhance renal elimination. The liver is principally responsible for metabolic alterations as well as conjugation, and the kidneys excrete the biologically inactivated and solubilized products. Only a small amount of glucocorticoids, androgens, and estrogens are secreted via the biliary system. The predominant route of elimination is through the kidneys (85%) after hepatic metabolism. The kidneys eliminate steroid metabolites both actively (renal tubular transport) and passively (glomerular filtration), depending on the class of steroid.

Corticosteroids, androgens, and progestins usually are metabolized significantly at ring A. The double bond is reduced, and 3-ketos are reduced to the hydroxy group. Subsequently, the hydroxy group is conjugated with either a sulfate or a glucuronide molecule (Fig. 2-17). Estrogens are a class of steroids that seem to be

FIG. 2-15. Estrone.

FIG. 2-16. 17β-Estradiol.

TABLE 2-4. *Metabolic alternatives for steroid elimination*

1. Ring A reduction
2. Oxidation or reduction of oxygen
3. Conjugation (sulfate, glucuronide)
4. Multiple events

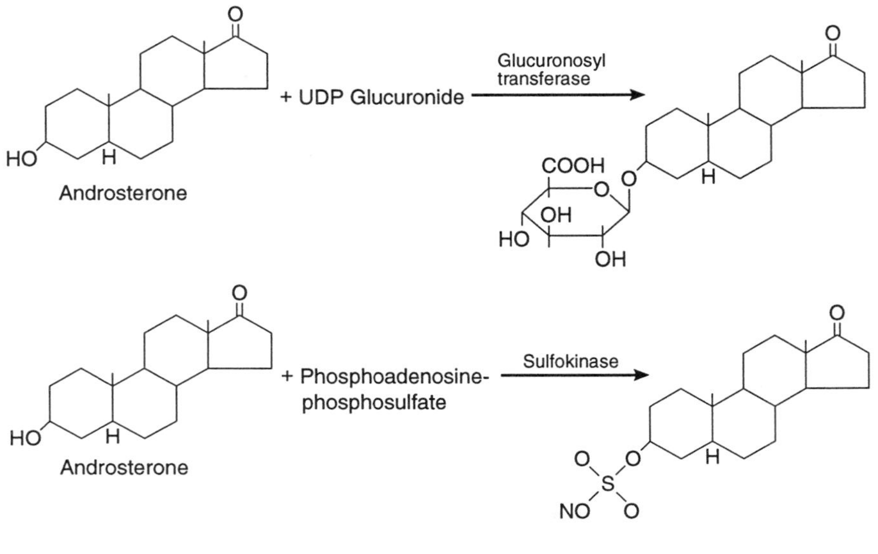

FIG. 2-17. Steroid conjugation.

uniquely metabolized. Two hydroxylation pathways modify the molecule, reduce biological activity, and increase solubility and renal excretion. One pathway involves hydroxylation at the 2 position of the A ring (termed catecholestrogen metabolism; Fig. 2-18) and the other pathway involves hydroxylation at carbon 16 to produce estriol. The hydroxy groups are then conjugated and the steroid excreted.

MECHANISMS OF STEROID HORMONE ACTION

Steroid hormones enter target cells by diffusion. The steroid then traverses the cytoplasm and enters the nucleus where it is bound by a nuclear protein called the receptor (Fig. 2-19). Steroid receptors are relatively large proteins that have high affinity for a specific hormone. Steroid receptors have a limited number of steroid binding sites (usually one per protein molecule) and are present in trace quantities within the nucleus. The affinity constants of steroid receptors range from 10^{-10} to 10^{-12} M. Such affinity constants are considered "specific" when compared to the nonspecific steroid binding seen in molecules such as albumin. The binding affinity of albumin for steroids is in the range of 10^{-4} to 10^{-6} M. Thus, these proteins exert their biological effects by binding steroids very specifically and tightly. Receptor binding of "heterologous" steroids occurs only within the same class of hormones (eg, estrogens) as well as their synthetic agonists and antagonists. Progestins and glucocorticoids share chemical similarity, and the progesterone and glucocorticoid receptors cross-bind these structures. However, the receptor usually prefers the target steroid by a factor of 10.

After the steroid binds to the receptor, the steroid–receptor complex is "activated." This activated complex binds to another nuclear protein called the acceptor protein, which is present on the DNA. The binding of the receptor steroid complex to the acceptor site on the DNA in the nucleus is thought to alter gene expression. Presumably, the acceptor sites are located near the DNA sequences that are transcribed after hormonal stimulation of the cell. In general, cell activation after steroid stimulation results in new mRNA transcription, and ultimately the mRNA is translated into specific proteins that alter cell function, growth, or differentiation.

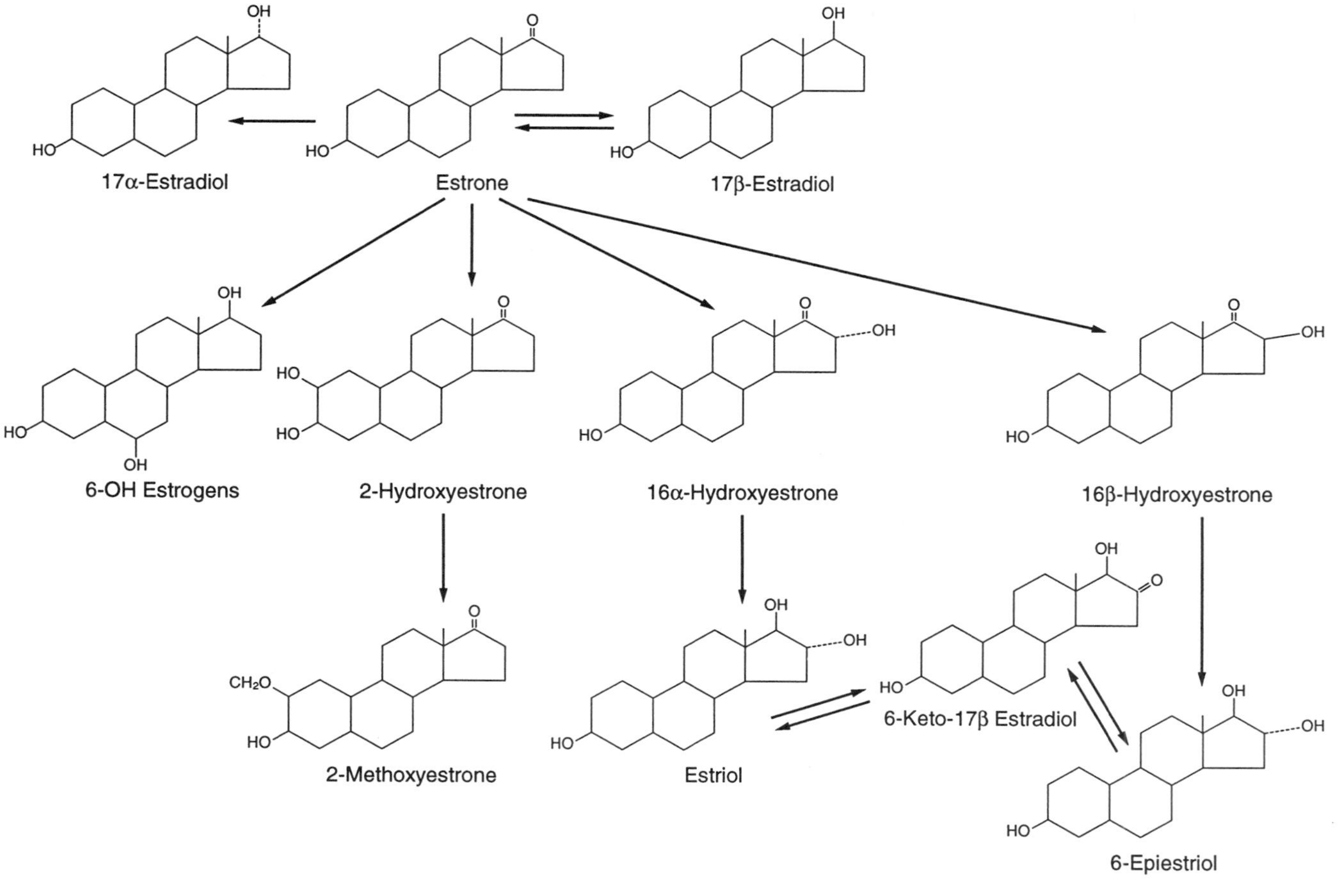

FIG. 2-18. Catecholestrogen.

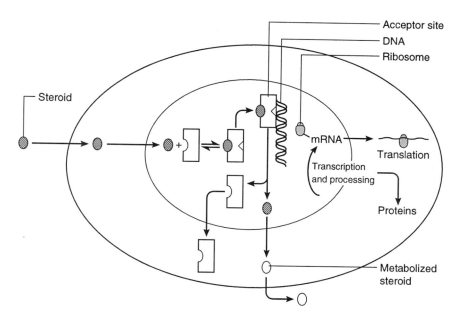

FIG. 2-19. General model for steroid–target tissue interactions.

The classic formulations that describe equilibrium kinetics also describe the physical nature of the association between receptor and steroid (Fig. 2-20). From this formula, the number of receptor sites and association constants can be derived. The dissociation/association constant of the steroid (K_d) is the concentration at which 50% of the receptor sites are bound. The number of molecules required to saturate the receptor is equal to the number of receptor sites (n). This is derived from the Scatchard mathematical transformation, which plots the ratio of bound steroid to free steroid against bound steroid (Fig. 2-21).

The intact nuclear form of the estrogen receptor has a molecular weight of 130,000 and has two subunits (Table 2-5). The principal ligand is estradiol-17β. The receptor optimally binds the synthetic ligand diethylstilbestrol and also binds the antagonists clomiphene citrate and tamoxifen. The receptor has been purified from human breast tumor cells, and the typical cellular abundance of the molecule is estimated to be 10,000 molecules per cell. The progesterone receptor optimally binds progesterone in vivo but has the highest binding affinity for the synthetic steroid promegestone. It also binds the antagonist mifepristone (RU 486). It has an estimated molecular weight of 225,000 and is composed of two subunits. The typical density of the progesterone receptor in target cells is 50,000–100,000 molecules per cell. The glucocorticoid receptor is the largest of the

$$[RS] = \frac{[R_t]\,[S]}{K_d + [S]}$$

FIG. 2-20. Classic formulation of rapid equilibrium kinetics (Michaelis–Menton equation). RS, bound receptor; S, steroid; K_d, dissociation constant; R_t, total receptor.

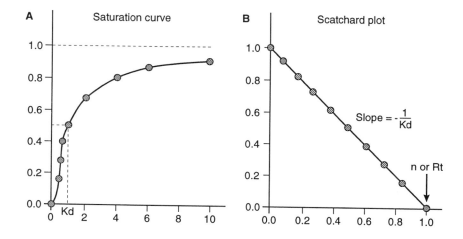

FIG. 2-21. Scatchard transformation of binding data. The intercepts and slope determine the dissociation constant (K_d) and the number of binding sites (n).

TABLE 2-5. *Molecular characterization of steroid hormone receptors*

Receptor	In vitro ligand	Synthetic ligand	Antagonist	Molecular weight	Subunits
Estrogen	Estradiol	DES	Tamoxifen	130,000	2
Progesterone	Progesterone	Promestone	RU 486	225,000	2
Glucocorticoids	Cortisol	DEX	Cortexolone	350,000	4
Androgen	Dihydrotestosterone	Methyltrienolone	Flutamide	120,000	1
Mineralocorticoids	Aldosterone	—	—	—	—

known receptors; it has an estimated molecular weight of 350,000 and possesses four subunits. It is present in the same approximate cellular density as the progestin receptor. The androgen receptor has an estimated molecular weight of 120,000 and is present at a concentration of only 5000 molecules per cell. The mineralocorticoid receptor has not been purified. It is the rarest of the receptors and is present at an estimated concentration of 1000 molecules per cell.

During the course of eukaryotic gene transcription, RNA polymerase must initiate and terminate at specific sites on the DNA. To initiate RNA polymerase action, a special region of DNA termed the "promotor" is usually attached near the critical area of DNA to be transcribed. The purpose of the promotor is to establish the accuracy of the start point for transcription. Additional "regulatory" elements are located adjacent to the promotor region and act as activators or switches to the promotor.

The acceptor molecule appears to be integrated within the regulatory site of the chromatin material. The promotor is initiated when the regulatory site is activated by the receptor–steroid complex (Fig. 2-22).

SUGGESTED READING

Berger FG, Watson G. Androgen-regulated gene expression. *Annu Rev Physiol* 1989;51:51.

Gharib SD, Wierman ME, Shupnik MA, Chin WW. Molecular biology of the pituitary gonadotropins. *Endocr Rev* 1990;11:177.

Greene GL, Press MF. Structure and dynamics of the estrogen receptor. *J Steroid Biochem* 1986;24:1.

Grigging GT. Editorial: Dinosaurs and steroids. *J Clin Endocrinol Metabol* 1993;77:1450.

Gustafsson JA, Carlstedt-Duke J, Poellinger L, et al. Biochemistry, molecular biology, and physiology of the glucocorticoid receptor. *Endocr Rev* 1987;8:185.

Gwynne JT, Strauss JF III. The role of lipoproteins in steroidogenesis and cholesterol metabolism in steroidogenic glands. *Endocr Rev* 1982;3:299.

Litwack G, Schmidt TJ, Miller-Diener A, et al. Steroid receptor activation: the glucocorticoid receptor as a model system. *Adv Exp Med Biol* 1986; 196:11.

Miller WL. Molecular biology of steroid hormone synthesis. *Endocr Rev* 1988;9:295.

Mooradian AD, Morley JE, Korenman SG. Biological actions of androgens. *Endocr Rev* 1987;8:1.

Mortel R, Satyaswaroop PG, Clarke CL, Zaino RJ. Sex steroid receptors in normal and malignant endometrium. *Ann Pathol* 1986;6:109.

Pasqualini JR, Sumida C. Ontogeny of steroid receptors in the reproductive system. *Int Rev Cytol* 1986;101:275.

Pinsky L, Kaufman M. Genetics of steroid receptors and their disorders. *Adv Hum Genet* 1987;16:299.

Power RF, Conneely OM, O'Malley BW. New insights into activation of the steroid hormone receptor superfamily. *Trends Pharmacol Sci* 1992;13: 318.

Walters MR. Steroid hormone receptors and the nucleus. *Endocr Rev* 1985; 6:512.

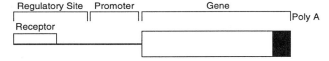

FIG. 2-22. Transcriptional control regions of a hormone-induced gene. The promotor site establishes the accuracy of RNA polymerase activity so that proper transcription of the gene occurs. The regulatory portion acts as a switch to control the timing or "induction" of the transcription. The regulatory region contains the acceptor protein, which binds to the steroid–receptor complex. Through this interaction, the regulator controls the timing of transcription.

Clinical Reproductive Medicine,
Edited by Bryan D. Cowan and David B. Seifer
Lippincott-Raven Publishers, Philadelphia © 1997

CHAPTER 3

Reproductive Peptide Hormones

Bryan D. Cowan

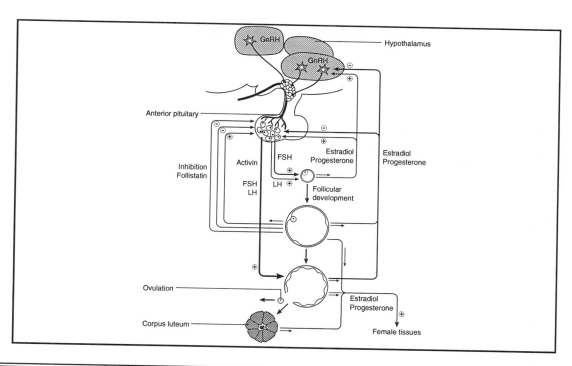

Chemistry of Circulating Gonadotropins	**Circulating Gonadotropins**
Biosynthesis of Human Chorionic Gonadotropin	**Mechanism of Action of Gonadotropins**
Pituitary Synthesis; Storage and Release of LH and	**Inhibins, Activins, and Follistatins**
FSH	**Suggested Reading**

B. D. Cowan: Division of Reproductive Endocrinology, Department of Obstetrics and Gynecology, University of Mississippi, Jackson MS 39216

Gonadal sex steroid synthesis and germ cell maturation is controlled by two gonadotropic hormones secreted by the adenohypophysis in men and nonpregnant women, and one placental hormone produced during pregnancy. The pituitary glycoproteins *follicle-stimulating hormone* (FSH) and *luteinizing hormone* (LH) exert effects on both the ovary and the testis. *Human chorionic gonadotropin* (hCG) stimulates steroid production in the ovary during early gestation. FSH is primarily responsible for the regulation of germ cell development in both sexes and ovarian estrogen synthesis in women. LH and hCG stimulate synthesis of androgenic sex steroids in both the testis and ovary, and progesterone production by the corpus luteum. LH, FSH, and hCG have no clinically important actions outside the reproductive tract.

Sex steroids have been considered the only regulators of gonadotropin production. Recently, gonadal peptides have been characterized that are potent regulators of FSH secretion. Inhibin and follistatin suppress FSH release, and activin stimulates FSH release. Gonadal peptides that regulate LH have been detected, but such putative substances await definitive characterization. In this chapter, we will discuss the chemistry and actions of gonadotropins (LH, FSH, and hCG) and gonadal peptides (inhibin, follistatin, and activin) that regulate reproduction.

CHEMISTRY OF CIRCULATING GONADOTROPINS

The three gonadotropins (LH, FSH, and hCG) along with thyroid-stimulating hormone (TSH) are classified together because of their biochemical similarity (Table 3-1). These hormones are glycoproteins composed of two polypeptide subunits that are associated with noncovalent but high-affinity binding (Fig. 3-1). One of the subunits (α) of these trophic hormones is common to each glycoprotein. Within each species, the a subunit possesses essentially the same amino acid sequence. The other subunit (β) differs considerably between these glycoproteins in its amino acid sequence. It is the β subunit that is responsible for hormone specificity, whereas the α subunit designates species specificity.

These trophic hormones are modified within the cell after amino acid assembly. Carbohydrate residues are attached to the protein backbone at specific locations

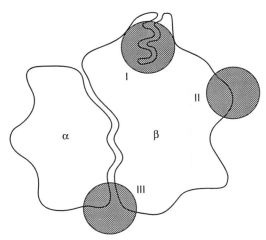

FIG. 3-1. Schematic illustration of the two subunits (α and β) of human chorionic gonadotropin (hCG). Additionally, the hatched circles illustrate three preferred antigenic sites on hCG. Antisera raised against hCG preferentially recognize antigenic determinants in these areas.

within the molecule (glycosylation). *Glycosylation* alters two biological characteristics of these molecules (Table 3-2)(Table 3-3). Increasing the carbohydrate content of the molecule extends the circulatory half-life, and glycosylation affects their biological actions. Curiously, removing the carbohydrate moieties does not affect the affinity of the protein for its receptor but reduces the ability of the hormone to stimulate target cell responses after binding to the receptor.

The approximate molecular weight of LH is 28,000, FSH is 33,000, and hCG is 39,000. The molecular weight of the common α subunit is about 14,000. The entire amino acid sequences of the common α and β chains for each individual hormone are known. During chemical separation, considerable "microheterogeneity" is observed in these molecules. This is principally because of wide variations in the charged sialic content of the molecules. These acidic glycoproteins thus acquire isoelectric points ranging from 3 to 3.5 for hCG, 4.5 to 5 for FSH, and 5.5 to 6.0 for LH.

The three-dimensional structure of the final molecule is maintained by internally crosslinked disulfide bonds within the α and β subunits. Five bonds exist in the α subunit and six exist in each β subunit. There are no interchain disulfide bonds or other covalent linkages between the α and β subunits.

The gene structures for the α and β subunits have been determined, and it appears that a single gene is responsi-

TABLE 3-1. *Characteristics of gonadotropins and FSH*

	Molecular weight	Chromosome	Gene copies
Common alpha subunit	14,000	6	1
LH-β	14,000	19	6
FSH-β	19,000	11	1
hCG-β	25,000	19	6
TSH-β	15,000	1	1

TABLE 3-2. *Glycosylation of peptides*

1. Posttranslational modification of amino acid structure
2. Extends circulatory half-life of hormone
3. Affects hormone action

TABLE 3-3. *Sialic acid content and circulatory half-life of gonadotropins*

	Sialic acid (%)	Circulation half-life
LH	2	0.5–1 h
FSH	5	3–4 h
hCG	10	6–24 h

TABLE 3-4. *Major steps in hCG biosynthesis*

Step	Probable Site
Apoprotein synthesis	Ribosome
Cleavage of signal protein	ER membrane
Initial glycosylation	ER membrane
Trimming of high-mannose intermediate	ER membrane
N-linked glycosyl addition	Golgi
O-linked glycosyl addition	Golgi
Disulfide bridges	Golgi
Assembly	Plasma membrane
Secretion	Secretory granule

ble for coding all of the α subunits within a species. There is a single gene encoding human LH-β and FSH-β, but there are six genes for hCG-β. Only three of the human hCG-β genes appear to be active. The gene encoding the α subunit is contained on chromosome 6. The genes that encode the β subunits for LH, FSH, hCG, and TSH are contained on chromosomes 19, 11, 19, and 1, respectively (see Table 3-1).

BIOSYNTHESIS OF HUMAN CHORIONIC GONADOTROPIN

The biosynthesis of hCG is known in greater detail than the corresponding synthesis of LH, FSH, or TSH. It is believed that the synthesis of the pituitary hormones occurs in a fashion similar to that for hCG and that the general principles of hCG synthesis apply to these hormones as well. Conceptually, nine major events occur during the synthesis of hCG, and these events occur sequentially in the intracellular compartments of the ribo-

some, endoplasmic reticulum membrane, Golgi, secretory granule, and plasma membrane (Table 3-4).

1. *Apoprotein synthesis* occurs for each of the α and β subunits (Fig. 3-2). Both subunits contain a *signal segment* of approximately 24 amino acids. Translation of the message occurs on the ribosome, and the signal segment is removed by an endopeptidase shortly before completion of the amino acid assembly. The fundamental α peptide has a molecular weight of 14,000 and the β peptide 18,000. These molecular weights are increased during subsequent addition of carbohydrate moieties.
2. *Glycosylation* occurs in three phases. In the first phase, oligosaccharides high in mannose content are attached (*N-linked*) to specific sites en bloc to the respective subunits. The α subunit is glycosylated at amino acids 52 and 75, whereas the β subunit is gly-

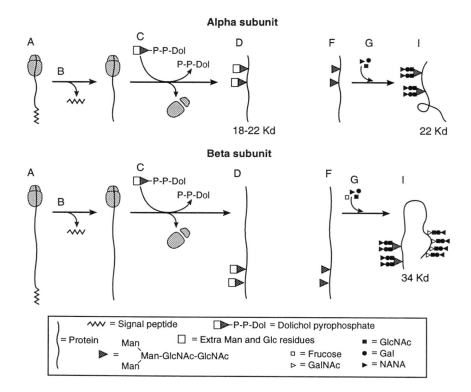

FIG. 3-2. Sequential steps of human chorionic gonadotropin (hCG) synthesis. For both α and β subunit synthesis, an apoprotein **(A)** is transformed to the mature element by the elimination of the signal segment **(B)**. Subsequently, glycosylation occurs **(C, D)**, and the initial glycosylation sites are modified **(F)**. The original glycolsylation sites are further modified in the α subunit **(G)** to produce the mature 22-Kd α monomer **(I)**. A similar modification occurs in the β subunit (G) but additional carbohydrate residues are attached to produce the mature 34-Kd β monomer (I).

cosylated at amino acids 13 and 30. During the second phase of carbohydrate modification, excess mannose and glucose residues are enzymatically *trimmed* from the oligosaccharide moieties. Finally, the N-linked oligosaccharide residues undergo sequential addition of other carbohydrate residuals, including sialic acid. Uniquely, the β subunit serine residues at 121, 127, 132, and 138 undergo *O-linked* glycosylation. The fully glycosylated α subunit has a molecular weight of 22,000 and the mature β subunit is 34,000. In all probability the five α and six β interchain disulfide bonds are formed within the Golgi.

3. *Assembly* of the mature α and β subunits into a biologically active hCG molecule occurs after the mature peptides have been secreted by the Golgi into a secretory granule. The secretory granule associates closely with the plasma membrane, and the mature hormone is secreted by *exocytosis*. In this process, the membrane of the secretory granule fuses with the cell membrane, and the cell membrane ruptures and releases the hormone.

PITUITARY SYNTHESIS; STORAGE AND RELEASE OF LH AND FSH

In the human, gonadotropes are present as angular cells distributed singly throughout the pituitary. In general, most cells will stain for both LH and FSH, but approximately 20% of the gonadotropes stain uniquely for FSH or LH. Gonadotropins are synthesized under the influence of episodic hypothalamic gonadotropin-releasing hormone (GnRH). The intracellular events that are responsible for release of gonadotropins involve two divergent pathways mediated by common activation of the receptor by GnRH (Fig. 3-3). The "common phase" of GnRH receptor activation involves stimulation of a receptor-associated guanosine nucleotide–binding protein (G). This activates phospholipase C (an enzyme that cleaves phospholipids at the 3 position of glycerol) to hydrolyze inositol phospholipids to diacylglycerol (DG) and inositol triphosphate (IP_3). DG is further metabolized to phosphatic acid (PA) and arachidonic acid (AA). The "rapid phase" of gonadotropin release is mediated by IP_3 and arachidonic acid derivatives, which cause an immediate increase in intracellular calcium and activate calmodulin. The "synthesis phase" is regulated by DG. In this pathway, activated protein kinase C phosphorylates endogenous cellular proteins. Protein phosphorylation then leads to synthesis of new LH and FSH.

Gonadotropins are initially synthesized as larger prehormones from which the unnecessary amino acid sequences are enzymatically cleaved. Oligosaccharides are added to the proteins after synthesis, and finally the oligosaccharides themselves are modified. Assembly of the α and β subunit produces the final hormone product. Curiously, α and β subunit assembly occurs optimally when the α subunit is produced in excess. The reasons for the excess production requirements of the α subunit are unknown, but certain disease conditions (trophoblastic disease) and abnormal gestations (ectopic pregnancy) are associated with unusually high α-subunit production.

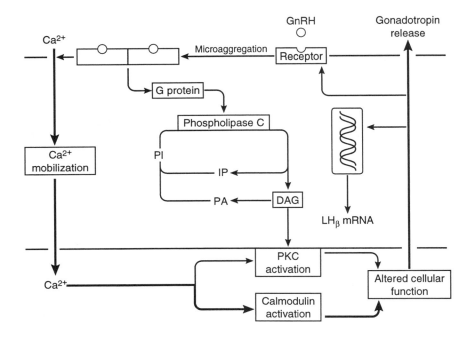

FIG. 3-3. Mechanism of action of gonadotropin-releasing hormone (GnRH). GnRH binds with the plasma membrane receptor and activates two pathways. Calcium is mobilized to the cytoplasm, and this mobilization appears to be coupled to the microaggregation of GnRH-bound receptors. Additionally, the G protein of the membrane receptor stimulates phospholipase C hydrolysis of lipids to form inositol triphosphate (IP), diacylglycerol (DAG), phophatidic acid (PA), and phophatidylinositol (PI). Calcium mobilization prompts immediate release of gonadotropins, and DAG activates protein kinase C (PKC). After PKC activation a cascade of protein phosphorylations occur and new gonadotropin synthesis is initiated.

CIRCULATING GONADOTROPINS

In general, the pituitary and placental gonadotropic hormones are not modified once they reach the circulation. They exist in the same molecular form in which they were synthesized and secreted by the pituitary. Circulating concentrations of LH and FSH have been evaluated extensively by specific radioimmunoassay. The plasma concentrations of LH and FSH are usually expressed in terms of standard biological units established by the National Institutes of Health. The circulating half-life of these molecules is proportional to the sialic content (Table 3-3).

The final metabolic pathway for gonadotropin elimination is not known. However, only 10–20% of administered hormone is excreted in the urine. Approximately 80–90% of the molecule is degraded in vivo.

MECHANISM OF ACTION OF GONADOTROPINS

Like steroids, gonadotropins exert specific biological effects on target tissues through activation of a unique receptor. Unlike the steroid hormone receptors, the gonadotropin receptors are bound to the membrane of the target cell (Fig. 3-4). After binding the gonadotropin, the membrane receptors stimulate the production of soluble intracellular "second" messengers. It is the second messenger that stimulates cellular responses.

The cell surface receptors for the glycoprotein peptide hormones are all integral proteins of the cell membrane and are insoluble in aqueous media. When activated by LH, FSH, or hCG, these membrane-associated receptors induce an intracellular second messenger of cyclic adenosine (cAMP). Three intrinsic proteins of the plasma membrane are required for hormone-mediated induction of cAMP. These are recognized as the hormone receptor, the regulatory component of the adenylate cyclase enzyme (G), and the catalytic component (C), which actually converts ATP to cAMP (see

Fig. 3-4). Interestingly, the three components of the receptor can be combined with components from different tissues or different species and yield a fully functional unit. This suggests that these important regulatory units have been genetically conserved throughout the different species.

The three components are unassociated physically and are free to float within the membrane to interact with each other. The receptor binds to the hormone at the cytoplasmic membrane. The regulatory component of the complex is referred to as the G protein because it binds guanine nucleotides. Binding of hormone to the high-affinity receptor is accompanied by activation of the G protein and G-protein binding to GTP. The activated G-GTP protein then stimulates the catalytic protein (C). The catalytic unit (C) (which ultimately converts ATP to cAMP) has little affinity for its physiologic substrate (ATP). However, when the catalytic component binds with activated G-GTP, the C component binds ATP. ATP is then converted to cAMP, which regulates intracellular processes.

Analogous to the stimulatory cascade described above, there exists a similar but unique set of membrane proteins that *decrease* cAMP production. The difference in the three-protein signaling mechanism of the inhibitory cascade is the G protein. The stimulator G-protein (G_s) is a different molecule from the inhibitor G protein (G_i). Both forms of the G protein (G_s or G_i) interact with only one pool of C proteins (Fig. 3-5). The cellular response depends on the ligand bound by the specific receptor molecule (R).

INHIBINS, ACTIVINS, AND FOLLISTATINS

The concept that peptides of gonadal origin play a role in the inhibition of gonadotropin secretion was proposed more than 65 years ago. However, the existence of these molecules was not proven until recently. The establishment of radioimmunoassay for gonadotropins and the development of monolayer culture of pituitary cells pro-

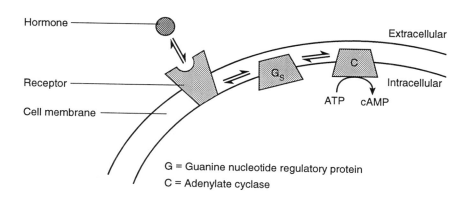

G = Guanine nucleotide regulatory protein
C = Adenylate cyclase

FIG. 3-4. Components of the membrane-bound adenylate cyclase-dependent hormone receptor system. Three plasma membrane proteins are required for hormone-mediated effects. The hormone receptor binds the hormone at the extracellular membrane. After binding the hormone, the receptor protein stimulates the G protein (G_s) to bind GTP. The activated G-GTP protein stimulates the catalytic protein (C). The catalytic protein ultimately converts ATP to cyclic AMP. Cyclic AMP then initiates a cascade of cellular protein phosphorylations.

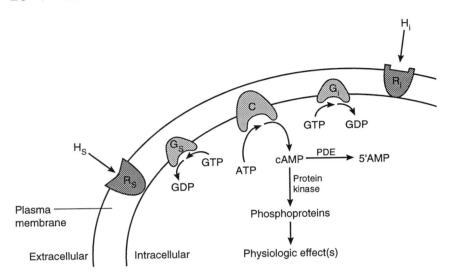

FIG. 3-5. Stimulatory or inhibitory receptor responses occur through a common C protein, which has an association with an inhibitor or stimulatory G protein. The hormone receptor binds either the inhibitory hormone (H_i) or the stimulatory hormone (H_s).

vided the fundamental tools necessary to isolate and characterize these molecules. The reagent used to characterize the inhibitory effect of water-soluble proteins on pituitary gonadotropin secretion was porcine follicular fluid (pFF). pFF inhibits the unregulated secretion of FSH from monolayer pituitary cell cultures but has no effect on LH (Fig. 3-6). In 1985, inhibin was isolated from pFF and characterized by four independent laboratories. Inhibin from pFF has a molecular weight of 32 kd and is composed of two subunits. The α subunit has a molecu-

lar weight of 20 kd and the β subunit has a molecular weight of 14 kd (Fig. 3-7). Human, porcine, bovine, and murine inhibins are closely related in structure and highly conserved. Two β subunits have been recognized, and these are termed βA and βB. In humans, the α and β B genes are found on different ends of chromosome 2, while the β A gene is encoded on chromosome 7. Two forms of inhibin (inhibin A and inhibin B) are formed by combination of the two different β subunits with an α chain. Like many peptides, the β and α subunits are

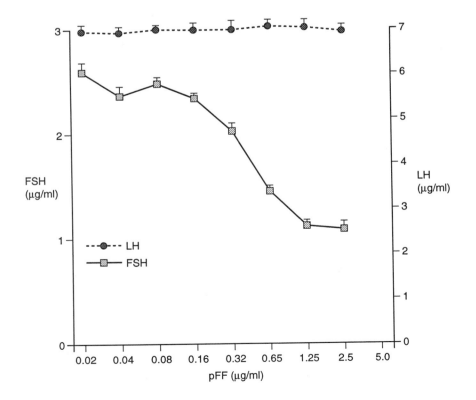

FIG. 3-6. Porcine follicular fluid (pFF) inhibits unregulated secretion of follicle-stimulating hormone from pituitary cell cultures. Luteinizing hormone is not inhibited by this reagent.

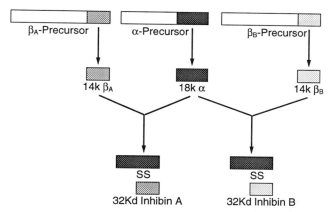

FIG. 3-7. Inhibins are formed from α and β precursors. Each precursor is clipped to form the mature 14-Kd β subunit and 18-Kd α subunit. The combination of βA with the α subunit forms the 32-Kd inhibin A, whereas α combined with βB forms the inhibin B molecule. The α and β subunits are bound together by two disulfide bridges.

formed from precursors, and the two subunits are covalently linked with disulfide bonds. The bioactivity of inhibin A is nearly equal to the bioactivity of inhibin B. FSH also participates in the feedback loop of inhibin by stimulating inhibin synthesis and production. Inhibin is produced in the granulosa and luteal cells of the ovary,

Sertoli cell of the testis, and cytotrophoblast of the placental villus.

The discovery of activins was linked to the isolation and characterization of inhibin. The in vitro bioassay using the pituitary monolayer culture was fundamental to the recognition of this new class of peptides. In the course of protein purification, certain fractions of pFF stimulated FSH secretion rather than inhibited its release. Purification and amino acid sequence characterization revealed that the stimulator was formed exclusively from the β subunits of the inhibin molecule. Three activin molecules were recognized (activin, homoactivin A, and homoactivin B). Thus, two classes of FSH regulators (inhibitor and stimulator) are synthesized by the granulosa and luteal cells of the ovary (Fig. 3-8). The combination of the α subunit with a β subunit leads to FSH suppressors, and combination of two β subunits leads to FSH stimulators (Fig. 3-9).

Follistatin is a novel single-chain glycosylated peptide with no structural relationship to inhibins or activins also exhibits potent and specific inhibition of pituitary FSH release. This molecule has been isolated from pFF using the same in vitro pituitary monolayer culture system. Follistatin has a molecular weight of 42 kd and is composed of a single polypeptide chain. This molecule was named follistatin to signify its ability to suppress release of FSH but not LH and to recognize its structural difference from inhibin. Follistatin is a binding protein for activin, and this decreases the levels of free activin.

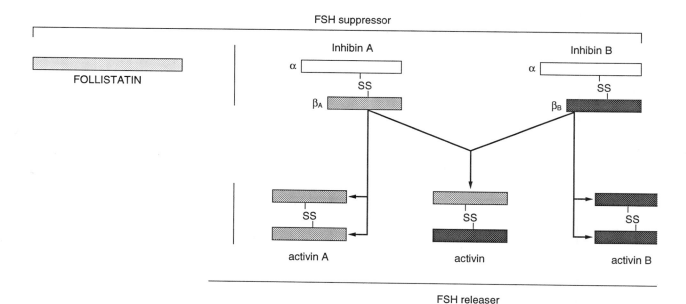

FIG. 3-8. Gonadal protein hormones that modify the secretion of follicle-stimulating hormone (FSH). Inhibins are formed by the combination of an α and a β subunit. Three activin molecules are formed by the combinations of βA homodimer, βB homodimer, and βA with βB. Follistatin is a noninhibin class molecule that inhibits FSH secretion.

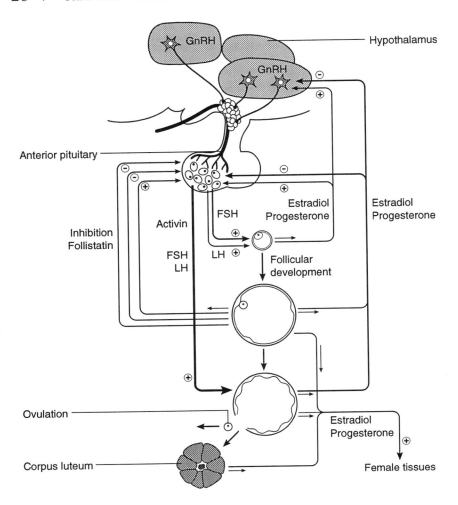

FIG. 3-9. Steroid and gonadal peptide regulation of ovarian function. The hypothalamus produces gonadotropin-releasing hormone (GnRH), which stimulates the release of pituitary luteinizing hormone and follicle-stimulating hormone (FSH). These pituitary peptides stimulate steroidogenesis and follicular maturation. Estradiol and progesterone regulate both pituitary and hypothalamic signals. Pituitary peptides (activin, inhibin, and follistatin) regulate pituitary release of FSH alone.

SUGGESTED READING

Adashi EY. Intraovarian peptides. Stimulators and inhibitors of follicular growth and differentiation. *Endocrinol Metabol Clin North Am* 1992;21: 1–17

Burger HG. Clinical utility of inhibin measurements. *J Clin Endocrinol Metab* 1993;76:1391–1396.

Conn PM, Crowley WF Jr. Gonadotropin-releasing hormone and its analogues. *N Engl J Med* 1991;324:93.

Fiddes JC, Talmadge K. Structure, expression, and evolution of the genes for the human glycoprotein hormones. *Recent Prog Horm Res* 1984;40: 43.

Findlay JK, Xiao S,Shukovski Z, Michel U. Novel peptides in ovarian physiology: inhibitin, activen, follistatin. In: *The Ovary.* Eds: Adashi KY, Leung PCK. New York: Raven Press, 1993.

Hillier SG, Miro F. Inhibin, activin, and follistatin. Potential roles in ovarian physiology. *Ann NY Acad Sci* 1993;687:29–38.

Hussa RO, ed. *The Clinical Marker hCG.* New York: Praeger, 1987.

Jameson JL, Lindell CM. Isolation and characterization of the human chorionic gonadotropin β subunit (CG β) gene cluster: regulation of transcriptionally active CG β gene by cyclic AMP. *Mol Cell Biol* 1988;8: 5100.

Kelley KM, Johnson TR, Gwatkin RB, Ilan J, Ilan J. Transgenic strategies in reproductive endocrinology. *Mol Reprod Dev* 1993;34:337–347.

Layman LC. Molecular biology in reproductive endocrinology. *Curr Opin Obstet Gynecol* 1995;7:328–339.

Naylor SL, Chin WW, Goodman HM, Lalley PA, Grzeschik KH, Sakaguchi AY. Chromosome assignment of genes encoding the alpha and beta subunits of glycoprotein hormones in man and mouse. *Somat Cell Genet* 1983;9:757.

O'Malley BW, Tsai M-J. Molecular pathways of steroid receptor action. *Biol Reprod* 1992;46:163.

Rabinovici J. The differential effects of FSH and LH on the human ovary. *Baillieres Clin Obstet Gynaecol* 1993;7:263–281.

Schreiber JR. Advances in ovarian physiology. *Semin Reprod Endocrinol* 1991;9:283–372.

Thotakura NR, Blithe DL. Glycoprotein hormones: glycobiology of gonadotrophins, thyrotrophin and free alpha subunit. *Glycobiology* 1995;5: 3–10.

Wierman ME, Gharib SD, Chin WW. The structure and regulation of the pituitary gonadotrophin subunit genes. *Bailliers Clin Endocrinol Metab* 1988;2:869.

Williams GR, Granklyn JA. Physiology of the steroid-thyroid hormone nuclear receptor superfamily. *Baillieres Clin Endocrinol Metab* 1994;8: 241–266.

Clinical Reproductive Medicine,
Edited by Bryan D. Cowan and David B. Seifer
Lippincott-Raven Publishers, Philadelphia © 1997

CHAPTER 4

Ovarian Phylogeny

Halina P. Wiczyk

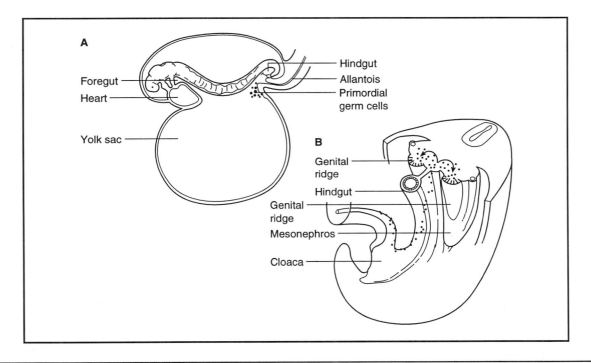

Historical Perspective
Embryogenesis
Meiosis
Follicular Formation
  Gonadotropin-Independent Follicle Formation

Gonadotropin-Dependent Follicle Formation
Atresia
  Follicular Depletion
Suggested Reading

H. P. Wiczyk: Department of Obstetrics and Gynecology, Bay State Medical Center, Springfield, MA 01199

The ovary is truly a unique organ. The constant changes and activities that occur over a span of almost 50 years are an intricate interplay of extraovarian and intraovarian influences. The generation of a mature fertilizable ovum each month is the primary goal of the ovary. However, only about 500 oocytes are ovulated during the reproductive life span of a woman. The majority of oocytes undergo fated atresia before ovulation. With aging, few follicles are left and atresia becomes complete. Estrogen production ceases and the menopause ensues. The growth and changes that occur throughout fetal life affect the function of the ovary irreversibly.

HISTORICAL PERSPECTIVE

The ovary was identified in the third century B.C. by the Greeks and further described in some detail by Soranus of Ephesus in the first century A.D. In the 17th century, Reiner de Graaf concluded incorrectly that the entire follicle (Graafian follicle) was an egg. It was early in the 19th century that Karl Ernst von Baer identified the presence of a distinct egg and was able to describe the exact relationship between an oocyte and the follicle. Prior to this, Leeuvenhoek had discovered mammalian spermatozoa in 1677. With the identification of the sperm and egg it was possible to understand the theory of fertilization. Although Waldeyer (latter half of the 19th century) believed that the sexually mature female was born with a finite number of oocytes, this theory was not fully accepted until the 1950s.

EMBRYOGENESIS

Genetic sex is determined at conception. Although development of the gonads occurs early in fetal life, sexual differences are not seen until development of the gonads (Chapter 5). Within 5 weeks of conception, the bipotential gonadal analgen can be identified. This can give rise to either the ovary or testis. The paired gonads form the genital ridge, which is a coelomic prominence overlying the mesonephros.

There are three different cell types that are essential to the development of the ovary. The first are the coelomic epithelial cells, which are derived from the gonadal ridge and later differentiate into granulosa cells. These granulosa cells are a heterogeneous cell population whose function depends on where they are located in relation to the oocyte. The granulosa cell compartment is avascular and separated from the surrounding stroma by a basal lamina membrane. The granulosa cells are interconnected by extensive intercellular gap junctions allowing for metabolic exchange and transport of small ions. Also, gap junction-like connections are made between the granulosa cells and the plasma membrane of the oocyte. These gap junctions are crucial in the regulation of oocyte maturation.

Ovarian stroma arises from the second cell type, the mesenchymal cell of the gonadal ridge. These become the theca-interstitial cells, which represent a heterogeneous cell population and have the ability to undertake de novo synthesis of androgens.

Primordial germ cells arise from the endoderm of the yolk sac and are the third cell type. The yolk sac is found at the caudal end of the embryo and these cells can be identified there as early as the third week of gestation. Migration of primordial cells can be traced with alkaline phosphatase staining. With the aid of pseudopodia, these cells migrate toward the genital ridge by amoeboid movements (Fig. 4-1). It is unknown precisely which cellular mechanisms control this movement, but chemotaxic sub-

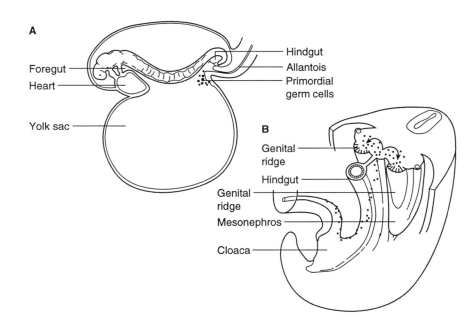

FIG. 4-1. Three-week-old embryo showing the primordial germ cells **(A)** and the migrational path along the wall of the hindgut into the genital ridge **(B)**.

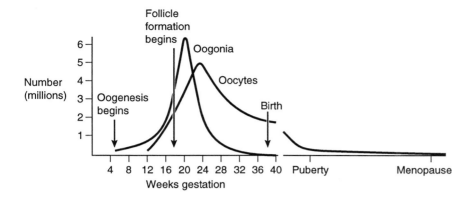

FIG. 4-2. Chronologic time line of germ cell populations in the ovary.

stances secreted at the gonadal ridge may play a role. Migration occurs between 4 and 6 weeks of gestation and proliferation of the germ cells begins during this movement. The germ cells are unable to survive outside the gonadal ridge and are mandatory for the induction of gonadal development. If germ cell migration does not occur, a functional gonad will not develop.

Once the germ cells arrive at the gonadal ridge (fifth week of gestation), the gonad enters a 2-week period referred to as the "indifferent stage." The indifferent gonads now contain germ cells and supporting cells that are derived from the coelomic epithelium and mesenchyme of the gonadal ridge.

In the female germ cells, one X chromosome is inactivated during migration to the gonadal ridge. However, two normal X chromosomes are necessary for structural and functional development of the ovary.

At about 8 weeks of fetal life, the germ cells undergo persistent mitosis, and three processes begin to occur simultaneously. Oogonial mitosis is counterbalanced by meiosis and atresia such that by 20 weeks of gestation the number of germ cells peaks at 6–7 million. This is the maximum and finite number of germ cells that now begin an irreversible process of attrition that results in the menopause some 50 years later (Fig. 4-2).

MEIOSIS

Meiosis is a complex process that begins between the 8th and 13th week of fetal life and is completed at the time of fertilization by a spermatozoan entering the oocyte. Meiosis I spans the time from initiation of the process in utero until the resumption and completion of the first meiotic division at ovulation. Up until that time the oocyte maintains a 46-chromosome complement. An oocyte progresses from the resting diplotene stage of prophase I (meiotic) to metaphase II by a process called meiotic maturation. This is characterized by dissolution of the oocyte's nuclear (germinal vesicle) membrane, condensation of chromatin, separation of homologous

chromosomes, and then emission of the first polar body. With the extrusion of the first polar body, the primary oocyte becomes a secondary oocyte with 23 chromosomes. This "mature oocyte" and its surrounding granulosa cells are released from the ovary at the time of follicle rupture. Sperm penetration (fertilization) initiates the second meiotic division. The second polar body is extruded after separation of the chromatids, thus completing the meiotic process (Fig. 4-3).

As meiosis begins, some of the oogonia leave the mitotic cycle and initiate nuclear changes that appear similar to prophase of the first meiotic division. As the oogonia enter the first meiotic division, they are transformed from oogonia to primary oocytes and this occurs before actual follicle formation. It is thought that this process begins in response to a factor originating from the rete ovarii or simply that contact with the rete ovarii induces oogonia to enter meiosis. Meiosis provides temporary protection from oogonial atresia and allows the germ cells to become surrounded by granulosa cells (primordial follicles). Oogonia that have not entered meiosis by the seventh month of gestation will undergo atresia and are usually not present at birth.

The primary oocyte is arrested in prophase of the first meiotic division until the time of ovulation. Progression from the leptotene stage to the diplotene stage occurs throughout gestation and is completed at birth. Arrest of meiosis is probably controlled locally in the ovary and has been the focus of in vitro experiments. The following factors have been implicated in maintaining meiotic arrest: cyclic adenosine monophosphate (cAMP) as well as enzyme systems involving intracellular levels of cAMP, calcium, calmodulin, steroids, hypophyseal hormones, purine bases, and putative polypeptide inhibitors (Chapter 1). The exact interplay between these factors in the regulation of meiotic arrest and subsequent maturation is not understood. It has been shown that a decrease in intracellular cAMP can signal reentry of oocytes into meiotic progression suggesting that cAMP maintains meiotic arrest. Gap junctions are intercellular communications that are present between cumulus cells and the oocyte

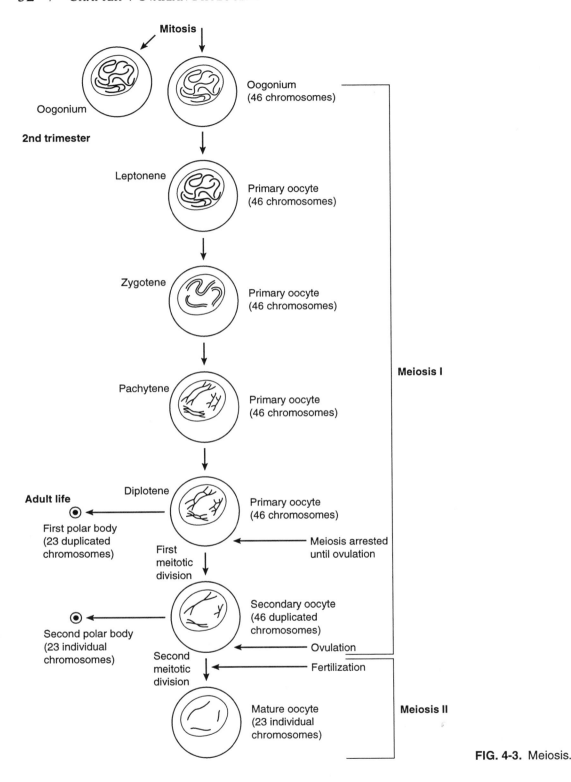

FIG. 4-3. Meiosis.

(Fig. 4-4). The cells are coupled metabolically and ionically. In vitro studies demonstrate that these gap junctions are necessary for oocyte growth. Denuded oocytes become necrotic because they appear to depend on granulosa cells to provide certain nutritional needs. A signifi-

cant decrease in the number of gap junctions is seen just prior to ovulation, and following ovulation the oocyte and surrounding cumulus are no longer coupled. Oocyte maturation inhibitor (OMI), a granulosa cell product, may also be involved in meiotic arrest. OMI is a polypeptide

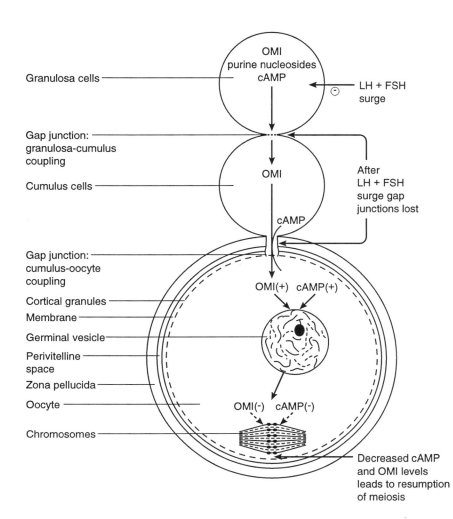

FIG. 4-4. Regulators of arrested meiosis in the oocyte.

found in the follicular fluid from ovaries of different mammals and has been shown in vitro to prevent oocytes from undergoing spontaneous meiotic maturation. In order for OMI to exert its inhibitory action, it requires the presence of cumulus cells. The *c-mos* proto-oncogene is another peptide factor that may control expression of a regulatory protein that maintains meiosis. Overall it is the intact follicle that maintains the oocyte in meiotic arrest.

FOLLICULAR FORMATION

Gonadotropin-Independent Follicle Formation

At about 16 weeks of gestation, the primary follicle is first seen. This is a complex of a primary oocyte arrested in prophase of meiosis encased in spindle-shaped granulosa cells and surrounded by a basal lamina. Although oogonial meiotic divisions cease and meiosis is arrested by about 7 months gestation, primordial follicles continue to be generated (until about 6 months postpartum).

This stage of follicular development is entirely gonadotropin-independent.

During this time, the highly cellular cortex becomes perforated by vascular channels that originate in the deeper medullary areas. The invading blood vessels divide the solid cortical cell mass into smaller segments. Mesenchymal cells not incorporated into primordial follicle formation begin to form the primitive ovarian stroma seen between the follicles. Oocytes not incorporated into follicles degenerate.

The next phase of follicular development, called the preantral growth phase, converts the primordial follicle into a secondary follicle. This conversion process continues without interruption for the next 50 years until the time of menopause. Mucopolysaccharides are secreted by the granulosa cells to give rise to the zona pellucida that surrounds the oocyte. The zona pellucida maintains contact with the granulosa cells via gap junctions. Granulosa cell proliferation then occurs resulting in multiple layers and an enlarged secondary follicle. By the sixth month of gestation preantral follicles are found, and a small number of antral follicles are found at birth. As the total granulosa cell mass increases, thecal differentiation begins. However, it is only during the third trimester that theca cells can be seen surrounding the follicles.

Gonadotropin-Dependent Follicle Formation

The fetal pituitary becomes functional by 12 weeks. Follicle-stimulating hormone (FSH) peaks in the circulation at 28 weeks, reaching levels seen in postmenopausal women. Fetal follicles begin to grow in response to gonadotropin influence at about 20 weeks. The important relationship between gonadotropins and normal ovarian development is demonstrated in two different situations. Hypophysectomy in the fetal rhesus monkey and anencephaly result in reduced follicular development. In both cases gonadotropin-independent meiosis and primordial follicle formation progresses but further growth ceases.

With the formation of a secondary follicle, granulosa cells develop receptors for FSH, estrogens, and androgens that become physiologically coupled by gap junctions. The differentiating secondary follicle acquires a thecal component as it migrates into the medulla. When thecal development begins a follicular blood supply and lymphatics arrive. One or two arterioles terminate in a network of capillaries next to the basal lamina. This blood supply does not penetrate the basal lamina and granulosa cells, and the oocyte remain avascular. With capillary formation, the theca cells acquire luteinizing hormone (LH) receptors and the capacity for steroidogenesis. Thus, the formation of a functional follicular unit with the presence of an oocyte, granulosa FSH receptors, and thecal LH receptors is completed. It is now ready to respond to appropriate stimulations that will occur at the time of puberty and throughout the reproductive years.

ATRESIA

Gonadotropin-independent atresia begins during fetal life. Atresia is a Greek word used to describe the closure of a natural opening. Using strict definition, atresia refers to antral follicles undergoing degenerative changes before the rupture that occurs during ovulation. But the word is also used to describe degenerative changes taking place during ovarian development. Germ cell content peaks at 20 weeks gestation. At birth, the germ cell number is reduced to 1–2 million. Thus, a substantial depletion of germ cells occurs in only 20 weeks. Because the female has a fixed number of germ cells, the newborn enters life having already lost 80% of her oocytes. With the onset of puberty, the germ cell mass has been further reduced to 400,000 oocytes. Of these, only about 500 of the original 6–7 million oocytes will mature under gonadotropic stimulation and ovulate.

Apoptosis is an active, orderly event that takes place in tissues undergoing developmental changes or responding to alterations in physiologic stimuli. This process takes place in normal cells and requires mRNA and protein synthesis. Cells shrink, chromatin condenses, and small spherical bits of membrane are formed, called apoptotic bodies, containing nuclear fragments. These cells are phagocytized by neighboring cells and before plasma membrane integrity is lost. There is no leakage of cytoplasmic components and thus no inflammatory reaction. Theca cells are outside the basal lamina and do not die during the process. The ovarian interstitial cells reabsorb these thecal cells.

Apoptosis is thought to be programmed cell death and is involved in follicle atresia. The factors that trigger apoptosis are cell-specific and are mediated by endonuclease activation, which specifically cleaves cellular DNA. There are ovarian growth factors, regulatory peptides, including the inhibin family of proteins, gonadotropins, and steroids that can be suppressive or stimulatory to apoptosis. Gonadotropins, estrogens, and several growth factors are follicle survival factors, whereas androgens promote atresia. Hormonal control and molecular mechanisms of follicle atresia demonstrate this as an active process that may be genetically predetermined.

Follicular Depletion

Repeated cycles of ovulation and atresia deplete the ovary of its follicles. During the reproductive years, the typical cycle of follicle maturation, ovulation, and corpus luteum formation occurs. This complex process progresses in a sequence of hypothalamic-pituitary-gonadal interactions resulting in an integration of ovarian steroids, pituitary gonadotropins, and autocrine/paracrine factors. Eventually, all of the oocytes are exhausted. The stroma becomes hyperplastic and dominates the ovary. In the last 10–15 years before menopause there is an acceleration of follicular loss accompanied by decreased reproductive potential. Ovarian responsiveness to gonadotropin stimulation is reduced and FSH begins to increase. With the cessation of cyclic ovarian function, estrogen production is diminished and the changes associated with menopause are manifested.

Thus ends an extraordinary process that began in the earliest stages of fetal development. Throughout gestation, childhood, puberty, and the span of the reproductive years, the ovary constantly grew, changed, and then eventually ceased follicular activity.

SUGGESTED READING

Adashi EY, ed. Putative intraovarian regulators. *Semin Reprod Endocrinol* 1989;7:1.

Gondos B, Hobel CG. Interstitial cells in the human fetal ovary. *Endocrinology* 1978;93:736.

Gondos B, Westergaard L, Byskov A. Initiation of oogenesis in the human fetal ovary: ultrasound structural and squash preparation study. *Am J Obstet Gynecol* 1986;155:189.

Guylas BJ, Hodgen GD, Tullner WW, Ross GT. Effects of fetal and maternal hypophysectomy on endocrine organs and body weight in infant monkey (*Macaca mulatta*) with particular emphasis on oogenesis. *Biol Reprod* 1977;16:216.

Hseuh AJW, Adashi EY, Jones PBC, Welsh TH Jr. Hormonal regulation of the differentiation of cultured ovarian granulosa cells. *Endocr Rev* 1984;5:76.

Hseuh AJ, Billig H, Tsafriri A. Ovarian follicle atresia: a hormonally controlled apoptotic process. *Endocr Rev* 1994;15:707.

Hurwitz A, Adashi EY. Ovarian follicular atresia as an apoptotic process: a paradigm for programmed cell death in endocrine tissues. *Mol Cell Endocrinol* 1992;84:C19.

Magner LN. *A History of Medicine.* New York: Marcel Dekker, 1992.

Pal SK, Torry D, Serta R, et al. Expression and potential function of the *c*-mos proto-oncogene in human eggs. *Fertil Steril* 1994;61:496.

Schreiber JR, Beckman MW, Polarek D, Davies PF. Changes in gap junction connexin-43 messenger ribonucleic acid levels associated with rat ovarian follicular development as demonstrated by in situ hybridization. *Am J Obstet Gynecol* 1993;168:1094.

Thatcher SS, Naftolin F. The aging and aged ovary. *Semin Reprod Endocrinol* 1991;9:189.

Tornell J, Hillensjo T. Effect of cyclic AMP on the isolated human oocyte–cumulus complex. *Hum Reprod* 1993;8:737.

Tsafriri A, Dekel N, Bar-Ami S. The role of oocyte inhibitor in follicular regulation of oocyte maturation. *J Reprod Fertil* 1982; 63:541.

Warikoo PK, Bavister BD. Hypoxanthine and cyclic adenosine 5'-monophosphate maintain meiotic arrest of rhesus monkey oocytes in vitro. *Fertil Steril* 1989;51:886.

Clinical Reproductive Medicine,
Edited by Bryan D. Cowan and David B. Seifer
Lippincott-Raven Publishers, Philadelphia © 1997

CHAPTER 5

Normal and Abnormal Sexual Development

Patricia E. Bailey

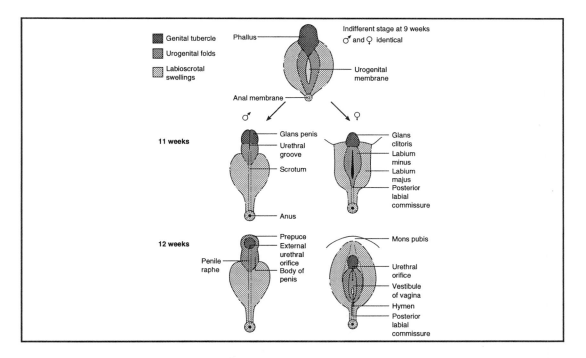

Embryology
  Development of the Gonads
  Development of the Genital Ducts
  Development of the External Genitalia
Disorders of Sexual Development

Male Pseudohermaphroditism
Female Pseudohermaphroditism
Ambiguous Genitalia
Suggested Reading

P. E. Bailey: Pediatric and Adolescent Gynecology Services, Department of Obstetrics and Gynecology, Bay State Medical Center, Springfield, MA 01199

The diagnosis of a disorder of sexual development is usually made during one of two stages of the life cycle. The first is at birth, when an infant is found to have ambiguous genitalia. The second is at puberty, when a child fails to proceed through a normal pubertal sequence. Even under the most normal of circumstances, birth and puberty are emotion-charged times. When compounded by a diagnosis that calls into question a fundamental such as gender, the anxiety and distress to the parents and to the patient can be overwhelming. These patients and their parents must be evaluated promptly and thoroughly; they must be counseled extensively and with exquisite sensitivity.

EMBRYOLOGY

Development of the Gonads

The first indication of gonadal development occurs during the fifth week after conception, with the development of the gonadal ridge, which is a bulge on the medial side of the mesonephros. The primordial germ cells then migrate from the yolk sac to the gonadal ridge by amoeboid movement during the sixth week after conception. At this point, the structure is referred to as the indifferent gonad.

Although the exact mechanism for testicular development has not been elucidated, development appears to occur in the presence of the testis-determining factor (TDF) (Fig. 5-1), the gene that is located in the SRY (sex-deter-

mining region Y) on the short arm of the Y chromosome. The Sertoli cells appear at 6–7 weeks of gestation and begin to secrete Mullerian inhibiting substance (MIS). At 8 weeks gestation, the Leydig cells differentiate and androgen synthesis begins. Testosterone secretion peaks between 15 and 18 weeks. The testes are morphologically identifiable 7–8 weeks after conception.

Whereas development of fetal ovaries begins at 50–55 days of embryonic development, the ovary as such is not identifiable until about the tenth week after conception. Although many oogonia degenerate before birth, the 2 million or so that remain at birth enlarge to become primary oocytes. They become surrounded by a layer of cuboidal cells and are then called the primary follicle. They remain quiescent until puberty.

Development of the Genital Ducts

In the indifferent state, the mesonephric ducts drain the mesonephric kidneys and the paramesonephric ducts develop on the lateral aspects of the mesonephroi. In the male, testicular androgens stimulate the mesonephric ducts to form male genital ducts, whereas MIS involutes the paramesonephric ducts (Fig. 5-1).

In embryos with ovaries or no gonads (ie, in the absence of testosterone and MIS), the mesonephric ducts regress and the paramesonephric ducts develop into most of the internal female genital tract. The cranial, unfused portions of the paramesonephric ducts develop into the uterine tubes. The caudal, fused potions of the para-

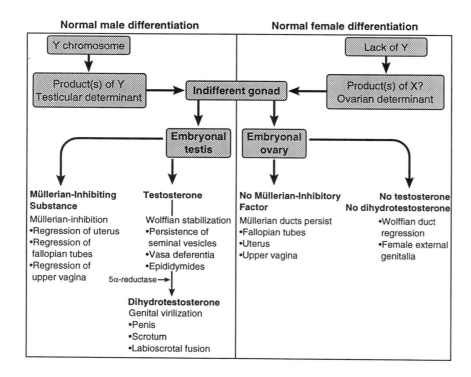

FIG. 5-1. Schematic diagram of normal male and female differentiation.

mesonephric ducts form the uterovaginal primordium, which gives rise to the uterus, cervix, and superior part of the vagina (Fig. 5-2). Contact of the uterovaginal primordium with the urogenital sinus induces the formation of the sinovaginal bulbs, which subsequently fuse to form a solid vaginal plate. Later the central cells of the plate break down, forming the lumen of the vagina. Until late fetal life, the lumen of the vagina is separated from the cavity of the urogenital sinus by the hymen, which usually ruptures during the perinatal period.

Development of the External Genitalia

The indifferent stage of the development of the external genitalia begins early in the fourth week when the genital tubercle develops at the cranial end of the cloacal membrane (Fig. 5-3). Labioscrotal swelling and urogenital folds then develop on each side of the cloacal membrane. The genital tubercle soon elongates to form a phallus. At the end of the sixth week, the urorectal septum fuses with the cloacal membrane, dividing the cloacal

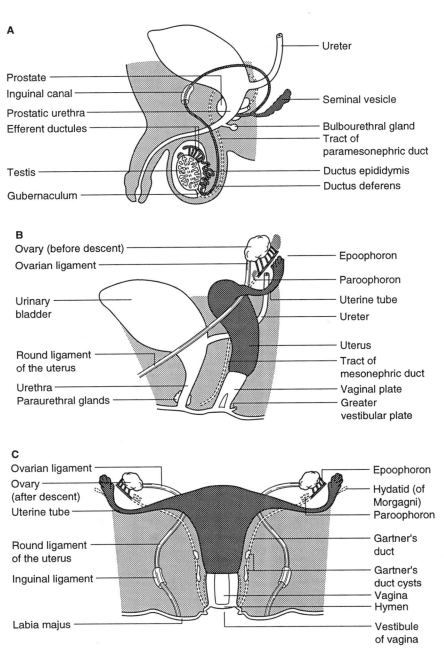

FIG. 5-2. Development of the male and female reproductive systems from the genital ducts and the urogenital sinus.

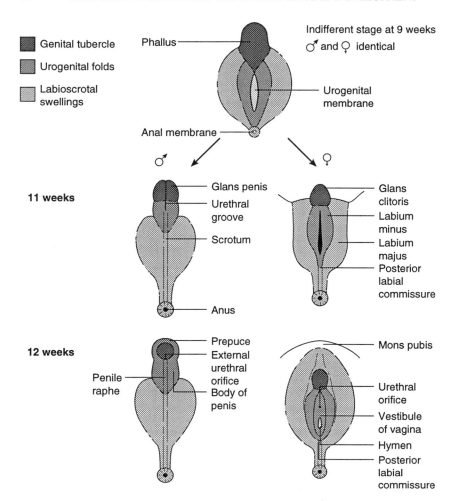

FIG. 5-3. Development of the external genitalia.

membrane into a dorsal anal membrane and a ventral urogenital membrane.

In the male fetus, development of the male external genitalia occurs under the influence of androgens produced by the fetal testes. The external genital target tissue cells convert testosterone to dihydrotestosterone (DHT) by the intracellular enzyme 5α-reductase. The phallus elongates to form the penis, pulling the urogenital folds ventrally (see Fig. 5-3). The urogenital folds soon fuse along the ventral surface of the penis to form the spongy urethra. The penile raphe is formed and the urethra is enclosed within the penis, moving the external urethral orifice progressively toward the glans. The labioscrotal swellings grow toward each other and fuse to form the scrotum. The line of fusion is visible as the scrotal raphe.

In the absence of androgens, the female external genitalia develop. Growth of the phallus ceases and the clitoris is formed. It develops like the penis, except that the urogenital folds fuse only posteriorly to form the frenulum of the labia minora. The unfused parts of the urogenital folds form the labia majora. The labioscrotal folds fuse posteriorly to form the posterior labial commissure and anteriorly to form the anterior labial commissure and the mons pubis. The unfused parts of the labioscrotal folds form the labia majora. The phallic part of the urogenital sinus gives rise to the vestibule of the vagina.

DISORDERS OF SEXUAL DEVELOPMENT

From the above discussion of normal male and female sexual development, it becomes a matter of intuition that genital ambiguity occurs *only* when there is too much androgen in the female fetus or too little androgen in the male fetus (Table 5-1). For logical considerations a few developmental/genetic defects are commonly discussed under the heading of disordered sexual development (eg, 45,XO, MIS deficiency, female 17-hydroxylase deficiency), but there is no "disorder" of sexual differentiation related to the genital sex of these patients. The term

TABLE 5-1. *Causes of disordered sexual development*

Male	Too little androgen
Female	Too much androgen

"pseudohermaphroditism" indicates that the gonadal sex is at variance with the genital sex. The term "male" or "female" denotes the gonadal (genetic) sex of the individual. The following will discuss the gonadal and hormonal defects associated with genital ambiguity.

Male Pseudohermaphroditism

In male pseudohermaphrodites (Table 5-2), the gonads are testes, the karyotype is XY, but the phenotype is feminized (to varying degrees). There are five basic alterations encountered: deficient androgen formation, deficient responses to androgen, deficient conversion of testosterone, defects in MIS, and gonadal formation errors.

Deficient Androgen Formation

Five enzymes are involved in the stepwise conversion of cholesterol to testosterone: cholesterol desmolase (P450$_{scc}$), 3β-hydroxysteroid dehydrogenase, 17α-hydroxylase (P450$_{c17}$), 17:20-desmolase(P450$_{c17}$), and 17β-hydroxysteroid dehydrogenase. A deficiency of any of these enzymes will lead to deficient androgen synthesis and thus to incomplete virilization of a male fetus. Depending on the location of the block in the steroidogenic pathway (Fig. 5-4), these disorders may also affect glucocorticoid and mineralocorticoid biosynthesis. It should be noted that internal female genital structures (uterus, tubes) are not found in these patients because the testes produce MIS. The pattern of inheritance appears to be autosomal recessive.

TABLE 5-2. *Male pseudohermaphroditism (karyotype = 46XY, gonad = testis)*

Defect	Inheritance
Deficient androgen formation	
Cholesterol desmolase deficiency	Auto recessive
3β-Hydroxysteroid dehydrogenase deficiency	Auto recessive
17α-Hydroxylase deficiency	Auto recessive
17:20-Desmolase deficiency	X-linked recessive, auto dominant
17β-Hydroxysteroid dehydrogenase deficiency	Auto recessive
Androgen insensitivity	
Complete	X-linked recessive/ X-linked dominant
Partial	X-linked recessive
5α-Reductase deficiency	Auto recessive
Lack of Mullerian duct regression	Auto recessive/X-linked recessive
Defective gonadal formation	
XY gonadal dysgenesis	
Mixed gonadal dysgenesis	
True hermaphrodite	
Leydig cell hypoplasia	Auto recessive

Auto, autosomal.

Cholesterol Desmolase (P450scc) Deficiency

This condition, also known as congenital lipoid adrenal hyperplasia (CLAH), is usually not compatible with life. Approximately 30 cases have been reported. Cholesterol desmolase is the enzyme that converts cholesterol to pregnenolone (see Fig. 5-4). Therefore, in this syndrome, there is a very early block in steroid biosynthesis, and consequently cortisol, aldosterone, and testosterone are not pre-

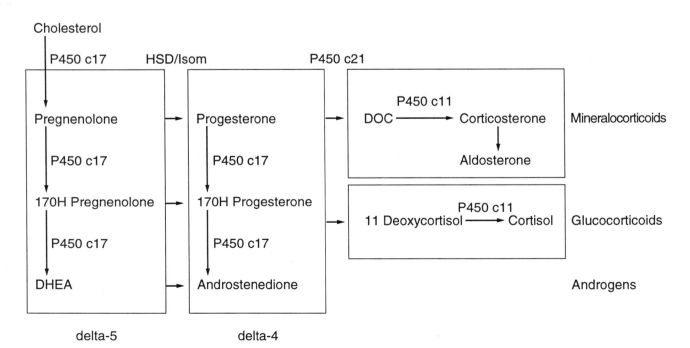

FIG. 5-4. Ovarian and adrenal biosynthesis.

sent in the circulation. Affected XY infants have female external genitalia or ambiguous genitalia, severe sodium wasting, and adrenals that are markedly enlarged and characterized by foamy-appearing cells filled with cholesterol. Laboratory studies show decreased serum and urinary levels of all adrenal and gonadal steroids and their metabolites, even after adrenocorticotropic hormone (ACTH) or human chorionic gonadotropin (hCG) stimulation. In those infants who survive, treatment of this disease includes mineral corticosteroids and glucocorticoids.

3β-Hydroxysteroid Dehydrogenase Deficiency

The enzyme 3β-hydroxysteroid catalyzes the conversion of D5 steroids to the D4 configuration (pregnenolone to progesterone, 17-hydroxypregnenolone to 17-hydroxyprogesterone (OHP), and dehydroepiandrosterone (DHEA) to androstenedione) (see Fig. 5-4). In the XY fetus, an enzymatic block at this level is characterized by incomplete masculinization of the external genitalia in the presence of normal internal male genital ducts and the absence of Mullerian ducts. In the XX fetus, there is increased DHEA secretion, which causes masculinization of the female external genitalia. This is the only enzyme defect that produces genital ambiguity (pseudohermaphroditism) in both males and females. Because aldosterone and cortisol are decreased, there is severe sodium wasting. Treatment includes glucocorticoids, mineralocorticoids, and appropriate hormone replacement at puberty.

17α-Hydroxylase Deficiency

17α-hydroxylase catalyzes the conversion of pregnenolone to 17-hydroxypregnenolone and progesterone to 17-hydroxyprogesterone (see Fig. 5-4). 17α-hydroxylase deficiency in 46XY individuals encompasses a spectrum of disorders from normal-appearing female external genitalia with a blind pouch to hypospadias and a small phallus. The degree of abnormality reflects the severity of the block. Cortisol production is impaired resulting in the excess secretion of the nonhydroxylated precursors deoxycorticosterone (DOC), corticosterone, and 18-hydroxycorticosterone. Despite impaired cortisol production, evidence of glucocorticoid deficiency is unusual, possibly because corticosterone has weak glucocorticoid activity. While affected females show hypertension, affected males usually display normal blood pressure. Treatment with physiologic doses of glucocorticoids suppresses ACTH production, which reduces levels of DOC, corticosterone, and 18-hydroxycorticosterone, resolving the hypertension and hypokalemia.

17:20-Desmolase Deficiency

17:20-Desmolase deficiency is an autosomal dominant or X-linked recessive, and affects only androgen (and subsequently estrogen) formation. Glucocorticoid and mineral corticoid production remain normal because the enzymatic block is distal to these pathways. There may be ambiguous external genitalia, with inguinal or intraabdominal testes, and severe hypospadias with male-type urethra and male duct development. If the diagnosis is made in infancy, treatment with testosterone should result in adequate growth of the penis and development of male secondary sex characteristics.

17β-Hydroxysteroid Dehydrogenase Deficiency

The enzyme 17β-hydroxysteroid dehydrogenase is needed for the conversion of androstenedione to testosterone and for the conversion of estrone to estradiol. Affected males show ambiguous genitalia, bilateral testes, and no Mullerian structures. The testes secrete androstenedione and estrone at an increased rate. Androstenedione is converted to testosterone at extratesticular sites in sufficient quantities to cause virilization, which can be marked at puberty. Peripheral conversion of estrone to estradiol can cause gynecomastia depending on the estrogen-to-testosterone ratio.

Deficient Responses to Androgen

Complete Androgen Insensitivity

Complete androgen insensitivity, also known as testicular feminization, is the most common form of male pseudohermaphroditism. It may be X-linked recessive or X-linked dominant, and is characterized by a female habitus, an XY karyotype, and functional testes. Typically, these patients present in late adolescence with primary amenorrhea. On physical examination, these patients have abundant breast tissue, scant or absent pubic hair and axillary hair, female external genitalia, and a vagina that ends in a blind pouch. The internal female genital structures are missing. The testes may be located in the pelvis or in an inguinal hernia.

In this disorder there is a target organ insensitivity to the androgens produced by the testes and therefore androgen induction of the Wolffian duct does not occur. Because these testes are normal and also produce MIS, Mullerian regression occurs. Although the testosterone is in the normal male range, virilization does not occur at puberty because of the target organ receptor defect. The concentration of LH is increased, presumably as a result of resistance in the hypothalamic-pituitary system to androgen inhibition. In contrast to gonadal dysgenesis with a Y chromosome, the occurrence of gonadal tumors in androgen insensitivity syndromes is relatively late, rarely before age 25, and the overall incidence is less, about 5%. For these reasons, gonadectomy can be performed after puberty at approximately age 16–18. After surgery, estrogen replacement should be instituted. Additionally, family members should be investigated carefully to screen for undiagnosed individuals.

Counseling of the patients should begin from the understanding that the patient is phenotypically, anatomically, legally, and socially female and should build on that understanding. Relating the patient's condition to "genes" is more helpful than telling her that she is "male." Patients and their parents must be counseled regarding the fact that the patient will not menstruate, nor will she have children. Additionally, with the parents out of the room, it is important to discuss the patient's sexual history with her. Often these girls have attempted intercourse and the results have been so dismal that their ability to function sexually may be impaired. Patients should be informed that there are several methods, both surgical and nonsurgical, which can be used to create a vagina and that she should be able to achieve normal sexual function. Psychiatric evaluation may be helpful.

Partial Androgen Insensitivity

In patients with partial androgen insensitivity, a degree of androgen responsiveness is present. Eponyms that have been used in the past for partial androgen insensitivity include Reifenstein, Gilbert-Dreyfus, and Lubs. These disorders have been shown to represent different spectrums of a single disorder. Partial androgen insensitivity is one tenth as common as complete androgen insensitivity. Clinically, a wide spectrum of genital findings occur, from almost complete failure of virilization with mild clitoromegaly and labial fusion to almost complete masculinization. The mode of inheritance is X-linked recessive.

Deficient Conversion of Testosterone

5α-Reductase Deficiency

Formerly known as pseudovaginal perineoscrotal hypospadias, this autosomal recessive syndrome is characterized by severe hypospadias, variable fusion of the labioscrotal fold, and variable development of a urogenital opening. The Wolffian structures, ie, the epididymis, vas deferens, and seminal vesicles are normal. The karyotype is XY. Because of the intracellular 5α-reductase deficiency, DHT cannot be formed adequately and therefore those structures that develop embryologically under the influence of DHT (the urogenital sinus, urogenital fold, tubercle, and swelling) do not develop. The testes secrete MIS and thus the Mullerian structures regress. At birth, the external genitalia are described as above and these individuals are usually assigned a female gender if the phallus is deemed inadequate. At puberty, they undergo marked although not complete masculinization. It should be noted that this is in contrast to androgen insensitivity syndromes in which virilization does not occur at puberty. The diagnosis can be made in infancy by demonstrating an elevated testosterone/DHT ratio, especially after hCG stimulation.

Defects in MIS

Also known as hernia uterine inguinale, this disorder is the result of abnormal synthesis or secretion of MIS (Mullerian inhibiting substance) by the fetal Sertoli cells or by the inability of the Mullerian ducts to respond appropriately to AMH. Because androgen production, utilization, and peripheral conversion are normal, it is characterized by otherwise normal male external genitalia with bilateral cryptorchidism and inguinal hernias. In the inguinal canal, uterus, and fallopian tubes are found. The gonads are testes and normal virilization occurs at puberty. These disorders can be autosomal or X-linked recessive. The individuals are fertile males.

Gonadal Formation Errors

XY Gonadal Dysgenesis

Loss of testicular tissue before 43 days of embryogenesis results in a female phenotype in spite of the XY chromosome complement. These individuals have normal female external genitalia, a uterus, and fallopian tubes (Swyer's syndrome). The diagnosis is made when they fail to enter puberty. They are of normal height and lack Turner's stigmata. These individuals are at high risk of developing a dysgerminoma or a gonadoblastoma (20–30%) and for this reason the gonads of these individuals should be extirpated. The uterus and tubes should not be removed, as pregnancy is possible through the use of donor oocytes or embryos.

In rare individuals, testicular degeneration occurs between 60 and 84 days of embryologic development (fetal gonadal atresia). If degeneration occurs early (Swyer's syndrome or embryologic gonadal atresia), the external female genitalia are normal. If testicular degeneration occurs after there has been secretion of testosterone and MIS, the result will be ambiguous genitalia with rudimentary components of both Mullerian and Wolffian systems. The degree of ambiguity is determined by the extent of development achieved before fetal gonadal loss occurred. Thus, this syndrome of 46XY "pure" gonadal dysgenesis represents a spectrum of clinical presentations ranging from a phenotypically normal female (Swyer's) to a phenotypically agonadal male ("vanishing testes"), depending exclusively on the state of embryologic or fetal development that was achieved prior to gonadal loss.

Mixed Gonadal Dysgenesis

The most commonly found karyotype associated with mixed gonadal dysgenesis is 45,X/46XY, although other forms of mosaicism are also found. The physical findings can range from ambiguous genitalia in males to normal females with streak gonads. Typically, the gonadal pattern is a streak gonad on one side of the pelvis and a normal or dysgenetic gonad on the opposite side.

Mullerian or Wolffian structures may be present, depending on the character of the ipsilateral gonad. Because of the very high incidence of gonadal tumors (25%), intraabdominal gonads should be removed.

True Hermaphroditism

The diagnosis of true hermaphroditism is made only when the coexistence of ovarian and testicular tissue can be demonstrated. There may be ovarian and testicular tissue within the same gonad (ovotestis) or in opposite gonads, but germ cells of both sexes should be demonstrated. The internal structures correspond to the adjacent gonad and absence of a uterine horn usually indicates an ipsilateral testis or ovotestis. The majority of true hermaphrodites are raised as males because of the size of the phallus, but most have an XX karyotype. Three fourths of these individuals develop gynecomastia and half menstruate after puberty.

Leydig Cell Hypoplasia

Leydig cells are the site of testicular testosterone production and in this syndrome, due to Leydig cell hypoplasia or a Leydig cell receptor defect for LH and hCG, testosterone is not produced. This syndrome is also called gonadotropin-resistant testes. These individuals are characterized by a male karyotype, a predominantly female phenotype, sexual infantilism, immature testes, and no Mullerian duct derivatives. Wolffian duct structures are usually present, although they may be hypoplastic. The gonadotropin concentrations are increased; the testosterone concentrations are low and cannot be stimulated by hCG. An autosomal recessive inheritance has been postulated.

Female Pseudohermaphroditism (Table 5-3)

The term *female pseudohermaphroditism* encompasses individuals with an XX karyotype, ovaries, normal uterus and tubes, and varying degrees of external genital virilization. Reproductive function is often possible. Only two sources of excess androgen exposure in utero are recognized: endogenous production (CAH) and exogenous (maternal hormone injection, androgen-secreting tumors).

Congenital Adrenal Hyperplasia

In all forms of CAH, there is a decreased capacity to produce cortisol due to an enzyme block in the steroid

TABLE 5-3. *Female pseudohermaphrodism (karyotype = 46,XX, gonad = ovary)*

Defect	Inheritance
Endogenous androgen excess (congenital adrenal hyperplasia)	
21-Hydroxylase deficiency	Auto recessive
11β-Hydroxylase deficiency	Auto recessive
3β-Hydroxysteroid dehydrogenase deficiency	Auto recessive
Exogenous androgen excess	
Maternal androgen-secreting tumor	
Drugs, medications	
Gonadal defects	
XO monosomy (Turner's syndrome)	
45,X/46,XX and 45,X/47,XXX mosaicism	
Structural abnormalities	
Involving the second sex chromosome	
XX gonadal dysgenesis (pure gonadal dysgenesis)	Auto recessive

Auto, autosomal.

pathway of cortisol synthesis. The steroids immediately preceding the block are present in the circulation in increased concentration. These disorders are transmitted as autosomal recessive.

21-Hydroxylase Deficiency

This is the most common form of these disorders and composes approximately 90% of the cases. This enzyme defect is the most common cause of ambiguous genitalia in newborns and, because affected females have the capacity for an entirely normal female sex and reproductive life, assignment should always be female. The presentations can vary in severity from partial to complete absence of the 21-hydroxylase enzyme system. There are three different clinical forms recognized: the salt-wasting type, the simple virilizing type, and the late onset type. In all of these disorders the unifying factor is that cortisol cannot be made in normal amounts and the increased ACTH leads to adrenal hyperplasia, which in turn results in increased amounts of 17-hydroxyprogesterone, dehydroepiandrosterone, androstenedione, and testosterone.

The extent of masculinization is dependent on the state of intrauterine development of the external genitalia at which the effect of androgen excess is first manifested. If left untreated, there is an increased androgen concentration that will cause excessive long bone growth and heterosexual precocity. In childhood, the patient is taller than her peers, with early pubic and axillary hair development and phallic hypertrophy. With continued androgen excess, the epiphyses fuse prematurely, so that in adulthood the patient will be shorter than her peers, with a masculinized body habitus. In the untreated patient, androgen excess will suppress the pituitary gonadotropins and ovarian function will not be stimulated. Therefore the patient will have neither female secondary sexual development nor menses. In the most severe forms of the enzymatic defect, there is a deficiency of desoxycorticosterone (DOC) and aldosterone in addition to androgen excess. This "salt-wasting form" can be fatal if not treated.

11β-Hydroxylase Deficiency

The 11β-hydroxylase enzyme in humans is found only in the adrenal cortex. Its deficiency leads to an increase in biosynthesis and secretion of 11-deoxysteroids, which are shunted into androgen biosynthesis. Clinically, virilization and hypertension are encountered. Like 21-hydroxylase deficiency, somatic growth is rapid, and there is early closure of the epiphyses. Additionally, there is phallic enlargement, premature appearance of pubic and axillary hair, breast hypoplasia, amenorrhea, and hypertension from overproduction of DOC. Treatment consists of exogenous glucocorticoids.

3β-Hydroxysteroid Dehydrogenase Deficiency

These individuals are severely ill at birth and rarely survive. As mentioned, this is the only enzymatic defect that causes ambiguity in both sexes (too much androgen in the female from excess DHEA; too little androgen in the male from reduced testosterone production).

17α-Hydroxylase Deficiency

In this disorder, only the non-17-hydroxylated corticoids, DOC and corticosterone, are formed. Androgen and estrogen formation do not occur. The syndrome is composed of hypertension, hypokalemia, infantile female internal genitalia, and failed puberty. Because androgens are not produced, this syndrome is not considered historically as a defect in sexual differentiation. No heterosexual ambiguity is observed in the female but, as noted earlier, this is not the case in the male.

Disorders of Gonadal Development

Although disordered gonadal development in the 46,XX female is not associated with genital ambiguity, the presentation of these syndromes here follows the logical understanding of defective sexual differentiation. In contrast, disordered gonadal development in 46,XY individuals is often associated with pseudohermaphroditism.

XO Monosomy (Turner's Syndrome)

The XO karyotype occurs in an estimated 0.8% of zygotes and is the most common chromosomal abnormality associated with spontaneous abortions. In liveborn phenotypically female newborns, the incidence of XO karyotype is approximately 1 in 2700 births.

The clinical features of Turner's syndrome (Turner's stigmata) are well known and include short stature (<58 in. tall), webbed neck (pterygium colli), high-arched palate, low-set and prominent ears, low posterior hairline, epicanthal fold, tendency of micrognathia, increased carrying angle of the arms (cubitus valgus), shield-like chest, wide-set nipples, cardiovascular anomalies, and renal anomalies. In these patients, the normal gonad is replaced by a white fibrous streak, 2–3 cm long and about 0.5 cm wide, which is located in the position normally occupied by the ovary. Germ cells are present in 45,XO embryos but are usually absent in 45,XO adults. This would indicate that the pathogenesis of germ cell failure is increased atresia, not failure of germ cell formation or migration to the gonadal ridge.

The diagnosis of Turner's syndrome is often made at adolescence, when the patient fails to enter puberty. Hormonal evaluation reveals elevated gonadotropins (in the postmenopausal range). The chromosomes are then evaluated, revealing the XO chromosome complement. Because of the high incidence of associated somatic anomalies, patients diagnosed with Turner's syndrome should undergo a careful evaluation at the time of diagnosis. This evaluation should include thyroid function testing and thyroid antibodies, evaluation of the renal system (either by intravenous pyelogram or renal ultrasound), echocardiogram, and audiometry. Additionally, the following evaluation should be performed annually: thyroid function testing, lipid profile and glucose metabolism, and blood pressure evaluation. Treatment with estrogen (Chapter 6) is usually instituted when the bone age is approximately 12 years to avoid epiphysial closure and to allow for a longer period of long bone growth. The initial dose of estrogen used should be very low. Starting with high doses of estrogen can result in tubular breast formation which is cosmetically unattractive. Growth hormone treatment has been used to increase adult height, but such treatment is expensive and controversial.

Mosaicism

Genetic mosaicism (45,X/46,XX and 45,X/47,XXX) is responsible for the majority of cases of gonadal dysgenesis variants and usually "dilutes" the frequency of abnormalities. These patients are not always short, may menstruate, and may even become pregnant. Treatment is similar to that of 45,XO.

Patients with deletion of the short arm of X have clinical findings that are similar to those of patients with an XO karyotype. Deletion of the long arm results in persons of normal stature and relatively few of the stigmata of Turner's syndrome. These patients have streak gonads, primary amenorrhea, and sexual infantilism.

There are many other X abnormalities including centric fragments, dicentric fragments, and ring X chromosomes. In these abnormalities, it is the deficient loci rather than the rearrangement that are responsible for the associated abnormalities.

XX Gonadal Dysgenesis

In chromosomally normal patients in whom gonadal dysgenesis (pubertal failure with elevated gonadotropins) has been diagnosed clinically, the term XX gonadal dysgenesis ("pure" gonadal dysgenesis) is used. In these patients, the Turner stigmata are missing and stature is normal. Their external genitalia are infantile and they have streak gonads with the associated hormonal abnormalities of gonadal dysgenesis. XX gonadal dysgenesis is inherited in an autosomal recessive fashion. The term "gonadal dysgenesis" may be a misnomer as this may

represent a form of ovarian failure rather than a true dysgenesis. The etiology of this failure is uncertain; however, in some subjects there may be an associated autoimmune disorder. These patients should be evaluated with thyroid studies, prolactin levels, and a serum cortisol level at the time of diagnosis. Additionally, these patients should be monitored periodically to screen for potential multiple endocrinopathy.

AMBIGUOUS GENITALIA

The diagnosis of ambiguous genitalia represents a social and medical emergency; prompt and thorough evaluation is required. Evaluation of such an infant requires a team approach, including a neonatologist, urologist, endocrinologist, geneticist, gynecologist, and a psychiatrist. It is especially important that a skilled and knowledgeable member of the team be designated as the spokesper-

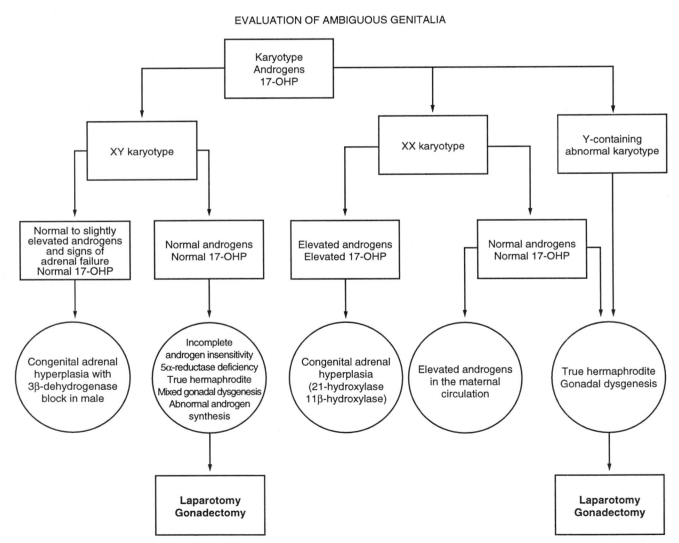

FIG. 5-5. Evaluation of ambiguous genitalia.

son and that this member provide the majority of the communication with the family. Speculation as to the sex of the baby should be avoided and the parents should be reassured that the baby will have a correct sex *assigned* within a finite length of time. Naming the child should be delayed until sex assignment has been accomplished. Sex assignment should occur once, and remove all uncertainty from the minds of parents and physicians. It is helpful for the physician to examine the baby in the presence of the parents and explain the common anlage for males and females.

An infant born with ambiguous genitalia should be considered to have adrenal hyperplasia until this has been excluded because adrenal hyperplasia is the only etiology of ambiguous genitalia that is life threatening. Electrolytes and blood glucose should be drawn. A history should be taken from the parents and should include use of virilizing medications during pregnancy, maternal virilization during the pregnancy, family history of similarly affected children, family history of previous unexplained neonatal deaths, and consanguinity.

A careful physical examination should then follow with particular attention paid to other anomalies besides those of the genitals. In evaluating the genitals, the following should be documented: length of the phallus, palpability of the gonads, position of the urethral meatus, degree of labioscrotal fusion, and presence of a vagina, vaginal pouch, or urogenital sinus. Radiologic evaluation of these patients is often unnecessary in the newborn period, but could include pelvic ultrasonography, retrograde injection of contrast media into the genital orifice to outline the urethral and/or vaginal anatomy, or magnetic resonance imaging (MRI).

Additional laboratory evaluation should include blood karyotype analysis, androstenedione, testosterone, dehydroepiandrosterone sulfate (DHEAS), DHEA, 17-OHP, ll-deoxycorticosterone, and ll-deoxycortisol.

The differential diagnosis includes female pseudohermaphroditism, male pseudohermaphroditism, true hermaphroditism, and gonadal dysgenesis. Any clinical signs of adrenal failure indicate that the newborn has a form of adrenal enzyme defect and must be aggressively evaluated. The flow diagram in Fig. 5-5 reviews the evaluation and establishment of a diagnosis in the case of ambiguous genitalia. Assignment of sex of rearing should be based on the following: future fertility, penile adequacy for coital function, and the projected appearance of the genitalia after puberty. The importance of parent counseling and close follow-up over the years cannot be overemphasized. Tragic anecdotes are often repeated about patients whose gender assignment was reversed.

SUGGESTED READING

Alquist JA. Gender identity in testicular feminization. Phenotypically, anatomically, legally, and socially female. *Br Med J* 1994;308:1041.

Delooz J, Van den Berghe H, Swillen A, Kleczkowska A, Fryns JP. Turner syndrome patients as adults: a study of their cognitive profile, psychosocial functioning and psychopathological findings. *Genet Couns* 1993;4;3;169.

Federman DD, Donohoe PK. Ambiguous genitalia: etiology, diagnosis, and therapy. *Adv Endocrinol Metabol* 1995;6:91.

Haqq CM, King CY, Ukiyama E, Falsafi S, Haqq TN, Donahoe PK, Weiss MA. Molecular basis of mammalian sexual determination: activation of mullerian inhibiting substance gene expression by SRY. *Science* 1994;266;1494.

Izquierdo G, Glassberg K. Gender assignment and gender identity in patients with ambiguous genitalia. *Urology* 1993;42;3;232.

Lim YJ, Batch JA, Warne GL. Adrenal 21-hydroxylase deficiency in childhood: 25 years' experience. *J Paediatr Child Health* 1995;31:222.

Meyers-Seifer CH, Charest NJ. Diagnosis and management of patients with ambiguous genitalia. *Semin Perinatol* 1992;16;5;332.

Page J. The newborn with ambiguous genitalia. *Neonatal Network* 1994;13:15.

Shah R, Woolley MM, Costin G. Testicular feminization: the androgen insensitivity syndrome. *J Pediatr Surg* 1992;27;6;757.

Sultan C, Lobaccaro JM, Belon C, Terraza A, Lumbroso S. Molecular biology of disorders of sex differentiation. *Horm Res* 1992;38;105.

Zajac JD, Warne GL. Disorders of sexual development. *Baillieres Clin Endocrinol Metab* 1995;9:555.

Clinical Reproductive Medicine,
Edited by Bryan D. Cowan and David B. Seifer
Lippincott-Raven Publishers, Philadelphia © 1997

CHAPTER 6

Disorders of Puberty

Cynthia H. Meyers-Seifer and David B. Seifer

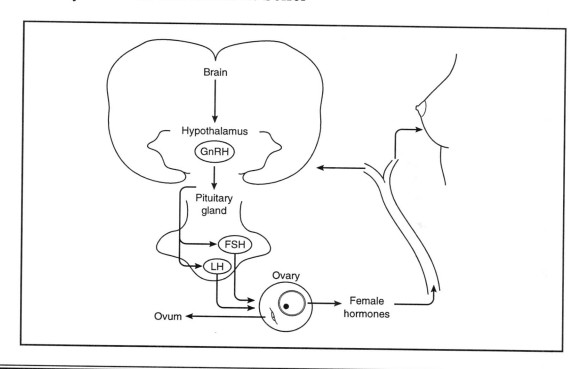

Factors Involved in the Onset of Puberty
Linear Growth in Puberty
Adrenarche
Physical Development During Puberty
Delayed Puberty
Differential Diagnosis for Delayed Puberty
Evaluation of Delayed Puberty
Precocious Puberty

Central Precocious Puberty
Peripheral Precocious Puberty
Combined Peripheral and Central Precocious Puberty
**Evaluation of Precocious Puberty (Central and
    Peripheral)**
Treatment
Summary
Suggested Reading

C. H. Meyers-Seifer: Department of Pediatrics, The Ohio State University, Children's Hospital,
Columbus, OH 43205, and D. B. Seifer: Department of Obstetrics and Gynecology, The Ohio State
University Medical Center, Columbus, OH 43210

Puberty or adolescence is the period of development from sexual immaturity to completion of physical and hormonal maturation (Fig. 6-1). The hormonal events during this transition result in secondary sex characteristics, a linear growth spurt, psychological changes, and potential fertility. The following chapter reviews the hormonal and physical features of normal puberty and subsequently offers an approach to evaluating abnormal puberty.

FACTORS INVOLVED IN THE ONSET OF PUBERTY

The hypothalamic-pituitary-gonadal axis is active in the fetus and becomes quiescent over the first 2 years of postnatal life. Puberty therefore represents the reactivation of pulsatile gonadotropin-releasing hormone (GnRH) secretion in late childhood (Fig. 6-2). An unknown signal results in decreased central inhibition of GnRH release, and episodic GnRH stimulation increases gonadotropin secretion. Changes in GnRH pulse frequency or amplitude are thought to be responsible for the changing follicle-stimulating hormone/luteinizing hormone (FSH/LH) ratio during puberty. The circulating FSH/LH ratio is elevated in early puberty and reverses in later puberty. In prepubertal girls there is a predominant FSH response to an exogenous dose of GnRH. The early ratio is probably due to less frequent GnRH pulses, which favors FSH release over LH. The predominance of FSH in early puberty appears to be important for ovarian follicle development at that time.

The timing of puberty is poorly understood. Several factors, including genetics, general health, nutrition, and psychological state, influence pubertal timing. Studies of mothers and daughters, sister pairs, and twins support the significance of genetics in achievement of menarche. Improved nutrition, health, and socioeconomic conditions are thought responsible for the decrease in age at menarche noted over the last century. A critical body weight or percentage of body fat may be essential for the initiation of the pubertal growth spurt and menarche. Moderately obese girls show an earlier age of menarche, whereas reproductive maturation appears delayed in states of malnutrition and decreased body fat. However, weight does not account for all menarcheal variations. For example, urinary gonadotropins increase concurrently with changes in body composition rather than as a response to these changes. Chronic illness, such as thyroid disease, may retard maturation timing. Delayed menarche is seen commonly in certain groups of athletes. This may reflect environmental causes of delayed menarche or a selection process that favors late maturation in athletics. In summary, there has been no specific metabolic "switch" identified that is responsible for decreasing the central inhibition of GnRH at puberty.

LINEAR GROWTH IN PUBERTY

Compared with prepubertal growth, pubertal height velocity is accelerated. The skeletal age correlates better than chronologic age with both pubertal stage and menarche. Accelerated pubertal growth is dependent on changes in sex steroid levels, growth hormone (GH), and

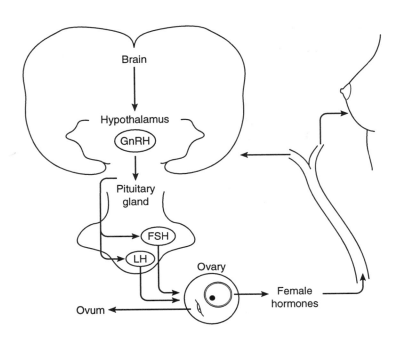

FIG. 6-1. The anatomic components of pubertal development. (Adapted from Rosenfield RL: The ovary and female sexual maturation. In: Kaplan SA, ed. *Clinical Pediatric Endocrinology,* 2nd ed. Philadelphia: WB Saunders, 1990.)

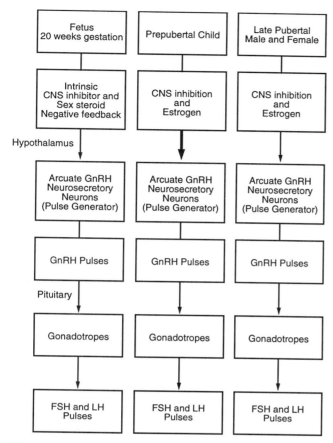

FIG. 6-2. Developmental changes in the hypothalamus and pituitary. In the fetus there is minimal CNS restraint and gonadotropins are high. There is low sensitivity to sex steroid–negative feedback. In the child there is decreased gonadotropin-releasing hormone (GnRH) due to increasing CNS restraint and supersensitive steroid-negative feedback, with decreased gonadotropins and sex steroids. With the onset of puberty, CNS inhibition and sensitivity to ovarian steroid–negative feedback lessens, with resulting increase in GnRH, gonadotropins, and estrogens. (Adapted from Reiter EO. Neuroendocrine control processes. *J Adol Health* 1987; 8:479.)

insulin-like growth factor (IGF-I) secretion. Understanding the interaction between sex steroids and GH during this period has important implications for the treatment of pubertal disorders.

Recent studies have attempted to sort out the contributions of gonadal sex steroids, GH, and IGF-I in pubertal growth and maturation. Although estrogen in girls and testosterone in boys rise throughout puberty, the peak growth velocity is lower in girls than boys and occurs at an earlier stage of puberty. During pharmacologic induction of puberty with pulsatile GnRH, the timing of the growth spurt recapitulates that of normal puberty. A large increase in GH pulse amplitude appears to coincide with peak growth acceleration in both girls and boys. Such observations underscore the uncertainty regarding the relative contributions of sex steroids and GH to adolescent development.

Pubertal growth in GH-deficient children is severely impaired, establishing GH as essential to achieve a growth spurt. Studies that compare sex steroid and/or GH therapy in hypopituitary, hypogonadal, and GH-deficient children suggest that a threshold level of GH is necessary for a growth spurt in all groups, and that the action of sex steroids and GH appear synergistic. In the absence of GH, gonadal steroids are thought to have limited growth promotion effects.

Evaluation of GH changes during spontaneous puberty has been difficult due to the episodic and predominantly sleep-associated secretion of hormones, and the need for prolonged sampling periods in healthy children. Studies in children with precocious, delayed, and pharmacologically induced puberty have increases in GH with pubertal growth. GH increases in normal boys are associated with growth velocity. Similar information is not yet available for girls.

The growth-promoting action of GH is dependent on an intermediate factor, somatomedin C or IGF-I. Circulating IGF-I is synthesized and released in response to GH, predominantly in the liver but also locally at the epiphyseal growth plate. IGF-I rises during puberty in association with the pubertal growth spurt, approximately one year earlier in girls than boys, and then declines in adulthood.

IGF-I concentration correlates with 24-hour mean GH concentration and pubertal stage in the study of normal boys mentioned earlier. In concordance with GH, IGF-I is elevated in children with precocious puberty and low in children with constitutional delay of growth and development. Normal growth in puberty thus appears dependent on an increase in GH, the effect of which is mediated via IGF-I.

The increase in growth factors during puberty is probably modulated by sex steroids. In girls estradiol is considered the main sex steroid associated with pubertal growth. Interestingly, although adolescent growth has generally been attributed to testosterone in boys, there is evidence to suggest that estradiol may play an important physiologic role in the male growth spurt. Testosterone may promote growth primarily after enzymatic conversion to estrogen.

ADRENARCHE

Preceding pubertal gonadal maturation (gonadarche) by 2–3 years is an increase in adrenal androgen production (adrenarche). In normal girls and boys, adrenarche occurs between the ages of 6 and 8 years. Before gonadotropins rise, plasma concentrations of dehydroepiandrosterone (DHEA), dehydroepiandrosterone sulfate (DHEAS), and other adrenal androgens increase. The zona reticularis is the source of the adrenal androgens, as this region of the adrenal gland develops in parallel with maturational increases in DHEA production.

The adrenal steroids continue to rise with progression of puberty, without a change in ACTH or cortisol secretion. Adrenal androgens, but not cortisol, show an increased response to pharmacologic doses of ACTH with adrenarche. Although many factors are being investigated, including pituitary hormones, estrogens, and intrinsic adrenal properties, the control of adrenarche is unidentified.

Adrenarche results in the appearance of axillary and pubic hair. A transient increase in long bone growth and maturation has also been noted between 6 and 8 years of age. There is speculation regarding the influence of adrenal androgens on maturation of the hypothalamic-pituitary-gonadal axis and the initiation of puberty. However, many clinical situations suggest that adrenarche and puberty occur independently and in parallel. For example, in girls with gonadal dysgenesis, adrenal androgen levels are appropriate for chronologic age and bone maturation.

Conversely, in children diagnosed with precocious puberty, adrenarche may not have occurred.

PHYSICAL DEVELOPMENT DURING PUBERTY

Although there may be some individual variation in timing, development of secondary sex characteristics proceeds through well-accepted stages (originally described by Tanner). Breast development results from adequate ovarian estrogen secretion. Stage I is prepubertal. Stage II involves elevation of subareolar breast buds. Stage III is characterized by increased breast size without change in contour. The areola and papilla form a secondary mound over the enlarging breast in stage IV. Stage V is attainment of mature female breast contour, with elevation of the papilla (Fig. 6-3). The appearance of breast buds is the first sign of puberty in most girls. Breast development (thelarche) is completed over an average of 4 years.

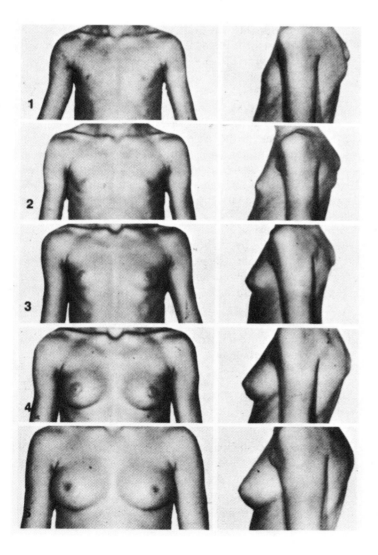

FIG. 6-3. Stages of breast development in girls. (With permission from Ross GT. Disorders of the ovary and female reproductive tract. In: Wilson JD, Foster DW, eds. *Williams Textbook of Endocrinology.* Philadelphia: WB Saunders, 1985;212).

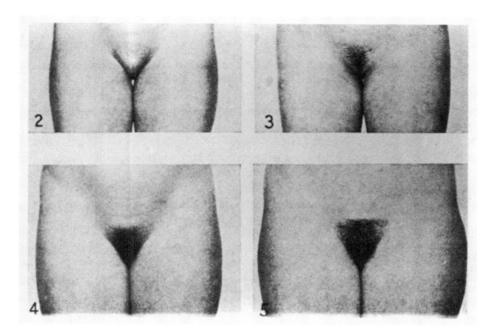

FIG. 6-4. Stages of pubic hair development in girls. (With permission from Ross GT. Disorders of the ovary and female reproductive tract. In: Wilson JD, Foster DW, eds. *Williams Textbook of Endocrinology*. Philadelphia: WB Saunders, 1985;212).

In general, pubic hair development (pubarche) begins shortly after thelarche, although in approximately 15% of normal girls, pubic hair appears before breast development. Pubic hair growth is stimulated during adrenarche. Tanner stage I is prepubertal. Stage II shows sparse, straight, slightly pigmented labial hair. Stage III begins to show dark, coarse, curly sexual hair which spreads to the pubis. The hair distribution is of adult type but decreased in stage IV, whereas in stage V the mature female escutcheon or inverted triangle pattern is attained (Fig. 6-4). The average duration of pubic hair development is 2.5 years.

Axillary hair development, also stimulated by adrenal androgens, appears approximately 2 years after the initiation of pubic hair and proceeds to completion over 15 months. Acne tends to occur coincidentally with axillary hair development.

The sequence of pubertal development is generally predictable but subject to individual variation in normal girls. The appearance of breast buds is accompanied by initial growth acceleration and is soon followed by the onset of pubic hair. Growth velocity usually peaks during stage II–III breast and stage II pubic hair development. Menarche, the first menstrual period, occurs approximately 2 years after the onset of breast development, most commonly during stage IV, as growth velocity wanes. Menstrual cycles are initially irregular and most frequently anovulatory. After 2 years, a pattern is usually established and by 21 years of age most menstrual cycles are ovulatory. Figure 6-5 shows the sequence of pubertal events for average girls in the United States. It is helpful to recall that in the individual the progression of puberty is better correlated with skeletal maturation or "bone age" than chronologic age.

Disorders of puberty may present as delayed or precocious onset of pubertal stages or as alterations in the normal temporal relationship of these stages. The following discussion focuses on the diagnosis and management of disordered puberty.

DELAYED PUBERTY

Delayed puberty should be considered when there is no evidence of breast development by age 13.5 or absence of menarche by age 16. These ages represent the mean +3 SD and describe the upper time limit for 99% of the female population in North America. Mean ages for particular female milestones ± 3 SD are as follows: breast buds 10.9 ± 3 years, sexual pubic hair 11.9 ± 3.3 years, and menarche 12.7 ± 3 years. Once breast buds develop in a young girl with delayed puberty, puberty will be completed >95% of the time. Generally, no more than 5 years should pass from breast budding until the onset of menarche.

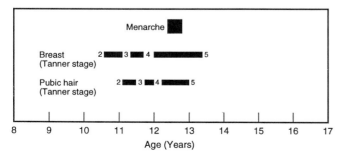

FIG. 6-5. Diagram of the normal sequence of pubertal events in girls. (From Copeland KC. Variations in normal sexual development. *Pediatr Rev* 1986;8:47.)

The great majority of young girls who are considered to have "delayed puberty" eventually prove to have no pathology and in fact have physiologic or constitutional delay of puberty. This benign variation of normal has an excellent prognosis with regards to eventual development of secondary sexual characteristics. However, constitutional delay is strictly a diagnosis of exclusion and therefore requires an appropriate workup to rule out the pathologic causes of delayed puberty.

DIFFERENTIAL DIAGNOSIS FOR DELAYED PUBERTY

The disorders responsible for delayed puberty may be grouped into three major diagnostic categories. They are eugonadotropic conditions, hypergonadotropic hypogonadism, and hypogonadotropic hypogonadism. These are summarized in Table 6-1.

Eugonadotropic conditions result from abnormal development of Mullerian structures. The most common example of this is Mullerian agenesis (Mayer–Rokitansky–Kuster–Hauser syndrome). Mullerian agenesis is the most common cause of primary amenorrhea in adolescent females with normal secondary sex characteristics. In contrast, individuals with androgen insensitivity syndromes present with a blind vaginal canal without a uterus. The gonads are testes. Testosterone production and serum gonadotropins are normal in these individuals. Breast development occurs because of peripheral aromatization of androgens to estrogens.

Even though young women with Mullerian agenesis or androgen insensitivity may be differentiated from one another by karyotype (ie, 46,XX versus 46,XY, respectively), two simpler clinical ways exist. Presence or absence of axillary and pubic hair and level of serum

TABLE 6-1. *Differential diagnosis of delayed puberty*

Eugonadotropic
  Mullerian agenesis
  Transverse vaginal septum
  Imperforate hymen
  Androgen-resistant syndrome
    Complete
    Incomplete
Hypergonadotropic Hypogonadism
  Gonadal dysgenesis
  Premature ovarian failure
  17α-Hydroxylase deficiency
Hypogonadotropic Hypogonadism
  Constitutional delay
  Hypothyroidism
  Anorexia nervosa
  Malabsorption
  Prolactinoma
  Kallman's syndrome
  Chronic illness
  Cushing's syndrome
  Craniopharyngioma
  Postsurgical hypopituitarism

testosterone can distinguish between these two diagnoses. Testicular feminization has normal to slightly elevated male levels of testosterone with absent to sparse sexual hair as compared to Mullerian agenesis with female levels of testosterone and normal sexual hair.

The most common cause of hypergonadotropic hypogonadism is gonadal dysgenesis. Examples include Turner's syndrome and Swyer's syndrome. Turner's 45,XO germ cell failure is believed to be due to accelerated atresia of primordial follicles. Mosaic forms of Turner's need to be identified in order to assure the absence of a Y chromosome. Buccal epithelial cells are unacceptable for detection of X chromosome mosaicism, because both 45,X and 45,X/46,XY individuals would be X chromatin–negative. Lymphocytes from peripheral blood are ideal sources of "tissue" to examine for mosaicism. The ability to detect mosaicism depends on the frequency of the minority cell lines, the number of cells analyzed per tissue, and the number of tissues analyzed. The most common form of a sex chromosomal mosaicism is 45,X/46,XX.

A female with Swyer's syndrome has a 46,XY karyotype. Even though the karyotype is the same as an individual with testicular feminization and both have sparse sexual hair, there are important differences that can be appreciated if examined from the perspective of the gonadal tissue. Swyer's syndrome individuals have gonadal dysgenesis represented by streaked gonads that failed to produce Mullerian inhibiting substance (MIS) and testosterone, therefore normal male development did not occur. A phenotypic female, complete with a Mullerian system, develops with low testosterone levels with elevated gonadotropins. Testicular feminization individuals produce MIS. Therefore no Mullerian system exists in these patients, and a blind vaginal pouch develops.

Turner's and Swyer's patients should receive hormone replacement to assure secondary sexual characteristic development. This replacement may begin at age 12–13 with low-dose estrogen, ie, ethinyl estradiol 5–10 µg or conjugated estrogens (Premarin) 0.3–0.625 mg daily for 3–6 months. If 0.3 mg of conjugated estrogens are started, then the dose can be raised by 0.3 mg every 4–6 months. Progestin, ie, medroxyprogesterone acetate (Provera) 5–10 mg, should be added in a cyclic fashion. If 0.625 mg of conjugated estrogen is started, the dose is not increased unless there is poor breast development, in which case the estrogen may be increased. Estrogen and progestins are administered in a cyclic fashion, ie, Premarin day 1 through day 25 of the calendar month and Provera day 13 through day 25. Days 25–30 are medication-free, allowing for a withdraw menses. If bleeding occurs earlier than day 23 of the month, the dose of Provera should be increased because a predominantly proliferative endometrium characteristically bleeds before 11 days of progestin therapy. If menses does not occur after three cycles, the dose of Provera may be lowered. Furthermore, there are well-designed clinical trials demonstrating the benefit of administering growth hormone in addition to estrogen prior to epiphyseal closure in girls with Turner's syndrome in order to optimize their adult height.

Another cause of delayed puberty presenting with hypergonadotropic hypogonadism is premature ovarian failure (POF). POF exists when amenorrhea is accompanied by elevated gonadotropins in a woman <35 years old. If POF occurs prior to age 30, a karyotype should be considered. Possible causes of POF include iatrogenic factors (including chemotherapy, radiotherapy), chromosomal disorders (ie, Turner's syndrome, Swyer's syndrome), pituitary tumor, and autoimmune diseases causing multiple endocrine gland failure syndrome. Endocrine manifestations include hyperthyroidism, hypothyroidism, hypoparathyroidism, thyroiditis, diabetes, adrenal insufficiency, myasthenia gravis, pernicious anemia, celiac disease, vitiligo, and alopecia. If an autoimmune etiology for POF is likely, associated autoimmune disorders should be excluded by measuring thyroid function tests, thyroid antibodies, rheumatoid factor, and antinuclear antibody. Hormone replacement is appropriate to avoid complications of long-term estrogen deprivation.

A deficiency of 17α-hydroxylase results in an impairment in the hydroxylation of progesterone and pregnenolone resulting in cortisol, estrogen, and androgen deficiencies. Patients with these conditions are rare, but they present with sexual immaturity, primary amenorrhea, hypertension due to increased mineralocorticoids, high serum gonadotropins and progesterone, but undetectable serum androgens and estrogens. The treatment of this form of congenital adrenal hyperplasia consists of glucocorticoid replacement and estrogen-progestin replacement.

Constitutional delay is the most common reason for hypogonadotropic delayed puberty. It is a diagnosis of exclusion, and attention should be directed to other pathologic reasons for delayed puberty presenting with low serum gonadotropins. Chronic systemic disease, including hypothyroidism, Cushing's syndrome, anorexia nervosa (AN), renal insufficiency, bowel disease, or central nervous system (CNS) disorders, may result in delayed puberty. Craniopharyngioma is a slow-growing tumor arising from squamous cells at the junction of the anterior and posterior pituitary. As it grows downward it compresses the pituitary gland and may produce hypogonadotropic hypogonadism as its initial presentation. Thus, patients with hypogonadotropic delayed puberty should have cranial floor imaging (MRI) to exclude destructive pituitary lesions.

EVALUATION OF DELAYED PUBERTY

A detailed history of the presenting complaint and a family history are critical to the initial evaluation (Fig. 6-6). The heights and pubertal timing of parents, grand-parents, aunts, uncles, and siblings are essential information. Physical exam should be performed with special attention to the patient's height, sense of smell, facial and body hair distribution, size of thyroid, axillary and/or pubic hair, breast contour, and evidence of galactorrhea. Confirmation of the presence of a patent vaginal orifice leading to a normal cervix and palpation of the uterus and adnexa are of importance in girls with mature secondary sex characteristics accompanied by primary amenorrhea. Specific laboratories are indicated based on the presence or absence of secondary sexual characteristics and can be reviewed in the algorithm summarized in Fig. 6-6 entitled "Assessment of Delayed Puberty."

PRECOCIOUS PUBERTY

Precocious puberty in girls is defined as the onset of puberty prior to age 8. This premature onset may be termed isosexual if the girl is feminized or heterosexual if virilized prior to this age. The mechanisms responsible for precocious puberty can be divided into central, peripheral, and combined peripheral and central.

Central precocious puberty is premature activation of the hypothalamic-pituitary-ovarian axis. This is an accelerated gonadotropin-dependent process similar to the normal process of puberty. Peripheral precocious puberty is gonadotropin-independent and secondary to elevated sex steroids from endogenous or exogenous sources. Combined precocious puberty is initiated by a peripheral cause that eventually leads to secondary activation of the hypothalamic-pituitary-ovarian axis.

Central Precocious Puberty

True or central precocious puberty results in a similar hormonal picture as observed with normal puberty. LH pulsatility increases in response to GnRH release. This results in increased ovarian steroid production. The premature production of these steroids leads to development of secondary sex characteristics, accelerated skeletal maturation and linear growth. This may lead to premature epiphyseal fusion and early cessation of growth.

In almost 50% of children with true precocious puberty the onset occurs before 6 years of age. Characteristic physical findings include breast development, enlarged labia minora, changes in vaginal mucosa, development of pubic hair, and cyclic menses. Seventy percent of patients with true precocious puberty have the idiopathic form. Diagnostic evaluation fails to identify an organic lesion. The most significant long-term complication of idiopathic central precocious puberty is adult short stature. Therefore, it is essential for the physician to recognize this situation early enough to initiate a workup and treat appropriately.

ASSESSMENT OF DELAYED PUBERTY

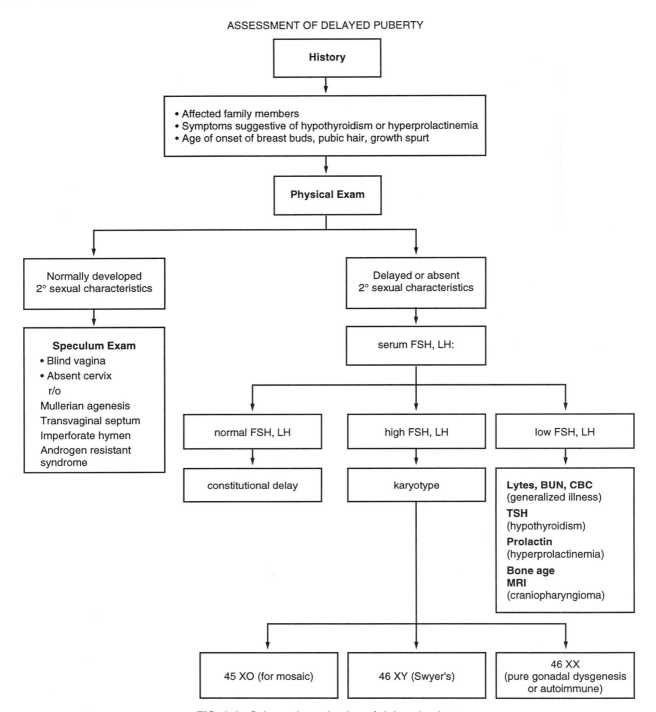

FIG. 6-6. Schematic evaluation of delayed puberty.

The most common organic etiology of central precocious puberty without addition symptoms is a hypothalamic hamartoma. This is usually localized in the floor of the third ventricle of the posterior hypothalamus. On CT, this tumor tends to be spherical and does not enhance after intravenous contrast administration. MRI offers the most sensitive diagnostic method for detection of this lesion. The majority of children are without neurologic signs or symptoms. However, a select group will suffer from seizure disorders and delayed speech or motor development. Other CNS lesions less commonly responsible for precocious puberty include astrocytoma, glioma, medulloblastoma, third ventricular cyst, pinealoma, prolactinoma, hydrocephalus, and trauma.

Peripheral Precocious Puberty

Peripheral precocious puberty is gonadotropin-independent pubertal development exclusive of hypothalamic-pituitary-ovarian axis activation. The etiology may be due to numerous sources, as outlined in Table 6-2.

Premature adrenarche is the most common cause of isolated early pubarche. It is the onset of pubic and axillary hair before age 8 without other signs of sexual development. Moderately elevated DHEAS levels are consistent with a benign increase in adrenal androgen secretion characteristic of premature adrenarche. Other adrenal androgens and testosterone remain in the prepubertal range. Premature adrenarche has no long-term sequelae and therefore only requires observation.

Congenital adrenal hyperplasia (CAH) leading to excessive adrenal androgen secretion may be a cause of peripheral precocious puberty. 21-hydroxylase, 11-hydroxylase, and 3-hydroxysteroid dehydrogenase deficiencies can occur. Girls with these enzymatic defects may present with virilization, short stature secondary to accelerated epiphyseal closure, and various degrees of adrenal insufficiency.

Virilizing adrenal tumors responsible for heterosexual precocious puberty are more common than feminizing tumors leading to isosexual precocious puberty. They are usually accompanied by markedly elevated DHEAS serum levels. Ultrasound, computed tomography (CT), and MRI are all useful for making a diagnosis. Selective venous catheterization or an iodomethyl cholesterol scan may prove helpful if CT or MRI does not demonstrate a discrete lesion. These tumors require surgical excision.

Feminizing tumors of the ovary such as theca cell and granulosa cell tumors may lead to isolated premature thelarche or menses. These tumors are usually unilateral and require oophorectomy. Arrhenoblastoma is the most common virilizing ovarian tumor. Eighty-five percent are palpable on pelvic exam. Similar to feminizing tumors of the ovary, they are generally unilateral and require surgical removal.

McCune–Albright syndrome is a triad of café-au-lait spots or irregular areas of skin pigmentation, polyostotic fibrous dysplasia of the skull and long bones, and GnRH-independent sexual precocity. The pathogenesis of this syndrome is due to a constitutively active mutation in a G-protein subunit located within the cell membrane of target endocrine organ(s). Other endocrine disorders are associated with this syndrome including hyperthyroidism, hypercortisol secretion, hyperprolactinemia, and increased GH secretion. Intermittent periods of breast development and uterine bleeding may be secondary to ovarian cysts and fluctuating elevations of serum estradiol. Although unilateral ovarian cysts may be present into childhood, many women with the syndrome will have normal fertility.

Combined Peripheral and Central Precocious Puberty

Activation of the hypothalamic-pituitary-ovarian axis resulting in central precocious puberty can result in association with peripheral precocious puberty. Examples of this can be noted in congenital adrenal hyperplasia or in McCune–Albright syndrome. The mechanism responsible for activation of the central axis is unclear. Treatment must address both the cause of the peripheral precocious puberty and the central precocious puberty.

EVALUATION OF PRECOCIOUS PUBERTY (CENTRAL AND PERIPHERAL)

A thorough workup for suspected precocious puberty consists of a history that includes chronologic timing of pubertal milestones with attention to the presence of oily skin, hair, acne, increased body odor, or lowering of the voice (Fig. 6-7). Family history of pubertal events is essential. History of the girl's height and weight will help determine interval growth and increase in growth velocity. Physical exam includes attention to neurologic exam, visual fields, thyroid size, distribution of sexual hair, contour of breast, presence of galactorrhea, general appearance of external genitalia, and presence of adnexal masses.

An essential laboratory test to obtain is a radiograph of the left hand and wrist for determination of bone age. Accelerated bone age may indicate central precocious puberty, McCune–Albright syndrome, or an adrenal or ovarian abnormality. Normal bone age probably indicates premature adrenarche or thelarche or ingestion of steroids. Additional specific laboratories are indicated as described in the algorithm summarized in Fig. 6-7 entitled "Assessment of Precocious Puberty."

TABLE 6-2. *Differential diagnosis of precocious puberty*

Central Precocious Puberty (gonadotropin-dependent)
  Idiopathic true precocious puberty
  Hypothalamic hamartoma
  Other CNS lesions: optic glioma, astrocytoma, head trauma, cranial irradiation
Peripheral Precocious Puberty (gonadotropin independent)
  Premature adrenarche
  Ingestion of steroids
  Congenital adrenal hyperplasia: 21-OH deficiency, 11-OH deficiency, 3-OH dehydrogenase
  Virilizing or feminizing adrenal neoplasm
  Virilizing or feminizing ovarian neoplasm
  McCune–Albright syndrome
  Human chorionic gonadotropin–secreting tumors: hepatoblastomas, dysgerminomas, pinealomas
Combined Peripheral and Central Precocious Puberty
Unknown Mechanisms
  Hypothyroidism
  Premature thelarche

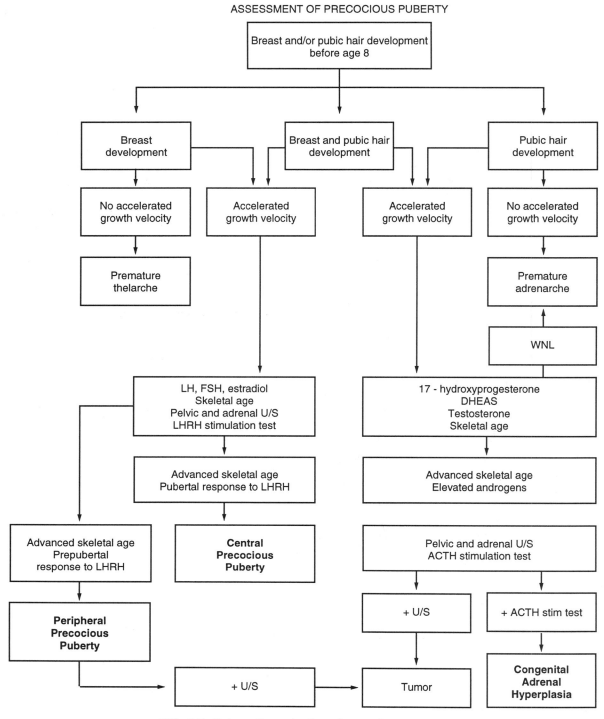

FIG. 6-7. Schematic evaluation of precocious puberty.

TREATMENT

Treatment is directed to cessation of the progression of secondary sexual characteristics and a retardation in accelerated bone growth and maturity. Specific treatment depends on the etiology of precocious puberty. Idiopathic central precocious puberty and hypothalamic hamartomas are generally treated with GnRH agonists. GnRH agonists can be given by subcutaneous, intramuscular, or intranasal routes. A single intramuscular injection of a depot form of agonist (ie, depot leuprolide acetate) has been shown to be effective in the treatment of idiopathic central precocious puberty. Central precocious puberty due to other brain tumors may require appropriate surgery, radiation, or chemotherapy.

Treatment of gonadotropin-independent peripheral precocious puberty has included medroxyprogesterone acetate in the past. Testolactone, an aromatase inhibitor that blocks estrogen synthesis, has been useful more recently in the treatment of patients with McCune–Albright syndrome. Treatment of late-onset congenital adrenal hyperplasia requires corticosteroids to suppress central ACTH production. Tumors of ovarian and adrenal origin require surgical removal.

On occasion ovarian cysts will be present in a young child with primary hypothyroidism or McCune–Albright syndrome. It is important to realize that surgical treatment is rarely indicated in either situation. Treatment of the underlying disease often results in regression of these functional cysts.

SUMMARY

Adolescent development involves changes in neuroendocrine function, linear growth, skeletal maturation, and physical characteristics. Sex steroids, GH, and IGF-I orchestrate the pubertal growth spurt and, ultimately, epiphyseal closure and cessation of linear growth. Pubertal milestones show wide variability in normal girls. However, girls suspected of having abnormally delayed or advanced adolescence require diagnostic evaluation. Treatment will vary with respect to the underlying cause but is directed at restoring normal maturation sequence and preserving adult height and function.

SUGGESTED READING

Hypothalamic-Pituitary-Ovarian Axis and the Menstrual Cycle

Koopman P, Gubbay J, Vivian N, Goodfellow P, Lovell-Badge R. Male development of chromosomally female mice transgenic for Sry. *Nature* 1991;351:117.

Kulin HE, Muller J. The biological aspects of puberty. *Pediatrics Rev* 1996; 17(3):75–86.

Meyers-Seifer CH, Seifer DB. The neuroendocrinology of the menstrual cycle. In: Collins RL, ed. *Ovulation Induction.* New York: Springer-Verlag, 1991:1.

Rosenfield RL. The ovary and female sexual maturation. In: Kaplan SA, ed.

Clinical Pediatric Endocrinology, 2nd ed. Philadelphia: WB Saunders, 1990:259.

Stanhope R, Adams J, Jacobs HS, Brook CGD. Ovarian ultrasound assessment in normal children, idiopathic precocious puberty, and during low dose pulsatile gonadotropin releasing hormone treatment of hypogonadotropic hypogonadism. *Arch Dis Child* 1985;60:116.

Stanhope R, Brook CGD. An evaluation of hormonal changes at puberty in man. *J Endocrinol* 1988;116:301.

Linear Growth and Onset of Puberty

Bourguignon J. Linear growth as a function of age at onset of puberty and sex steroid dosage: therapeutic implications. *Endocr Rev* 1988;9:467.

Brooks-Gunn J. Antecedents and consequences of variation in girls' maturational timing. *J Adol Heal* 1988;9:365.

Martha PM, Reiter EO. Pubertal growth and growth hormone secretion. *Endocrinol Metab Clin North Am* 1991;20:165.

Stanhope R, Preece MA, Grant DB, Brook CGD. New concept of the growth spurt of puberty. *Acta Paediatr Scand* 1988;347:30.

Adrenarche and Physical Development

Parker LN. Adrenarche. *Endocrinol Metab Clin North Am* 1991;20:71.

Wheeler MD. Physical changes of puberty. *Endocrinol Metab Clin North Am* 1991;20:1.

Delayed Puberty

Albanese A, Stanhope R. Investigation of delayed puberty. *Clin Endocrinol* 1995;43(1):105–110.

Kaplan SA. Growth and growth hormone. In: Kaplan SA, ed. *Clinical Pediatric Endocrinology*, 2nd ed. Philadelphia: WB Saunders, 1990:36.

Reindollar RH, Byrd JR, McDonough PG. Delayed sexual development: a study of 252 patients. *Am J Obstet Gynecol* 1981;140:371.

Rosenfield RL. Diagnosis and management of delayed puberty. *J Clin Endocrinol Metab* 1990;70:559.

Shalet SM. Treatment of constitutional delay in growth and puberty. *Clin Endocrinol* 1989;31:81.

Precocious Puberty

Kaplan SL, Grumbach MM. Pathophysiology and treatment of sexual precocity. *J Clin Endocrinol Metab* 1990;71:785.

Kappy M, Stuart T, Perelman A, et al. Suppression of gonadotropin secretion by a long-acting gonadotropin-releasing hormone analog (leuprolide acetate, lupron depot) in children with precocious puberty. *J Clin Endocrinol Metab* 1989;68:1087.

Parker KL, Lee PA. Depot leuprolide acetate for treatment of precocious puberty. *J Clin Endocrinol Metabol* 1989;69:689.

Pescovitz OH. Precocious puberty. *Pediatr Rev* 1990;11:229.

Pescovitz OH, Comite F, Hench K, et al. The NIH experience with precocious puberty: diagnostic subgroups and response to short-term luteinizing hormone releasing hormone analogue therapy. *J Pediatrics* 1986; 108:47.

Clinical Reproductive Medicine,
Edited by Bryan D. Cowan and David B. Seifer
Lippincott-Raven Publishers, Philadelphia © 1997

CHAPTER 7

Regulation of the Ovarian Menstrual Cycle

Victoria Sopelak

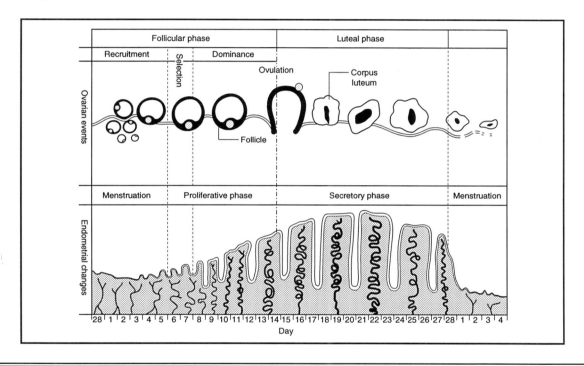

Phases of the Menstrual Cycle
    Early Follicular (Follicular Recruitment)
    Midfollicular (Dominant Follicle Selection)
    Late Follicular (Gonadotropin Surge and Ovulation)
    Early Luteal Phase (Postovulatory)
    Late Luteal Phase (Premenstrual)
Uterine and Endometrial Changes Associated with
    the Ovarian Menstrual Cycle
    Menstruation (Uterine Events)

Postmenstrual Endometrium
Late Proliferative Endometrium
Luteal Phase Uterine Changes
    (Early Secretory Phase)
Late Luteal Phase Uterine Changes
    (Late Secretory Phase)
Conclusion
Suggested Reading

V. Sopelak: Division of Reproductive Endocrinology, Department of Obstetrics and Gynecology,
University of Mississippi Medical Center, Jackson, MS 39216

The cyclic vaginal bleeding that characterizes the menstrual cycle is reflective not only of endometrial and stromal changes taking place in the uterus but of events occurring in the hypothalamus, pituitary, ovary, and other reproductive tissues (Fig. 7-1). Gonadotropic hormones produced by the pituitary stimulate follicular development, ovarian hormone biosynthesis and secretion,

oocyte maturation, ovulation, and luteal function. Hormonal changes occurring at different points during the menstrual cycle affect reproductive tissues important for sperm transport, fertilization, and conception. Synchronization of these events depends on appropriate pulsatile stimulation from the hypothalamus and an intricate system of feedback mechanisms. This chapter will focus on

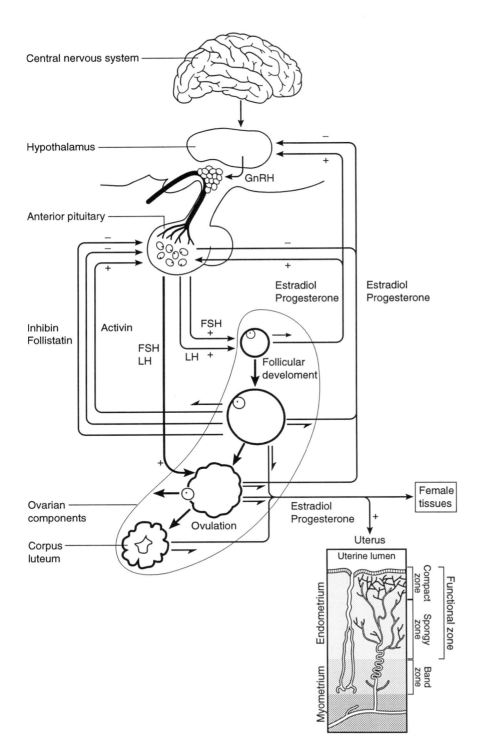

FIG. 7-1. Components of the normal menstrual cycle.

follicular and pituitary hormonal events that regulate the idealized 28-day menstrual cycle.

PHASES OF THE MENSTRUAL CYCLE

Early Follicular (Follicular Recruitment)

Just prior to the onset of vaginal bleeding, levels of estrogen, progesterone, and inhibin (all hormones produced by the granulosa cells) are low in the circulation (Fig. 7-2). These low hormone levels stimulate high-frequency low-amplitude gonadotropin-releasing hormone (GnRH) pulses (one pulse every 60–90 minutes) from the hypothalamus that result in a premenstrual rise in follicle-stimulating hormone (FSH) (see Fig. 7-2). FSH secretion provides the fundamental signal for recruitment of a cohort of follicles from the ovarian pool (Chapter 15). Initially, these follicles are <4 mm in diameter (Fig. 7-3) and contain high levels of luteinizing hormone (LH)-stimulated aromatizable androgens in their theca cells but low concentrations of estradiol and low aromatase activity in the granulosa cells. However, the granulosa cells of these follicles contain a highly responsive FSH-stimulable aromatase system. When FSH binds to granulosa cell receptors, granulosa cell mitosis and proliferation increases, aromatase is produced (facilitating the conversion of an-

drogens into estradiol), and more FSH receptors are induced. Thus, the more FSH, the greater the FSH receptor concentration, the higher the aromatase activity, and the more estrogen is produced. Estrogen, in turn, also stimulates granulosa cell proliferation and synthesis of more FSH receptors. These additive effects of estrogen and FSH lead to an increase in the receptor density of individual granulosa cells.

Granulosa cells contain androgen receptors within their cytoplasm, and these may regulate follicular development. Low concentrations of non-5α-reduced androgens enhance aromatase activity and estrogen production, but high concentrations of 5α-reduced androgens inhibit aromatase activity and lead to follicular atresia. Thus androgens, even though they are the precursors of estrogen production, also contribute to the fate of the follicle.

As intrafollicular and circulating levels of estrogen increase, follicular fluid is produced and accumulates in the intercellular spaces between the granulosa cells to form an antrum (see Chapter 15, Fig. 15-4). The granulosa cells of these secondary follicles contain LH, prolactin, and prostaglandin receptors and they produce the protein hormone inhibin. Inhibin preferentially suppresses pituitary production of FSH (see Fig. 7-1) and its circulating levels increase in parallel with estrogen secretion as the follicles increase in size. This leads to a shift in the LH/FSH ratio. FSH secretion diminishes but LH is aug-

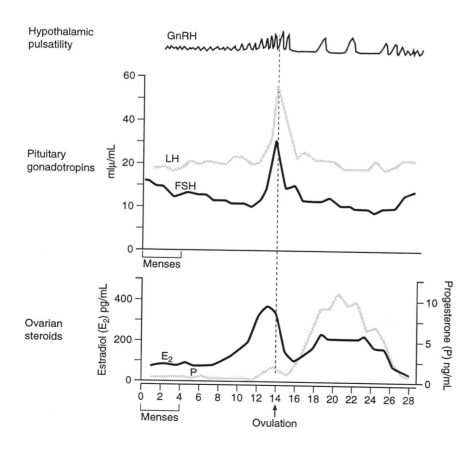

FIG. 7-2. Interrelationships between hypothalamic-pituitary and ovarian hormone patterns during the menstrual cycle.

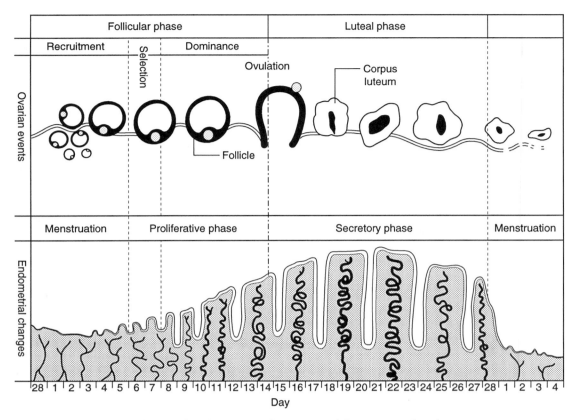

FIG. 7-3. Ovarian and uterine events of the menstrual cycle.

mented by cycle day 5 (see Fig. 7-2). These coordinated hypothalamic-pituitary-ovarian (HPO) events in the early follicular phase result in early gonadotropin-dependent development of several (cohort) follicles (see Fig. 7-3).

Midfollicular (Dominant Follicle Selection)

The midfollicular phase is characterized by "selection" of a dominant or lead follicle from the cohort of initial growing follicles that were stimulated by FSH (see Fig. 7-3). The exact mechanism whereby one or more follicles are chosen to continue their maturation and ovulate (selection) rather than undergo atresia is complex. Selection of the dominant follicle is probably related to the density of FSH receptors, the ability of the follicle to produce estrogen, and the intraovarian vascular support.

The increase in number of granulosa cells within the dominant follicle is accompanied by neovascularity within the theca interna. By day 9, the vascularity of the dominant follicle is twice that of other follicles. This augmentation in vascularity leads to increased delivery of FSH to the granulosa cell receptors, LH and low-density lipoproteins to the theca, increased proliferation of granulosa cells, increased estrogen production, antrum development, and the induction of LH, prolactin, and prostaglandin receptors.

Increased circulating levels of estrogen (see Figs. 7-1 and 7-2) and inhibin have a negative feedback effect on pituitary secretion of FSH. This results in diminished circulating levels of FSH. FSH deprivation leads to atresia of the entire follicular cohort with the exception of the dominant follicle. The dominant follicle continues development to the preovulatory state in spite of decreasing FSH levels because it has now acquired increased sensitivity to FSH. Thus, the cardinal feature of follicular dominance is its ability to synthesize estrogen before any other follicle. Estrogen then modulates mechanisms that increase the dominant follicles' survival while eliminating all other follicular candidates.

Late Follicular (Gonadotropin Surge and Ovulation)

The late follicular phase is characterized by rapid follicular growth, the development of a positive (stimulatory) feedback effect of estradiol on gonadotropin secretion, a surge of LH and FSH, meiotic maturation of the oocyte, ovulation, and formation of the corpus luteum (Figs. 7-3 and 7-4). The length of time from selection of the dominant follicle to ovulation is variable. Thus, the onset of the midcycle LH surge is generally used to provide a reference point for discussing the timing of hormonal and intrafollicular dynamics associated with ovu-

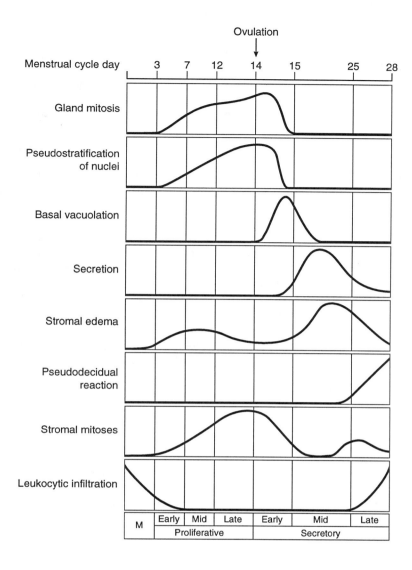

FIG. 7-4. Patterns of histologic changes throughout the menstrual cycle.

lation. As the preovulatory follicle continues to secrete increasing levels of estradiol, an estrogen-FSH synergy initially promotes the ability of FSH to increase and maintain FSH receptors followed by an enhancement of the ability of FSH to increase and maintain LH receptors on the granulosa cells. Following the appearance of LH receptors in the granulosa cells, small preovulatory amounts of progesterone and 17-hydroxyprogesterone are produced. This rise in progestins occurs during the last 2–3 days before the onset of the midcycle surge (see Fig. 7-2). The preovulatory rising estradiol and progesterone act on the pituitary gonadotrope to enhance its responsiveness to GnRH. It is hypothesized that the parallel rise of progesterone may induce the progressive increase in basal LH levels seen during this time period. However, premature luteinization of the granulosa cells is inhibited by the presence of the oocyte within the follicle.

The midcycle gonadotropin surge results from activation of positive estradiol feedback at the level of the pituitary and hypothalamus. When concentrations of estradiol are persistently elevated above a threshold of 300–500 pg/ml for roughly 48 hours, an LH and FSH surge is initiated. The midcycle LH surge (see Fig. 7-2), with a total duration of approximately 48 hours, not only triggers events leading to oocyte extrusion but stimulates resumption of meiosis (reduction division) in the oocyte, luteinization of the granulosa cells, and synthesis of progesterone and prostaglandins. Ovulation (the release of the oocyte) takes place 36–40 hours after the onset of the LH surge. Changes within the oocyte itself are observed within 16 hours from the initiation of the LH surge. During this time, the oocyte completes prophase 1 of the first meiotic division as it passes from the diplotene stage into diakinesis (see Chapter 15, Fig. 15-7). The second meiotic division generally begins 30–34 hours after the onset of the LH surge. The gamete reaches the haploid stage, referred to as the metaphase 2 oocyte, approximately 32–36 hours from the onset of the LH surge and 1–2 hours prior to follicular rupture (ovulation). This mature oocyte is now capable of being fertilized.

The mechanism whereby the oocyte resumes meiosis involves LH-mediated alterations in receptors and hormones. An initial stimulation in LH receptors concomitant with the onset of the LH surge is followed by a refractory stage where the LH receptors are desensitized and "downregulated." This desensitization is associated with a decrease in both the number and the sensitivity of the LH receptors leading to decreased levels of cAMP and oocyte maturation inhibitor (OMI) (Chapter 15), decreased estradiol production, and disruption of the gap junctions connecting the oocyte to its surrounding granulosa cells. The LH surge also initiates luteinization of the granulosa cells and shifts steroidogenesis in favor of progesterone secretion through the induction of 3β-hydroxysteroid dehydrogenase (HSD) activity. The associated midcycle FSH surge appears to stimulate the production of a plasminogen activator that helps to detach the oocyte/cumulus mass from the follicle wall. In addition, FSH plays a role in the conversion of granulosa cells to functional luteal cells by facilitating LH receptor induction. Follicle rupture and oocyte extrusion, which generally occurs 38–42 hours from the onset of the LH surge, is evoked by LH-mediated stimulation of prostaglandin (PG) synthesis (primarily $PGF_{2\alpha}$ and PGE) and production of proteolytic enzymes such as collagenases. The oocyte-cumulus complex is extruded from the follicle at a weakened point in the follicle wall known as the "stigma." Expulsion of the oocyte and follicle fluid through the stigma is a gentle, nonexplosive process. This oocyte-cumulus mass is then "picked up" by the fimbriated end of the fallopian tube. Ciliated cells of the fallopian tube help propel the oocyte-cumulus complex through the ampullary portion of the tube where fertilization generally occurs.

Early Luteal Phase (Postovulatory)

The luteal phase is characterized by high concentrations of LH receptors on the granulosa and theca cells. The cellular response to LH is to change the enzymatic machinery of the granulosa cells from estradiol secretion to predominately progesterone production (see Fig. 7-2). Just prior to ovulation, the granulosa cells increase in size, vacuolate, and accumulate a yellow pigment called lutein. During the first 3 days following ovulation, these LH-transformed granulosa and theca cells luteinize and become a 2.5-cm structure known as the corpus luteum. The corpus luteum is composed of large and small luteal cells, endothelial cells, macrophages, pericytes, and fibroblasts. The large luteal cells produce relaxin and oxytocin and are most active in steroidogenesis, with greater aromatase activity and more progesterone synthesis compared to small cells. Interleukins and growth factors are produced by the on-luteal cells. Capillaries penetrate into the granulosa layer and antral cavity under the influence of angiogenesis-inducing factors.

Adequate progesterone production by the corpus luteum depends on the antecedent FSH and LH signals from the pituitary as well as maintenance of tonic LH secretion and development of an adequate blood supply. Progesterone production, which begins approximately 24 hours before ovulation, is maintained for 11–14 days following ovulation. Maximal production occurs 3–4 days after ovulation (see Fig. 7-2). Peak vascularization of the corpus luteum is reached by day 8 or 9 after ovulation and is associated with peak circulating levels of progesterone. The increased vascularity ensures that adequate amounts of low-density lipoprotein (LDL) cholesterol, the substrate for progesterone production, reaches the luteal cells. Most luteal phases are approximately 14 days in length with lengths between 11 and 17 days considered normal.

Progesterone from the corpus luteum acts both locally and centrally to suppress new follicular growth. Because ovulation in subsequent cycles tends to occur contralateral to the previous corpus luteum, progesterone is thought to suppress follicular growth locally. Follicular growth during the luteal phase is also inhibited by inadequate levels of gonadotropins that occur from the negative feedback of high luteal concentrations of estrogen, progesterone, and inhibin. Compared to the high-frequency and low-amplitude pulses of LH found during the follicular phase (resulting from pulses of GnRH), the luteal phase is characterized by low-frequency and high-amplitude pulses of LH (see Fig. 7-2). Whereas progesterone acts to lower the LH frequency, ovarian estradiol appears most effective in modulating the amplitude.

Late Luteal Phase (Premenstrual)

The secretory activity and functional lifespan of the corpus luteum is dependent on appropriate LH support. Unless implantation and human chorionic gonadotropin (hCG) from the developing embryo rescues the corpus luteum, involution occurs. Definitive luteolytic factors have been defined for some species (ruminants), but not for the human menstrual cycle. The demise of the corpus luteum in 14 days is due to an active luteolytic mechanism. It has been suggested that estrogen production by the corpus luteum itself, mediated by alterations in prostaglandin concentrations, is involved in luteolysis. During the last 4–5 days of the functional life of the corpus luteum, there is a precipitous decline in levels of progesterone, estradiol, and inhibin (see Fig. 7-2). The two principal enzymes involved in progesterone synthesis (cholesterol side chain cleavage and 3β-hydroxysteroid dehydrogenase) have continually declined throughout the luteal phase from their maximum at the time of ovulation. The loss of the highly steroidogenic large luteal cells and a decrease in the ability of the small luteal cells to respond to LH accompanies the late luteal phase decline in steroidogenesis.

The decline in steroids and inhibin results in a change in LH secretion, removal of the pituitary from negative feedback suppression, and an increase in circulating FSH concentration. The more dramatic rise in FSH compared to LH is due in part to removal of inhibin, which selectively suppresses FSH, and to removal of the negative feedback effects of estradiol at the pituitary level (see Fig. 7-1). The decrease in estradiol restores the ability of the pituitary to respond to GnRH signals from the hypothalamus (see Fig. 7-2). In addition, an increase in GnRH pulse frequency causes a predominance of FSH secretion. The increase in FSH during the later portion of the luteal phase is instrumental in initiating recruitment of a cohort of follicles for the ensuing cycle. Thus, the demise of the corpus luteum heralds the initiation of the next menstrual cycle.

UTERINE AND ENDOMETRIAL CHANGES ASSOCIATED WITH THE OVARIAN MENSTRUAL CYCLE

Menstruation (Uterine Events)

Low levels of hormones, specifically progesterone and estradiol, are thought to initiate the endometrial changes associated with the onset of menstrual bleeding (see Figs. 7-2 and 7-3). During the 4–24 hours before menstruation, vasoconstriction of the coiled arteries and arterioles of the endometrium results in ischemia and necrosis in the upper portion of the endometrium (see Fig. 7-1). Vessel and tissue necrosis is receded by vasospasms, possibly stimulated by prostaglandin F2-α and the release of lysosomal lytic enzymes. As the coiled arteries relax after this vasoconstriction (ischemia–reperfusion cycle), the endometrium becomes detached from the basal layer leading to multifocal and progressive exfoliation of cells and shedding of the vessels. This generally results in 4–6 days of menstrual bleeding with a loss of 25–60 ml of blood.

Although menstrual bleeding may continue for several days, endometrial regeneration generally begins within 2 days after the onset of menstruation. Because hormone levels are still low, this reparative process may be initiated in response to tissue loss rather than hormonal influence. The repair process lasts until the fifth or sixth day and involves reepithelialization of the spongiosum. Regeneration of the microvasculature is initiated from the remaining arteriolar stump in the basalis and is most likely controlled by several local tissue growth factors such as epidermal growth factor, angiogenic growth factor, transforming growth factor, or fibroblast growth factor.

Postmenstrual Endometrium

The endometrium contains estrogen and progesterone receptors and responds to the hormonal milieu emanating from the ovary. By day 5 or 6, when menstruation has ceased, the endometrium is 1–2 mm thick and consists mainly of the basal layer and a small amount of spongiosum (see Figs. 7-1 and 7-3). In response to rising levels of estrogen, there is proliferation (due to increased mitoses) of epithelial and stromal cells in the surface layer, or stratum functionale. During the early to midproliferative phase, the glands are initially tubular and straight but become more tortuous as estrogen levels increase. While only one fourth of the stromal and glandular cells stain positively for progesterone receptors at this time, estrogen receptor content is highest. The stroma appears fibrous and the stromal cells appear as naked nuclei due to containing limited amounts of cytoplasm.

Late Proliferative Endometrium

Under the influence of estrogen, proliferation of the epithelial and stromal cells of the endometrium continues as does glandular mitosis and nuclear pseudostratification. Glycogenesis and glycogen storage begins on approximately day 10 and this leads to increased lengthening and coiling of the endometrial glands. Maximal pseudostratification of glandular cells is found just prior to ovulation. Cell nuclei begin migrating toward the surface as glycogen storage increases in the glandular epithelium. The surface epithelium is composed of columnar cells at this time. The endometrial thickness at midcycle averages 10–12 mm in maximum diameter or 5 mm in height (see Fig. 7-3). This proliferation is mainly in the functionalis layer. Under this estrogen-dominant phase of endometrial growth, there is an increase in ciliated and microvillous cells that begins on days 7–8 of the cycle. Localization of these ciliated cells around gland openings and their pattern of movement influence the mobilization and distribution of endometrial secretions during the subsequent secretory phase. The concentration of progesterone receptors increases most notably in the glandular cells whereas estrogen receptors begin to decline.

Luteal Phase Uterine Changes (Early Secretory Phase)

The endometrium displays a combined reaction to estrogen and progesterone activity following ovulation (Figs. 7-2 and 7-3). Despite continued availability of estrogen, the endometrial height remains at 5–6 mm due to a decline in mitosis and DNA synthesis associated with progesterone interference with estrogen receptor expression and progesterone stimulation of 17β-hydroxysteroid dehydrogenase and sulfotransferase. Confinement of growing individual components to this area of fixed endometrial height leads to progressive tortuosity of the glands and coiling of the spiral vessels (see Figs. 7-1 and 7-3). Following ovulation the endometrium undergoes secretory differentiation under the influence of progesterone as evidenced by the appearance of subnuclear intracytoplasmic vacuoles in the basal portion of the glandular epithelium. Giant mitochondria and nucleolar channels appear in the gland cells due to an infolding of the nuclear membranes. By days 6–7 of the luteal phase, the secretory products have moved to the apex of the glands where they are extruded into the glandular space by apocrine-type secretion. In contrast, the nucleus becomes positioned at the base of the cell. Although a rising progesterone level arrests glandular proliferation, it supports continued growth of the arteriolar system. Peak production of endometrial secretions, including glycoproteins and peptides, plasma transudates, and immunoglobulins, coincides with blastocyst implantation during the midluteal phase. During this first half of the secretory phase, acid phosphatase and potent lytic enzymes are confined to lysosomes. Progesterone stabilizes the lysosomal membranes and inhibits their release.

Late Luteal Phase Uterine Changes (Late Secretory Phase)

Distended tortuous secretory glands with little intervening stroma characterize the endometrium 7 days postovulation (see Fig. 7-3). However, by 13 days postovulation the endometrium differentiates into three zones (see Fig. 7-1) as follows: (a) the basalis portion fed by straight vessels and surrounded by indifferent spindle-shaped stroma; (b) the middle lace-like stratum spongiosum composed of loose edematous stroma with tightly coiled spiral vessels and exhausted dilated glandular ribbons; and (c) the superficial stratum compactum layer with its large polyhedral stromal cells. The predominant morphologic feature of the endometrium at the time of implantation is edema of the endometrial stroma. This edema may result from increased capillary permeability as a consequence of estrogen- and progesterone- mediated prostaglandin production. Granulocytes, called K cells, become located perivascularly and probably play an immunoprotective role. During the last 2–3 days of the luteal phase, predecidual cells, characterized by cytonuclear enlargement, increased mitotic activity, and a basement membrane, can be identified surrounding blood vessels. In the absence of fertilization, estrogen and progesterone levels decline resulting in destabilization of the lysosomal membranes and release of lytic enzymes into the cytoplasm. Activation of these enzymes leads to prostaglandin release, extravasation of red blood cells, tissue necrosis, and vascular thrombosis culminating in vasomotor reactions, tissue loss, and menstruation. A summary of the histologic changes that occur in the endometrium throughout the menstrual cycle are depicted in Fig. 7-4.

CONCLUSION

The normal menstrual cycle is dependent on an appropriately functioning HPO axis. Gonadal steroids, most importantly estrogen and progesterone, exert negative and positive feedback action on gonadotropin secretion. Follicular growth and maturation relies on FSH-induced events whereas ovulation and luteal function depends primarily on LH secretion. The gonadal steroids then initiate cyclic changes in the endometrium necessary for implantation if fertilization occurs.

SUGGESTED READING

Lobo RA. The menstrual cycle. In: Mishell DR, Davajan V, Lobo RA, eds. *Infertility, Contraception and Reproductive Endocrinology,* 3rd ed. Boston: Blackwell Scientific, 1991;104–124.
Speroff L, Glass RH, Kase NG, eds. Regulation of the menstrual cycle. In: *Clinical Gynecologic Endocrinology and Infertility,* 5th ed. Baltimore: Williams and Wilkins, 1994;183–230.

Hypothalamus-Pituitary

Ferin M, Jewelewicz R, Warren M, eds. Hypothalamic- pituitary-ovarian communication. In: *The Menstrual Cycle; Physiology, Reproductive Disorders, and Infertility.* New York: Oxford University Press, 1993;42–61.
Yen SSC. The human menstrual cycle: neuroendocrine regulation. In: Yen SSC, Jaffe RB, eds. *Reproductive Endocrinology; Physiology, Pathophysiology and Clinical Management,* 3rd ed. Philadelphia: WB Saunders, 1991;273–308.

Ovary

Adashi EY. Endocrinology of the ovary. In: Edwards RG, ed. *New Concepts in Fertility Control. Human Reproduction,* vol 9, Supplement 2. New York: Oxford University Press, 1994;36–51.
Adashi EY. The ovarian life cycle. In: Yen SSC, Jaffe RB, eds. *Reproductive Endocrinology; Physiology, Pathophysiology and Clinical Management,* 3rd ed. Philadelphia: WB Saunders, 1991;181–237.
Erickson GF, Schreiber JR. Morphology and physiology of the ovary. In: Becker KL, ed. *Principles and Practice of Endocrinology and Metabolism.* Philadelphia: JB Lippincott, 1990;776–788.
Paulson RJ. Oocytes, from development to fertilization. In: Mishell DR, Davajan V, Lobo RA, eds. *Infertility, Contraception and Reproductive Endocrinology,* 3rd ed. Boston: Blackwell Scientific, 1991;140–149.

Uterus and Endometrium

Ferin M, Jewelewicz R, Warren M, eds. The genital tract. In: *The Menstrual Cycle; Physiology, Reproductive Disorders, and Infertility.* New York: Oxford University Press, 1993;62–69.
March CM. The endometrium in the menstrual cycle. In: Mishell DR, Davajan V, Lobo RA, eds. *Infertility, Contraception and Reproductive Endocrinology,* 3rd ed. Boston: Blackwell Scientific, 1991;125–139.
Hansard LJ, Walmer DK. Descriptive histology; the gold standard for clinically evaluating the endometrium. In: Metzger DA, ed. *Infertil Reprod Med Clin North Am* 1995;6(2):281–292.
Speroff L, Glass RH, Kase NG, eds. The uterus. In: *Clinical Gynecologic Endocrinology and Infertility,* 5th ed. Baltimore: Williams and Wilkins, 1994;109–139.
Strauss JF, Gurpide E. The endometrium: regulation and dysfunction. In: Yen SSC, Jaffe RB, eds. *Reproductive Endocrinology; Physiology, Pathophysiology and Clinical Management,* 3rd ed. Philadelphia: WB Saunders, 1991:309–356.

Clinical Reproductive Medicine,
Edited by Bryan D. Cowan and David B. Seifer
Lippincott-Raven Publishers, Philadelphia © 1997

CHAPTER 8

Dysfunctional Uterine Bleeding

Bryan D. Cowan

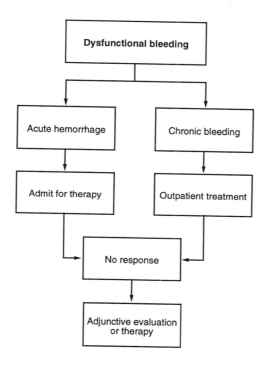

Diagnosis
Therapy

Conclusion
Selected Reading

B. D. Cowan: Division of Reproductive Endocrinology, Department of Obstetrics and Gynecology, University of Mississippi Medical Center, Jackson, MS 39216

Dysfunctional uterine bleeding (DUB) affects women from the adolescent years to the perimenopausal interval. DUB is a diagnosis of exclusion and requires a systematic check to eliminate other pathologic causes of genital tract bleeding. DUB is virtually synonymous with anovulatory bleeding and occurs in two forms. The most common and bothersome form of DUB is breakthrough bleeding. This pattern of bleeding occurs during steady-state, acyclic estrogen production. Bleeding may be light and intermittent or infrequent and associated with hemorrhage. It is thought that breakthrough bleeding occurs when the estrogen-stimulated endometrium proliferates beyond its inability to maintain integrity. Examples of breakthrough bleeding include estrogenized/androgenized chronic anovulation syndromes and following unopposed exogenous estrogen therapy. The second type of DUB is termed withdrawal bleeding. This form of DUB is the least bothersome and is seen when circulating estrogen concentrations fall. The estrogen-stimulated endometrium is no longer supported and bleeding occurs. Two common clinical presentations of estrogen withdrawal bleeding include preovulatory bleeding associated with a fall in estradiol at midcycle and the estrogen withdrawal bleeding associated with perimenopausal bleeding during the final phases of ovarian follicular depletion. Because DUB is not associated with the usual prostaglandin production and vasoconstriction seen with menstrual (progestin withdrawal) bleeding, the clotting and healing mechanisms that abate bleeding in DUB are probably different.

DIAGNOSIS

Clues to the etiology of abnormal uterine bleeding are derived by clinical and laboratory examinations. The clinical evaluation should include a systematic evaluation to exclude organic pathology (Table 8-1). The medical history should determine menarche, cycle intervals, and cycle frequency. Historical investigation should include medications. Commonly used drugs associated with abnormal vaginal bleeding include exogenous hormones, anticoagulants, salicylates, phenothiazines, and digitalis. Infrequently ingested medications associated with abnormal vaginal bleeding include monoamine oxidase inhibitors, anticholinergics, illicit drugs, reserpine, and diet pills (Table 8-2). The general physical examination is commonly unrevealing but will occasionally provide clues to the existence of systemic disease. A general examination should investigate blood pressure, pulse, body habitus, hair quality and distribution, ecchymosis and petechiae, adenopathy, and hepatosplenomegaly.

The most important portion of the examination in patients with abnormal genital bleeding is the pelvic examination. During this examination, the perineum, vagina, and cervix should be inspected for lesions or trauma. A Pap smear is generally included as a cytologic screen for dysplasia, but cervical cancer is usually detected by visualizing a tumor. Uterine palpation will determine the size and consistency of the uterus and provide clues to the possibility of pregnancy (enlarged and softened uterus) or the presence of uterine fibroids (enlarged, firm, and irregular uterus). Adnexal palpation usually will detect adnexal masses. Uncommonly, the pelvic examination is ambiguous and requires further evaluation. Transvaginal sonography provides excellent pelvic visualization, is readily available, and is cost-efficient for patients with ambiguous pelvic examinations. Additionally, transvaginal sonographic illumination of the endometrium can provide an indirect measure of the risk of endometrial hyperplasia and detect small transmural or submucosal leiomyomata that cannot be detected on pelvic examination. On occasion, office hysteroscopy may provide additional useful information by ruling out polyps or small submucosal fibroids.

Other tools that provide clues to the etiology of DUB are the menstrual calendar and the progestin withdrawal test. The menstrual calendar is a tabular document generated by the patient that marks the days of the year where bleeding occurs. The clinician can determine the pattern and duration of bleeding by scanning this document. The

TABLE 8-1. *Differential diagnosis of abnormal uterine bleeding*

1. Anovulation (dysfunctional uterine bleeding)
2. Primary coagulation disorder
3. Abnormal pregnancy
   a. Threatened abortion
   b. Spontaneous abortion
   c. Ectopic pregnancy
4. Systemic disease
   a. Hepatic dysfunction
   b. Renal dysfunction
   c. Thyroid dysfunction
   d. Leukemia
5. Genital tract lesions
   a. Trauma
   b. Tumor
   c. Infection
6. Exogenous hormone therapy
7. Concomitant medications

TABLE 8-2. *Medications associated with abnormal vaginal bleeding*

Commonly used medications
1. Exogenous hormones
2. Anticoagulants
3. Salicylates
4. Phenothiazines
5. Digitalis
Uncommonly used preparations
1. Monoamine oxidase inhibitors
2. Anticholinergics
3. Illicit drugs
4. Reserpine
5. Diet pills

purpose of the progestin withdrawal test is to establish the estrogen status of a patient. Progestin (100 mg progesterone in oil intramuscularly or 10 mg medroxyprogesterone acetate orally for 7–10 days) is administered to induce menstrual flow. If the patient has enough circulating estrogen (estrone and estradiol) to stimulate a proliferative response in the endometrium, bleeding will occur 2–14 days after cessation of progestin therapy. Any bleeding is considered a positive test. A positive response to this test indicates an estrogenized endometrium that is at risk to bleed in the future and confirms a patent outflow tract. Additionally, an estrogenized endometrium is considered at risk for the development of hyperplastic sequelae (adenomatous hyperplasia and endometrial cancer) if untreated.

Laboratory testing is designed to supplement the clinical evaluation and exclude disease processes that can produce abnormal bleeding. The laboratory evaluation is usually conducted in a three-tier process (Table 8-3). In general, patients with abnormal uterine bleeding are screened with a pregnancy test and complete blood count. The purpose of the pregnancy test is to exclude pregnancy as the source of bleeding. The purpose of the blood count is to determine the hemoglobin, hematocrit, and platelet count. The second tier of laboratory testing is based on positive findings of the clinical examination. If androgen excess is detected (facial hirsutism, acne, or signs of virilization), a clinically relevant androgen profile is obtained. The third tier of testing is reserved for patients who are refractory to conventional medical therapy for DUB. A bleeding time is obtained to measure hemostasis; thyroid hormones and prolactin are measured to exclude endocrinopathy and measurements of renal and hepatic function are commonly included.

A diagnostic algorithm for the systematic evaluation of abnormal bleeding is presented in Fig. 8-1. This algorithm is truncated to emphasize the pathway that leads to the diagnosis of DUB. The clues provided by history, physical examination, and laboratory testing will allow physicians to eliminate pathologic causes of abnormal genital bleeding (see Table 8-1). The diagno-

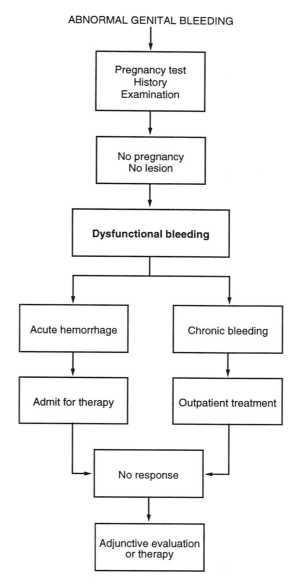

FIG. 8-1. Schematic algorithm to evaluate abnormal genital bleeding in adolescents and adults. Dysfunctional uterine bleeding is diagnosed by a negative pregnancy test, normal genital inspection, and negative endometrial biopsy. Adjunctive evaluations and treatments are indicated if bleeding persists after therapy.

TABLE 8-3. *Laboratory evaluation of dysfunctional uterine bleeding*

1. Basic tests
   a. Pregnancy test
   b. Complete blood count
2. Endocrine tests
   a. Prolactin
   b. Thyroxin and thyroid-stimulating hormone
   c. Testosterone
   d. Dehydroepiandrosterone sulfate
3. Coagulopathy/metabolic
   a. Bleeding time
   b. Creatinine
   c. Liver function tests
   d. Fibrinogen

sis of DUB can be confirmed only when pathologic causes have been excluded.

THERAPY

Treatment of DUB will be clued by hemoglobin concentration type of bleeding. The most important concern in the evaluation of a patient with hemorrhage associated with dysfunctional bleeding is to assess the clinical impact of the bleeding. Women with a hemoglobin >8 g % can be managed as outpatients. Hospitalization should be considered for women with lower hemoglobin concentrations. The goal of therapy for hemodynamically stable anovulatory bleeding is to halt estrogen-stimulated endometrial proliferation, induce endometrial maturation, and slough the endometrium (menses) in an orderly and scheduled fashion. Medical management is the primary therapy for the majority of cases of abnormal uterine bleeding. Therapeutic agents include hormones, nonsteroidal antiinflammatory preparations, and gonadotropin-releasing hormone agonists (GnRH-a) in addition to iron replacement therapy if indicated. Other preparations of historical interest are mentioned but their use is currently limited.

Progestational preparations are the most logical and common choices to treat DUB. Replacement with natural progestins was not practical until relatively recently. Vaginal suppositories (25–400 mg), intramuscular progesterone in oil (50–200 mg), and sublingual or buccal troches are now available. Few data exist to indicate the optimum dose of natural products. However, these preparations are commonly associated with unwanted administration (injection or suppository) or gastrointestinal (troches) effects. The traditional synthetic progestin replacement drugs, such as medroxyprogesterone acetate (MPA) and norgesterone, have had extensive clinical and metabolic evaluations. Both are effective in acute use, stable in pill form, and do not require special handling.

The suggested duration of administration of progestin hormones is taken from the literature reporting experience with postmenopausal hormonal replacement. The goals are the same, namely, to halt endometrial proliferation and induce its maturation but minimize the unwanted metabolic alterations associated with progestin therapy. The usual dose of MPA is 10 mg daily for 10 days. Many physicians use shorter courses of MPA or intramuscular progesterone to induce acute and rapid withdrawal bleeding. Although short-duration progestin therapy will induce menstrual flow, a minimum of 10 days of therapy is required to prevent hyperplastic changes of the endometrium in women receiving postmenopausal replacement therapy. After approximately 2–3 months of therapy, the endometrial lining becomes thin and the menstrual blood loss is reduced.

In general, MPA therapy should be provided on a monthly basis. It is helpful to provide each patient with a menstrual calendar to record the days of bleeding and the timing of hormone administration. Occasionally, patients may take MPA on alternate months. This is especially the case if scant or absent progestin-induced withdrawal bleeding occurs after withdrawal.

Women with hemodynamically stable acute bleeding may be treated by combination oral contraceptives. The goal of therapy is to provide high-dose estrogen in combination with progestin. In our experience, patients will have an adequate response to 4 pills taken daily for 3 days followed by 3 pills taken daily for 3 days. This is the equivalent of one pack of birth control pills. At the cessation of this therapy, a heavy menstrual flow is expected.

Women with hemodynamically unstable anovulatory bleeding (hemorrhage) require special attention. If the hemoglobin is <8 g % or the patient is orthostatic, hospitalization is required. The goal of therapy in these seriously ill women is to replace the intravascular losses and stop the bleeding. Transfusion may be necessary when severe anemia and hemodynamic instability are present. Because inadequate estrogen support of the proliferating endometrium (estrogen breakthrough) is the etiology of this type of hemorrhage, acute phase therapy should begin with high-dose estrogen. Conjugated equine estrogens (25 mg) should be administered intravenously every 4 hours for 4–6 doses. Nausea and emesis are common after intravenous administration of this amount of estrogen and antiemetic therapy is often required. Bleeding usually ceases within 4–24 hours (1–6 doses of estrogen). An alternative approach is the administration of a combination oral contraceptive pill 4 times a day for 5–7 days. The mechanism of estrogen-mediated control of bleeding is unknown but is probably related to vascular and not proliferative effects of estrogen on the endometrium. If significant bleeding continues after estrogen therapy, other diagnostic and therapeutic modalities are indicated.

Nonsteroidal antiinflammatory drugs (NSAIDs) block the conversion of arachidonic acid to prostaglandins and inhibit uterine bleeding. Two vasoactive substances are produced from arachidonate metabolism. One is a vasoconstrictor (thromboxane A2) and the other is a vasodilator (prostacyclin). Reduction of arachidonic acid conversion to prostaglandins by NSAIDs reduces vascular dilatation and enhances platelet aggregation. Suggested NSAIDs include mefenamic acid, ibuprofen, or naproxen sodium. In general, these preparations should be administered 24–48 hours prior to the anticipated onset of menses and continued throughout the days of heavy menstrual flow. These agents provide pain relief for dysmenorrhea and substantially reduce menstrual blood loss.

Reduction of fibrinolytic activity reduces menstrual blood loss. Inhibitors of fibrinolytic activity include ε-aminocaproic acid and transamic acid. Unfortunately, these agents commonly induce side effects such as nausea, dizziness, diarrhea, headaches, abdominal pain, and allergic manifestations. Additionally, intracranial thrombosis has been described in a few women in association with these drugs. Therefore, the potential benefits of these drugs commonly do not outweigh the risks and their use should be limited to special applications.

Ergot alkaloids induce uterine contractions but have little effect on abnormal uterine bleeding. Because other agents (hormones, NSAIDs) are far superior therapeutic agents, the use of ergot alkaloids has generally been abandoned. Additionally, these preparations are contraindicated in patients with hypertension.

The development of analogs to GnRH has provided the clinician with a specific tool to suppress ovarian function at the level of the pituitary. Long-acting GnRH-a has been developed that suppresses the ability of the pituitary to secrete gonadotropins. The effect of this therapy is to induce a hypogonadal state and stop DUB. After pituitary-gonadal suppression has been achieved, patients are usually treated with cyclic low-dose conjugated estrogen and progestin in a fashion similar to that for menopausal patients. This hormonal replacement therapy reduces hot flashes, protects against hypoestrogen-induced bone demineralization, and supports estrogen-dependent tissues (breasts, vagina, skin, uterus). This therapy has shown particular promise for estrogenized/androgenized chronic anovulation patients who suffer the effects of unopposed estrogen (DUB) and hyperandrogenism (hirsutism).

Surgical therapy of anovulatory uterine bleeding is reserved until medical options fail or the status of the patient deteriorates. Uterine curettage, hysteroscopy, endometrial ablation, and hysterectomy are often designed to be both diagnostic and therapeutic. Pathologic conditions may exist that were not detected during the initial evaluation of abnormal genital tract bleeding. Although medical therapy may have treated anovulatory uterine bleeding, other lesions may exist that contribute to the bleeding. These include endometrial polyps, submucous fibroids, endometrial hyperplasia, and adenocarcinoma of the endometrium.

Uterine curettage samples the endometrium and reduces acute hemorrhage in anovulatory uterine bleeding in 70–85% of cases. Additionally, examination under anesthesia may yield useful information that was not detected initially.

Hysteroscopy prior to uterine curettage can direct the physician to suspicious endometrial lesions or diagnose conditions that may be inapparent to the "blind" curette. After uterine curettage, repeat hysteroscopy will confirm that the lesion has either been removed or properly sampled. In a comparative study of hysteroscopy versus uterine curettage, hysteroscopy was shown to be superior for the diagnosis of pathologic conditions of the endometrium.

Endometrial ablation is an alternative treatment for women with refractory anovulatory bleeding. Techniques vary but the most commonly employed method utilizes the resectoscope to strip off the endometrium and superficial myometrium. This can be accomplished with a roller-ball electrocautery device or the resectoscopic loop electrode. Approximately 20–40% of patients who undergo endometrial ablation will continue to have cyclic bleeding but the bleeding is substantially reduced. The long-term effect of this therapy is unknown. Patients with anovulatory uterine bleeding probably should continue to be treated with cyclic progestin therapy to avoid continuous acyclic estrogen stimulation of residual nests of endometrium.

Hysterectomy is generally reserved as the final surgical treatment option for refractory genital tract bleeding. Excessive bleeding without pathologic causes or anemia can be treated by hysterectomy if the patient decides that her bleeding represents a significant burden to her life.

CONCLUSION

The efficient diagnosis of DUB requires the elimination of pathologic disorders that produce bleeding. A pregnancy test should be performed and each patient should have a genital inspection to exclude tumors and trauma. When DUB is diagnosed, treatment is usually medical. Chronic DUB can be treated with progestins, oral contraceptives, or combined estrogen/progestin preparations in combination with iron replacement therapy when indicated. Hemorrhage from DUB requires hospitalization, high-dose intravenous conjugated estrogen, and blood replacement for acute phase management. Adjunctive evaluations to exclude systemic disease and coagulation disorders are indicated if DUB is refractory to medical therapy. Surgery is reserved for recalcitrant DUB.

SELECTED READING

Anderson ABM, Guillebaud J, Haynes PJ, Turnbull AC. Reduction of menstrual blood-loss by prostaglandin-synthetase inhibitors. *Lancet* 1976;1: 774–776.

Barber HRK, Graber EA. Gynecologic tumors in children and adolescents. *Obstet Gynecol Surv* 1973;28:357–381.

Bayer SR, DeCherney AH. Clinical manifestations and treatment of dysfunction uterine bleeding. *JAMA* 1993;269:1823–1828.

Buttram VC, Reiter RC. Uterine leiomyomata: etiology, symptomatology, and management. *Fertil Steril* 1981;36:433–445.

Claessens EA, Cowell CA. Acute adolescent menorrhagia. *Am J Obstet Gynecol* 1981;139:277–280.

Cowan BD, Morrison JC. Management of abnormal genital bleeding in girls and women. *N Engl J Med* 1991;324:1710–1715.

DeVore GR, Owens O, Kase N. Use of intravenous premarin in treatment of dysfunctional uterine bleeding: a double-blind randomized control study. *Obstet Gynecol* 1982;59:285–291.

Fraser IS, McCarron G, Markham R, Resta T, Watts A. Measured menstrual blood loss in women with menorrhagia associated with pelvic disease or coagulation disorder. *Obstet Gynecol* 1986;68:630–633.

Goldstein SR, Nachtigall M, Snyder JR, Nachtigall L. Endometrial assessment by vaginal ultrasonography before endometrial sampling in patients with postmenopausal bleeding. *Am J Obstet Gynecol* 1990;163:119–123.

Hall P, MacLachlan N, Thorn N, Nadd MWE, Taylor CG, Garrioch OB. Control of menorrhagia by the cyclo-oxygenase inhibitors naproxen sodium and mefenamic acid. *Br J Obstet Gynaecol* 1987;94:554–558.

Jennings JC. Abnormal uterine bleeding. *Med Clin North Am* 1995;79: 1357–1376.

Jutras MA, Cowan BD. Abnormal bleeding in the climacteric. *Obstet Gynecol Clin North Am* 1990;17:409–426.

McLachlan RI, Healy DL, Burger HG. Clinical aspects of LHRH analogues in gynecology: a review. *Br J Obstet Gynaecol* 1986;93:431–454.

Mendenhall HW. Evaluation and management of dysfunctional uterine bleeding. *Semin Reprod Endocrinol* 1984;2:369–373.

Muram D. Vaginal bleeding in childhood and adolescence. *Obstet Gynecol Clin North Am* 1990;17:389–408.

Padwick ML, Pryse-Davies J, Whitehead MI. A simple method for determining the optimal dosage of progestin in postmenopausal women receiving estrogens. *N Engl J Med* 1986;315:930–934.

Siegler AM. Office hysteroscopy. *Obstet Gynecol Clin North Am* 1995;22: 457–471.

Steinkampf MP. Systemic illness and menstrual dysfunction. *Obstet Gynecol Clin North Am* 1990;17:311–319.

Taylor PJ, Gomel V. Endometrial ablation: indications and preliminary diagnostic hysteroscopy. *Baillieres Clin Obstet Gynaecol* 1995;9:251–260.

Wathen PI, Henderson MC, Witz CA. Abnormal uterine bleeding. *Med Clin North Am* 1995;79:329–344.

Whitehead MI, Hillard TC, Crook D. The role and use of progestogens. *Obstet Gynecol* 1990;75:59s–76s.

Clinical Reproductive Medicine,
Edited by Bryan D. Cowan and David B. Seifer
Lippincott-Raven Publishers, Philadelphia © 1997

CHAPTER 9

Amenorrhea

Bryan D. Cowan

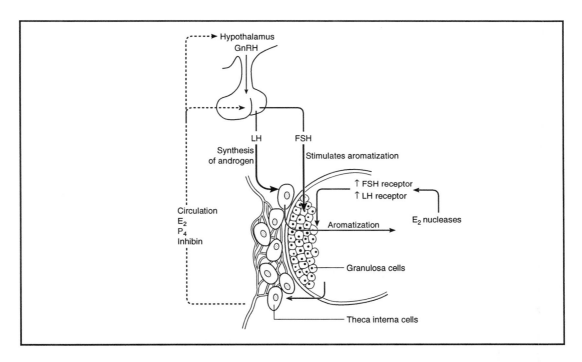

Classifications of Anovulation
  Chronic Anovulation
  Anovulation Due to CNS-Hypothalamic-Pituitary
    Dysfunction
  Gonadal Failure
  Mullerian and Outflow Tract Defects
Diagnosis
Interpretation of the Amenorrhea Evaluation
  Prolactin

Thyroid Function
Progestin Withdrawal
Gonadotropins
Estrogen-Stimulated Progestin Withdrawal
Danger Zones
  Modest Hyperprolectinemia
Hypogonadotropic Hypogonadism
Summary
Selected Reading

B. D. Cowan: Division of Reproductive Endocrinology, Department of Obstetrics and Gynecology, University of Mississippi Medical Center, Jackson MS 39157

The criteria for diagnosis of amenorrhea are satisfied when menarche has not occurred by 16 years of age (primary amenorrhea) or when a woman who previously experienced regular menses has absence of menstruation for three cycles (secondary amenorrhea). Historically, great significance has been assigned to the difference between primary and secondary amenorrhea because the incidence of genetic and anatomic abnormalities is higher in patients with primary amenorrhea. However, these terms represent an arbitrary assignment of a diagnosis based on the occurrence of menarche. It is more appropriate to assess the developmental maturation of secondary sex characteristics and the pathophysiologic changes that produce the symptoms of anovulation/amenorrhea than to classify the timing of amenorrhea. In general, the evaluations of primary and secondary amenorrhea follow the same diagnostic algorithms. The pathophysiologic causes of amenorrhea can be grouped into chronic anovulation syndromes, central nervous system (CNS) lesions or dysfunction, gonadal failure, or Mullerian abnormalities. Fortunately, only a few tests of endocrine function combined with proper clinical interpretation are necessary to diagnose the causes of amenorrhea/anovulation.

CLASSIFICATIONS OF ANOVULATION

The relative frequencies of the causes of amenorrhea/anovulation in women who present for evaluation are somewhat dependent on practice patterns. Our population distribution is shown in Table 9-1. Chronic anovulation is the most common etiology of disrupted menstrual function in our patients. Hypothalamic-pituitary dysfunction represents the second most common etiology of anovulation/amenorrhea and accounts for 40% of cases. Ovarian failure affects 5% of our patients with amenorrhea and only 3% of amenorrhea is due to end-organ defects.

Chronic Anovulation

Control of the ovarian-menstrual cycle is entrained in the "ovarian clock." In this model, estradiol represents the principal regulator of hypothalamic-pituitary responses. Low estrogen concentrations stimulate pituitary follicle-stimulating hormone (FSH) secretion and ovarian follicu-

logenesis. In response to FSH stimulation, rising follicular estrogen concentrations suppress FSH and select the dominate follicle. Finally, high concentrations of estradiol stimulate the midcycle release of the pituitary luteinizing hormone (LH) surge. Normally, this cycle is repeated throughout the reproductive life of a woman. Events that interfere with the proper estrogen signaling of the pituitary produce anovulation/amenorrhea.

Circulating estrogens are derived from gonadal (ovary) and extragonadal (adipose) sites. In the ovary, gonadotropin-dependent estrogen production (Fig. 9-1) is mediated by granulosa cell responses to FSH. Gonadotropin-dependent estrogen production is cyclic, and peak production occurs in the late proliferative phase and luteal phase of the cycle. The predominate ovarian estrogen is estradiol (E_2). In contrast, extraglandular gonadotropin-independent estrogens are derived from the conversion of circulating androgens to estrogens (Fig. 9-2). The peripheral conversion of androgens to estrogens occurs in a steady state. The predominant estrogen produced by peripheral conversion of androgens is estrone (E_1). Although the precise purpose for extraglandular conversion of androgens to estrogens is not clear, this may produce high concentrations of estrogens in target tissues without the need to deliver hormone through the systemic circulation.

Peripheral endocrine disorders that alter estrogen signaling of the pituitary and induce menstrual disturbances are the most common causes of anovulation/amenorrhea. Seven defects of peripheral endocrine function may influence circulating estrogen/androgen concentrations and result in aberrant feedback signals to the hypothalamic-pituitary-ovarian (HPO) axis (Table 9-2). Of these, polycystic ovarian syndrome (PCOS) is the most common cause of chronic anovulation. The term PCOS emphasizes the heterogeneity of this entity. Ovulatory failure, infertility, hirsutism, obesity, insulin resistance, and bilateral polycystic ovaries are common features of PCOS but are not unique to the syndrome. A variety of endocrine dysfunctions of diverse etiologic origins (Cushing's syndrome, congenital adrenal hyperplasia, virilizing tumors, hyperprolactinemia, and thyroid dysfunction) can present with clinical manifestations similar to those of PCOS.

Androgens significantly affect the ability of the HPO axis to respond properly to estrogen. Women have two sources of circulating androgens. Gonadotropin-stimulated ovarian stroma produces androstenedione and testosterone, and adrenocorticotropin (ACTH)-stimulated adrenal zona reticularis produces androstenedione, testosterone, dehydroepiandrosterone (DHEA), and DHEA sulfate (DHEAS). The most biologically important androgen produced by these two organs is testosterone. The ovary produces 25% of the circulating testosterone, 25% more is contributed by the adrenal glands, and a final 50% is derived from peripheral conversion of testosterone precursors (Fig. 9-3). Androstenedione is the principal precursor

TABLE 9-1. *Amenorrhea/anovulation*

Type	%
1. Chronic anovulation	52
2. Hypothalamic pituitary dysfunction	40
3. Ovarian failure	5
4. Uterine defect	3

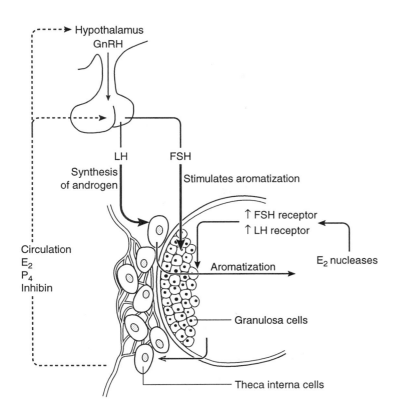

FIG. 9-1. Gonadotropin-ovarian interaction and the regulation of follicular maturation and steroidogenesis. E2, estradiol; prog, progesterone.

for peripheral testosterone synthesis. Typically, ovarian androgens (testosterone and androstenedione) and adrenal androgens (androstenedione, DHEA, DHEAS) are elevated in PCOS. Direct adrenal and ovarian vein catheterization studies suggest that PCOS patients have a combined adrenal and ovarian origin for androgen excess. Furthermore, "medical ovariectomy" with gonadotropin-releasing hormone (GnRH) agonists have helped to deter-

mine the relative contributions of ovarian and adrenal androgens to this syndrome. After suppression of ovarian function with GnRH agonist, ovarian androgens (androstenedione, testosterone) are reduced to castrate levels but adrenal androgens (DHEA and DHEAS) are unaffected. Thus, biglandular excess production of both ovarian and adrenal androgens is the signature of PCOS. If PCOS is untreated, altered carbohydrate, lipid, and androgen metabolism results in hypertension, diabetes, and cardiovascular disease.

Although sex hormones are the primary mediators of HPO responses, hormone-binding globulins modulate the effects of these steroids. In general, specific binding globulins exist for all biologically potent steroids and the bulk of steroid hormones that circulate in the plasma are bound by these proteins. Sex hormone-binding globulin (SHBG) (Table 9-3), also named testosterone-estradiol-binding globulin (TeBG), has a high affinity for testos-

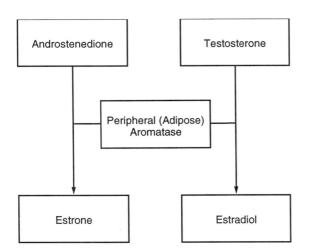

FIG. 9-2. Peripheral conversion of androgens (androstenedione, testosterone) to their respective estrogens (estrone, estradiol) by peripheral (adipose) aromatase.

TABLE 9-2. *Classification of chronic anovulation*

1. Polycystic ovary syndrome (PCOS)
2. Congenital adrenal hyperplasia (classic and adult-onset)
3. Hormone-secreting tumor (ovary or adrenal)
4. Hyperadrenalism (Cushing's)
5. Aging (increased peripheral aromatase activity)
6. Obesity (increased converting enzyme)
7. Thyroid dysfunction (SHBG alterations)

SHBG, sex hormone-binding globulin.

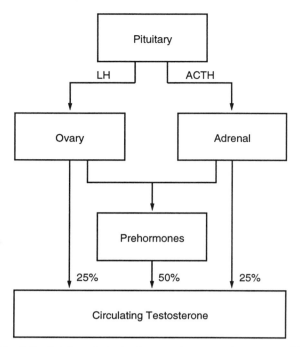

FIG. 9-3. Origin of testosterone in normal women. LH, luteinizing hormone; ACTH, adrenocorticotropin.

TABLE 9-3. *Characteristics of Sex Hormone-Binding Globulin (SHBG)*

1. Molecular weight = 90,000
2. Synthesized in the liver
3. Binds T, E_2, 5α-dehydrotestosterone with high affinity
4. Synthesis decreased by:
   progestins
   glucocorticoids
   androgens
   hypothyroidism
   hypoinsulinemia
   obesity
   hyperprolactinemia
5. Synthesis increased by:
   estrogens (oral contraceptives, pregnancy)
   hyperthyroidism
   anorexia nervosa

men. Potent synthetic progestins, glucocorticoids, growth hormone excess (acromegaly), and thyroxine deficiency (hypothyroidism) lower SHBG. Alternately, hyperthyroidism from either an endogenous or an exogenous source elevates SHBG. Thus, the level of circulating SHBG is a major regulator of the availability of sex steroids. This relationship represents an important factor in the interpretation of circulating hormone concentrations and biological actions at target tissues.

In addition to abnormal androgen/estrogen and SHBG metabolism, PCOS is associated with peripheral resistance to insulin and glucose intolerance. Both obese and nonobese women with PCOS demonstrate a positive correlation between hyperinsulinemia and hyperandrogenism, implying that androgen excess may somehow mediate peripheral insulin resistance. However, glucose intolerance is not exclusively related to androgen excess because normalization of androgens in these women does not alter hyperinsulinemia.

The genesis of PCOS can be summarized by the events described in Fig. 9-5. Here the defect is not the HPO axis. Anovulation is initiated and then sustained by elevated cir-

terone, estradiol, and 5α-dihydrotestosterone. In addition, albumin plays a major role in the binding of sex steroids. Approximately 58% of circulating estradiol is bound to albumin, 40% is bound to SHBG, and 2% is free in the circulation (Fig. 9-4). SHBG-bound steroids are generally not available for target tissue binding and are considered "inactive." In contrast, albumin-bound sex steroids are biologically active and available for both peripheral metabolism and target organ stimulation.

Hepatic production of SHBG is promoted by estrogen and inhibited by androgen. As such, adult women have about twice the plasma concentration of SHBG as adult

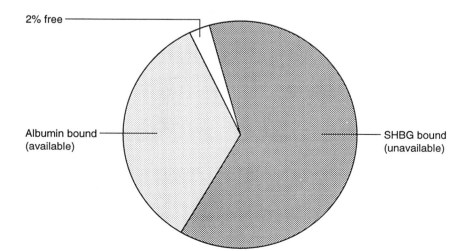

FIG. 9-4. The relative proportion of circulating estradiol that is albumin bound, sex hormone-binding globulin (SHBG) bound, and free.

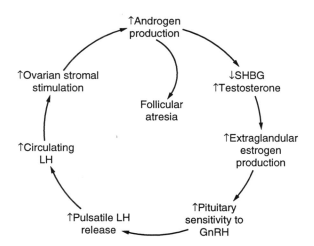

FIG. 9-5. Anovulation and polycystic ovary syndrome. Increased androgen production from either adrenal or ovarian sources leads to steady-state excess ovarian androgen production.

culating androgens (from any source). Increased androgen production leads to increased acyclic peripheral estrogen (E_1) formation. Estrogen then preferentially inhibits pituitary FSH secretion and establishes a high LH/FSH ratio that sustains acyclic nonincremental estrogen feedback on the HPO axis. LH stimulates excess secretion of androgens by the ovarian stroma cells. Excess production of androgens reduces SHBG production, and this alteration augments the biological activity of circulating androgens. Additionally, circulating androgens are more available for peripheral conversion to estrogen. Thus, elevated androgens induce an acyclic steady state of estrogen production that perpetuates chronic anovulation. Ovarian changes such as inadequate follicular maturation and increased follicular atresia are secondary events that occur from both inadequate FSH and excess LH stimulation to the follicle.

Other conditions that can mimic PCOS include congenital adrenal hyperplasia (CAH; classic and adult-onset), androgen- or estrogen-secreting tumors of the ovary and adrenal gland, hyperadrenalism of Cushing's syndrome, and thyroid dysfunction. The clinician also must consider that aging is associated with a two- to fourfold increase in extraglandular estrone formation (increased aromatase activity) and that obese women have excessive converting tissue (adipose tissue). Furthermore, the conversion of androgens to estrogens is uniquely modulated by thyroid dysfunction in that SHBG is increased in hyperthyroidism but conversely reduced in hypothyroidism.

Anovulation Due to CNS-Hypothalamic-Pituitary Dysfunction

Anovulation or amenorrhea secondary to CNS dysfunction can occur from aberrations of CNS-hypothala-

TABLE 9-4. *Dysfunction of the hypothalamic-pituitary unit*

1. Aberrations of CNS-hypothalamic interactions
   a. Pseudocyesis
   b. Anorexia nervosa
   c. Stress or nutritional anovulation
2. Defects of hypothalamic-pituitary interactions
   a. Hypothalamic lesions (reduced GnRH)
   b. Kallmann's syndrome (isolated GnRH deficiency)
   c. Sheehan's syndrome
   d. Pituitary or stalk tumors

mic function or from structural defects of the hypothalamic-pituitary axis. Factors responsible for chronic anovulation resulting from dysfunction of the hypothalamic-pituitary unit are presented in Table 9-4.

Aberrations of CNS-Hypothalamic Interaction

Emotional states influence menstrual and reproductive function in humans. Psychological influences are among the most potent and prevalent natural stimuli affecting the regulation of the reproductive system. The brain controls endocrine secretion and integrates feedback information from hormones derived from peripheral target organs. The limbic system is recognized as a crucial link between behavioral stimuli and the endocrine system. The functional state of the hypothalamus is inseparably related to the pattern of neural activity in the limbic circuit. Physical, emotional, and social stresses activate the sympathetic nervous system and stimulate pituitary release of stress hormones (prolactin, growth hormone, and adrenocorticotropic hormone, or ACTH). Central to this response is the release of corticotropin-releasing factor (CRF) from the hypothalamus. CRF stimulates ACTH and β-endorphin release by the anterior pituitary and reduces gonadotropin production. Thus, chronic activation of CRF from sustained stressful stimuli may downregulate LH and FSH secretion.

Pseudocyesis represents the classic example of willful or emotional alteration of reproductive function. This syndrome of "phantom pregnancy" has been recognized since ancient times. Women with pseudocyesis have hypersecretion of prolactin and pituitary LH. Circulating estradiol and progesterone levels are increased, and the levels of prolactin and LH are high enough to maintain luteal function and galactorrhea in affected women. It is postulated that reduced dopaminergic tone of the hypothalamic-pituitary axis is responsible for the hypersecretion of both prolactin and LH in this syndrome. Such patients show dramatic responses to GnRH and increased sensitivity to dopamine suppression.

Anorexia nervosa represents another extraordinary psychogenic reproductive disorder that affects adolescent girls. The salient features of anorexia nervosa are summarized in Table 9-5. Physical symptoms include hypothermia, hypotension, and amenorrhea. Specific hypothalamic

TABLE 9-5. *Features of anorexia nervosa*

1. Adolescent girls
2. Obsession with dieting
3. Morbid fear of losing control over body weight and body image
4. Amenorrhea
5. High achievement with intense and commonly obsessive-compulsive behavior
6. Distorted self-perception
7. Family history of sexual abuse with a domineering and/or insensitive parent

abnormalities described in this syndrome include amenorrhea, reduced frequency and amplitude of LH pulses, hypersecretion of cortisol, abnormal thermoregulation, and abnormal pituitary response to GnRH and thyrotropin-releasing hormone (TRH). Paradoxically, hypersecretion of adrenal cortisol is associated with suppression of adrenal androgen secretion.

Psychogenic amenorrhea (functional hypothalamic amenorrhea) represents the most common type of amenorrhea. In contrast to anorexia nervosa, psychogenic amenorrhea usually occurs in adult women. Affected women tend to be unmarried, engaged in intellectual occupations, report stressful life events, often consume sedatives or hypnotic drugs, practice weight control, and have a history of previous menstrual irregularities. An impairment of the hypothalamic GnRH pulse generator is the underlying cause of ovarian inactivity in women with hypothalamic amenorrhea. The frequency and amplitude of GnRH pulses are diminished and ovarian activity ceases. The function of the HPO system regresses to the prepubertal state. Under these conditions, progesterone withdrawal bleeding does not occur and treatment with clomiphene citrate for ovulation induction is usually not effective. Spontaneous reversal of hypothalamic amenorrhea following appropriate counseling or lifestyle changes provides strong evidence for the psychogenic cause of this disorder.

Exercise and menstrual dysfunction is occurring more frequently in association with the popularity of physical exercise. The type, duration, intensity of exercise, body composition, and stress factors of individual participants are confounding factors that must be considered in assessing exercise-related amenorrhea. Most women with exercise-induced amenorrhea participate in strenuous competition-type sports. The incidence of amenorrhea is higher in runners and ballet dancers than in swimmers and joggers. This difference is attributable mostly to the relatively high percentage of body fat among swimmers compared to the reduced body fat among runners and ballet dancers.

Defects of Hypothalamic–Pituitary Interactions

Hypogonadotropic hypogonadism associated with anosmia (Kallmann's syndrome) occurs more frequently in males than in females. Circulating levels of LH and FSH are undetectable or low. Puberty is delayed and physical examination typically shows eunuchoid proportions. This syndrome is often transmitted as an autosomal dominant trait but may occur sporadically. Anatomic evidence suggests that embryologic agenesis of the olfactory apparatus produces anosmia and defective neuronal control of GnRH release.

Pituitary tumors may be detectable in as many as 10% of normal patients. Most tumors are small, hormonally inactive, and cause no pituitary dysfunction. Inert tumors that affect pituitary function and hormonally active tumors compose the group of pituitary neoplasms that require medical or surgical treatment. Endocrinologically active tumors are rare. Hypersecreting pituitary adenomas secrete ACTH, growth hormone, prolactin, thyroid-stimulating hormone (TSH), FSH, LH, and β-endorphin. To confuse matters, hormonally inactive pituitary tumors are indistinguishable from their active counterparts by computed tomography (CT) or magnetic resonance imaging (MRI) studies. Most inactive tumors that compromise pituitary function are large. Such tumors produce signs and symptoms of neuropathy (visual field defects, headache) or endocrinopathy (hypopituitarism). Small inactive tumors that cause no pituitary dysfunction usually require no therapy. *Craniopharyngioma* is the most important hormonally inactive suprasellar tumor. It arises from embryologic remnants of Rathke's pouch. This neoplasm accounts for only 3% of intracranial tumors. Because it develops along the anterior surface of the infundibulum of the pituitary stalk, it commonly interferes with hypothalamic-pituitary endocrine function. Craniopharyngiomas are most common in the second decade. Important clinical features are visual impairment and delayed puberty. Dynamic pituitary testing (Chapter 13) shows some degree of hypopituitarism in almost all cases. Growth hormone and gonadotropin deficiency are invariably seen in association with this tumor. The usual endocrine presentation associated with this tumor is hypogonadotropic-hypogonadal amenorrhea.

Other neoplastic or infectious processes that produce hypothalamic hypopituitarism include germinoma, glioma, Hand–Schuller–Christian disease, midline dermoid cysts, tuberculosis, and sarcoidosis. In addition to primary neoplastic processes, metastatic diseases can affect the pituitary and produce amenorrhea. Occasionally, the *empty sella syndrome* is associated with defective hypothalamic-pituitary function. However, women with an empty sella usually show no endocrine impairment. Acquired hypopituitarism may result from surgical or radiologic ablation, or may occur as a result of infarction from a large pituitary tumor, granulomatous lesions, or hypotension in the postpartum period (Sheehan's syndrome). Panhypopituitarism is clinically expressed by amenorrhea, hair loss, fatigue, and hypotension. Hypothalamic releasing hormone challenge shows pituitary hypofunction for TRH, gonadotropins,

ACTH, and growth hormone. Prolactin deficiency is associated only with Sheehan's syndrome.

Gonadal Failure

Pathologic *gonadal failure* presents clinically in two forms: delayed or absent puberty (*gonadal dysgenesis*) or secondary amenorrhea (*premature ovarian failure*). In both instances, the defect is loss of gonadal function (Table 9-6). It is the timing of the gonadal loss that determines whether the defect is called gonadal dysgenesis or premature ovarian failure. The diagnosis of gonadal dysgenesis is suspected on a clinical basis when secondary sexual development (puberty) has not been initiated by age 13 (Chapter 6). Premature ovarian failure is defined as loss of previously established ovarian function prior to 35 years of age. Both are confirmed by an elevated FSH. The causes of gonadal dysgenesis are generally classified into *chromosomally competent* (pure gonadal dysgenesis) and *chromosomally incompetent* (gonadal dysgenesis). As such, a karyotype analysis is important for the complete evaluation of gonadal dysgenesis. Women with chromosomally incompetent causes of gonadal dysgenesis who bear a Y chromosome (or fragments) should have the ovaries removed to avoid the 25% risk of tumor development. The causes of premature ovarian failure are more complex than gonadal dysgenesis and include unknown causes, chromosomal incompetence, autoimmune endocrinopathy, galactosemia, chemotherapy, irradiation, or previous surgery.

Mullerian and Outflow Tract Defects

Mullerian or *congenital uterine anomalies* represent a unique cause of primary amenorrhea in young women with otherwise normal secondary development. The absence of menarche by age 16 or cyclic abdominal pain in sexually maturing girls indicates the need for evaluation and the high probability of obstructive uterine defects. It is important to recognize that some defects are associated with incomplete outflow (Chapter 19).

TABLE 9-6. *Causes of gonadal failure[a]*

Gonadal dysgenesis (failed puberty)	Premature ovarian failure (ovarian failure <35 yo)
Abnormal chromosome	Abnormal chromosome
Normal chromosome	Autoimmune
	Galactosemia
	Chemotherapy
	Radiation
	Surgery
	Environment (dioxin)

[a]Rule out presence of Y component in gonadal dysgenesis or in premature ovarian failure.

The classic defect associated with amenorrhea and normal secondary sexual development is congenital Mullerian aplasia (Mayer–Rokitansky–Küster–Hauser syndrome). In this syndrome, the uterus is absent and the vagina is fused or forms only a short pouch. Ovarian development is normal. This syndrome can be confused with complete androgen resistance syndrome (Chapter 5) and transverse vaginal septum (Chapter 19). Imperforate hymen produces a syndrome of amenorrhea, normal secondary development, and cyclic pain. Occasionally, an abdominopelvic mass is palpable (hematometra). Other acquired causes include surgically induced intrauterine synechia (Asherman's syndrome), cervical stenosis, and obstructing tumors.

DIAGNOSIS

Figure 9-6 illustrates the basic algorithm for the diagnostic evaluation of women with anovulation/amenorrhea. All algorithms proposed for the evaluation of anovulatory women consider the same elements, but there is variability in the sequence of some tests. The purpose of the basic algorithm is to determine the func-

BASIC DIAGNOSTIC ALGORITHM FOR AMENHORRHEA

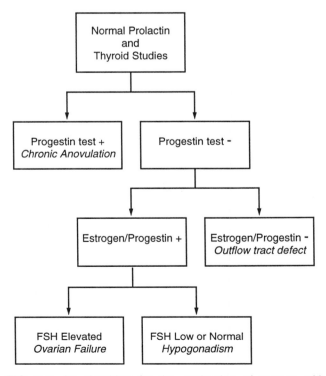

FIG. 9-6. An algorithm for the evaluation of women with amenorrhea. Progestin test = progestin withdrawal, estrogen/progestin P test = estrogen-stimulated progestin withdrawal, FSH = follicle- stimulating hormone.

tional "compartment" responsible for amenorrhea. Supplemental algorithms will further evaluate women with hyperprolactinemia, hypogonadotropic hypogonadism, ovarian failure, or uterine defect. Because the most common cause of secondary amenorrhea is pregnancy, it is important to make this diagnosis prior to any further evaluation. Currently, both serum and urine kit assays employ highly sensitive methods for the detection of low amounts of human chorionic gonadotropin (hCG) (10–25 mIU/ml). The cost of the pregnancy test is low in comparison with other hormonal assessments. In our program, all patients with a negative pregnancy test who fulfill the criteria of amenorrhea are evaluated by measuring serum prolactin, TSH, and gonadotropins (FSH, LH). Additionally, a progestin withdrawal test (P test) is initiated at that visit. These tests in the initial evaluation avoid ambiguous results induced by subsequent treatments and reduce the time required to establish a discriminate diagnosis.

INTERPRETATION OF THE AMENORRHEA EVALUATION

Prolactin

The purpose of the prolactin measurement is to exclude hyperprolactinemia as a cause of amenorrhea. Hyperprolactinemia in the anovulation/amenorrhea syndrome is a common occurrence that affects 35% of women. Its detection is significant since approximately 40% of patients with hyperprolactinemia have a pituitary adenoma. Treatment of anovulation/amenorrhea in women with hyperprolactinemia usually requires unique drugs (bromocriptine) or surgery (Chapter 10).

Thyroid Function

Thyroid dysfunction as a cause of anovulation/amenorrhea occurs in approximately 2–5% of patients. The most common thyroid dysfunction presenting with anovulation/amenorrhea is hypothyroidism. Hyperthyroidism typically produces menstrual dysfunction, such as hypermenorrhea or polymenorrhea, but anovulation is uncommon. An elevated TSH with a normal or subnormal T_4 indicates primary hypothyroidism and a low T_4 with a normal or low TSH supports secondary or tertiary hypothyroidism. An elevated T_4 associated with a normal TSH suggests hyperthyroidism.

Progestin Withdrawal

The progestin withdrawal test determines the estrogen status of the patient and establishes evidence of a normally functioning outflow tract. The test is positive (the patient is "estrogenized") if uterine bleeding occurs after discontinuation of the medication. Bleeding usually occurs 2–4 days after cessation of progestin. Occasionally, the progestin is administered concomitantly with the LH surge (or initiates the LH surge) and bleeding is delayed several days beyond the expected time of bleeding. Spotting is a positive test, but this alone should not be interpreted as a reassuring sign that no other endocrine dysfunction is present.

Gonadotropins

Gonadotropin measurements establish the functional capacity of the ovary. Ovarian failure is diagnosed when FSH is menopausal. Elevated LH can occur at the midcycle surge or can be seen in PCOS. However, FSH greater than menopausal levels is never demonstrated in these conditions.

Estrogen-Stimulated Progestin Withdrawal

This test determines the presence of a responsive endometrium in combination with a competent outflow tract. It is performed after a negative progestin withdrawal. We use 2.5 mg of conjugated estrogens for 25 days with medroxyprogesterone (10 mg) on days 16–25. Menstrual flow confirms the presence of both a hormonally responsive endometrium and an outflow tract. The failure of withdrawal after this test suggests an unresponsive or absent endometrium (Asherman's syndrome or hysterectomy), an obstructed outflow tract (Mullerian defects or cervical/vaginal lesions), or pregnancy (remember to test for pregnancy prior to drug administration).

DANGER ZONES

Structural lesions of the CNS represent the most serious conditions that produce amenorrhea. Tumors that affect endocrine function and produce amenorrhea are typically detected in one of two conditions. Recognition of these presentations will avoid erroneous diagnosis in women with tumors and eliminate unnecessary and expensive tests in unaffected women.

Modest Hyperprolactinemia

Modest hyperprolactinemia (<100 ng/ml) can occur when the dopaminergic tone of the pituitary is affected by structural lesions. As such, imaging studies of the cranium should be obtained when modest hyperprolactinemia (25–100 ng/ml) cannot be explained by drug use. Detected tumors usually do not secrete prolactin. They induce prolactin elevations by exerting structural inhibitory effects on the dopaminergic innervation of the pituitary (Chapter 10).

HYPOGONADOTROPIC HYPOGONADISM

Like modest hyperprolactinemia, hypogonadotropic hypogonadism can be induced by neoplasms of the hypothalamus, pituitary, or connecting stalk. Imaging studies of the pituitary should be obtained in women with this condition to exclude tumors. Although tumors are rare (<3% of cases with amenorrhea), craniopharyngioma is probably the most common lesion that produces amenorrhea with hypogonadotropic hypogonadism. It is insufficient to assume a diagnosis (in this case weight- or exercise-induced amenorrhea) prior to the exclusion of rare but serious structural lesions of the CNS.

SUMMARY

In this chapter, we reviewed the four major causes of the anovulation/amenorrhea syndromes (chronic anovulation, hypothalamic-pituitary disturbances, gonadal failure, and outflow tract defects). The basic diagnostic algorithm allows the physician to classify each patient affected with amenorrhea into an appropriate diagnostic category. Once properly classified, further testing may be required to determine the ultimate cause of amenorrhea. Special consideration should be provided to women with modest hyperprolactinemia or hypogonadotropic hypogonadism. Here the risk of serious CNS tumors is the greatest and should be excluded by imaging studies. Also, special consideration should be provided to women with hypergonadotropic hypogonadism. These women are at increased risk of having a Y chromosome and the development of a germ cell tumor. They are also at greater risk of short stature (Chapter 6).

SELECTED READING

Aron DC, Tyrrell JB, Wilson CB. Pituitary tumors. Current concepts in diagnosis and management. *West J Med* 1995;162:340–52.

Axelrod J, Reisine TD. Stress hormones: their interaction and regulation. *Science* 1984;224:452–459.

Bonen A. Exercise-induced menstrual cycle changes. A functional, temporary adaptation to metabolic stress. *Sports Med* 1994;17:353–357.

Brill AI. What is the role of hysteroscopy in the management of abnormal uterine bleeding? *Clin Obstet Gynecol* 1995;38:319–345.

Crosignani PG, Ferrari C, Malinverni A, Barbieri C, Mattei AM, Caldara R, Rocchetti M. Effect of central nervous system dopaminergic activation on prolactin secretion in man: evidence for a common central defect in hyperprolactinemic patients with and without radiological signs of pituitary tumors. *J Clin Endocrinol Metab* 1980;51:1068–1073.

Cumming DC, Rebar RW. Exercise and reproductive function in women. *Am J Ind Med* 1983;4:113–125.

Fraser IS. Vaginal bleeding patterns in women using once-a-month injectable contraceptives. *Contraception* 1994;49:399–420.

Goldzieher JW, Green JA. The polycystic ovary. I. Clinical and histologic features. *J Clin Endocrinol Metab* 1962;22:325–338.

Hergenroeder AC. Bone mineralization, hypothalamic amenorrhea, and sex steroid therapy in female adolescents and young adults. *J Pediatrics* 1995;126:683–689.

Hertweck SP. Anorexia nervosa: issues for the obstetrician and gynecologist. *Curr Opin Obstet Gynecol* 1995;7:371–374.

Jenkins JS, Gilbert J, Ang V. Hypothalamic-pituitary function in patients with cranio-pharyngiomas. *J Clin Endocrinol Metab* 1976; 43:394–399.

Kirschner MA, Zucker IR, Jesperson DL. Ovarian and adrenal vein catheterization studies in women with idiopathic hirsutism. In: James VHT, Serio M, Guisti G, eds. *The Endocrine Function of the Ovary.* New York: Academic Press, 1976;443–456.

Kleinberg DL, Noel GL, Frantz AG. Galactorrhea: a study of 235 cases, including 48 with pituitary tumor. *N Engl J Med* 1977;296:589–600.

Lieblich JM, Rogol AD, White BJ, Rosen SW. Syndrome of anosmia with hypogonadotropic hypogonadism. *Am J Med* 1982;73:506–519.

Rebar R, Judd HL, Yen SSC. Characterization of the inappropriate gonadotropin secretion in polycystic ovary syndrome. *J Clin Invest* 1976; 57:1320–1329.

Rosenfield RL, Moll GW Jr. The role of proteins in the distribution of plasma androgens and estradiol. In: Molinatti CG, Martini L, James BHT, eds. *Androgenization in Women.* New York: Raven Press, 1983; 25–45.

Rosenfeld JA. Update on continuous estrogen-progestin replacement therapy. *Am Fam Phys* 1994;50:1519–1523, 1527–1528.

Seifer DB, Collins RL. Current concepts of beta-endorphin physiology in female reproductive dysfunction. *Fertil Steril* 1990;54:757–771.

Yen SSC. Chronic anovulation caused by peripheral endocrine disorders. In: Yen SSC, Jaffe RB, eds. *Reproductive Endocrinology: Physiology, Pathophysiology, and Clinical Management.* Philadelphia: WB Saunders, 1986;441–449.

Yen SS. Female hypogonadotropic hypogonadism. Hypothalamic amenorrhea syndrome. *Endocrinol Metab Clin North Am* 1993;22:29–58.

Clinical Reproductive Medicine,
Edited by Bryan D. Cowan and David B. Seifer
Lippincott-Raven Publishers, Philadelphia © 1997

CHAPTER 10

Hyperprolactinemia

Vivian Lewis

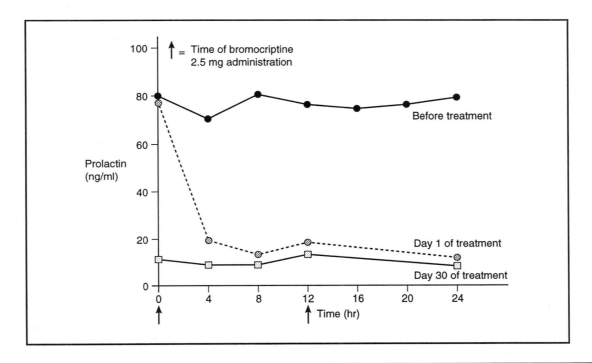

Normal Prolactin Secretion
Pathologic Causes of Hyperprolactinemia
Physiologic Causes of Hyperprolactinemia
Clinical Presentation
Imaging Studies of the Pituitary

Therapy
Surgery
Pregnancy
Selected Reading

V. Lewis: Division of Reproductive Endocrinology, Department of Obstetrics and Gynecology, University of Rochester Medical Center, Strong Memorial Hospital, Rochester NY 14642

In this chapter we will review the normal physiology of prolactin secretion and causes of abnormal secretion. Treatment modalities and guidelines for their use will also be discussed in depth.

NORMAL PROLACTIN SECRETION

Prolactin is secreted in a pulsatile fashion, approximately every 90 minutes. In addition, there are circadian patterns detectable in both men and women. Peak levels are seen between 3 a.m. and 5 a.m., and a modest increase is detectable in the afternoon (Fig. 10-1). Interestingly, these changes are also seen in lactating women.

The structure of prolactin is subject to significant variability. The majority of circulating hormone is monomeric, so-called small prolactin, which is considered the biologically active form. Dimeric ("big") and polymeric ("big-big") forms constitute 10–25% of circulating hormone. These forms usually have less affinity for the prolactin receptor and less biological activity. All are detected in immunoassay systems and contribute to the total mass of the hormone that is measured (Fig. 10-2). Normal monomeric prolactin has a half-life of 20 minutes and is present unbound to serum proteins. In contrast, polymeric prolactin is slowly cleared from the circulation.

There are certain patients with hyperprolactinemia consisting of disproportionate amounts of dimeric and polymeric forms. Because of the low bioactivity of these

forms, they are able to maintain normal reproductive function. While it is important to recognize that different forms of prolactin can exist, the need to identify such variants in clinical practice is rare. For example, women with pituitary adenomas sometimes secrete large quantities of polymeric prolactin during pregnancy. This form of prolactin is cleared very slowly from the circulation.

Control of prolactin secretion is principally tonic inhibition caused by dopamine. The neurons of the arcuate and ventromedial nuclei release dopamine into the portal circulation of the hypothalamus. These vessels supply the anterior pituitary and result in hypothalamic regulation of prolactin secretion. A proposed regulatory substance, gonadotropin-associated protein (GAP), could work in the same manner. GAP is a small peptide, encoded by the DNA sequence adjacent to sequence encoding gonadotropin-releasing hormone. Most of the evidence suggesting that this substance is a physiologic regulator comes from other species, although GAP has been isolated from human hypothalamic extracts. Injection of GAP into rats rapidly lowers prolactin levels. Administration of anti-GAP antisera to rabbits increases prolactin levels. The role of GAP in humans is uncertain (Table 10-1).

The physiologic need for other prolactin stimulators is poorly understood. Sleep, pregnancy, and stress cause prolactin release as does food (especially a tryptophan-rich meal). A variety of hormones can stimulate prolactin release. Thyrotropin-releasing hormone (TRH) increases prolactin release and this explains the association of primary hypothyroidism and galactorrhea. A variety of peptides can stimulate prolactin release. Vasoactive intestinal peptide (VIP) is synthesized in the hypothalamus as well as the anterior pituitary. It may in part mediate the prolactin response to suckling and stress and may also act as a autocrine regulator of prolactin release. The significance of the prolactin stimulatory properties of some peptides, such as opioid peptides, cholecystokinin, and the posterior pituitary hormones oxytocin and vasopressin, is unknown.

In addition to the anterior pituitary, another organ capable of prolactin production is the uterus. Explants of normal decidualized human endometrium and myometrium produce prolactin in vitro. Neither bromocriptine nor dopamine affects this synthesis. Placenta and amniotic membranes have similar capabilities, all of which are thought to play a role in electrolyte balance for the fetus.

PATHOLOGIC CAUSES OF HYPERPROLACTINEMIA

Since the primary regulation of prolactin secretion occurs via the inhibitory influence of dopamine, any mechanism that lowers pituitary dopamine will result in increased prolactin secretion. Tumors that compromise

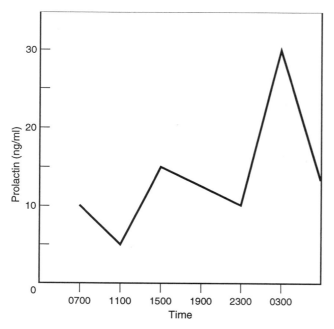

FIG. 10-1. Circadian pattern of prolactin secretion. Mean prolactin levels measured hourly in a group of normally menstruating women. (Modified from Kletsky and Davajan; see "Selected Reading.")

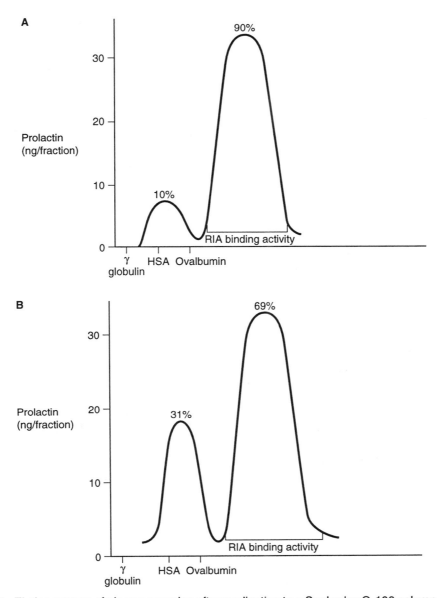

FIG. 10-2. Elution pattern of plasma samples after application to a Sephadex G-100 column. **A:** Plasma from a normal, non-pregnant woman. **B:** Plasma from a pregnant woman. Note that the preponderance of binding activity is seen in the fraction corresponding to "little" prolactin, with a MW of 21,000. A second peak is seen between the markers for ovalbumin and HSA corresponding to a MW of about 56,000. (Modified from Noel, Suh and Frantz; see "Selected Reading.")

portal circulation, or destructive lesions of the hypothalamus or pituitary, can result in diminished dopamine concentration in the anterior pituitary (Table 10-2).

Chromophobe adenomas are the most common pituitary tumor. They are found in 10–25% of the population in autopsy series. They are more common in women than men and are often asymptomatic. The common terminology *chromophobe adenoma* is based on the histologic staining properties of the lactotroph cells. Larger tumors are likely to secrete greater amounts of prolactin. Growth hormone secreting tumors also secrete prolactin in about 40% of

cases. By contrast, prolactin secretion is only rarely seen in adrenocorticotropic hormone (ACTH)-secreting tumors. Ectopic prolactin production has been reported as a feature of ovarian teratomas, a gonadoblastoma, and a renal cell carcinoma. However, such cases are rare.

Empty sella syndrome can mimic a pituitary tumor. It is caused by a congenital weakness in the sella diaphragm that enables cerebrospinal fluid to extend into the pituitary fossa. The increased pressure can interrupt normal portal blood flow, effectively lowering the concentration of dopamine in the anterior pituitary. A similar mecha-

TABLE 10-1. *Physiologic regulators of prolactin*

Stimulation	Inhibition
TRH	Dopamine
Serotonin	Acetylcholine
Estrogens	GAP
Progesterone	
Histamine	
Opioid peptides	
GnRH	
VIP	
Oxytocin	
Angiotensin II	
Exercise	
Pregnancy	
Food	
Stress	
Sexual intercourse	

TRH, thyrotropin-releasing hormone; GAP, gonadotropin-associated protein; VIP, vasoactive intestinal peptide.

nism of action is operative in infiltrative lesions. Diseases such as sarcoidosis, Hand–Schuller–Christian disease, and granulomatous diseases can also create a mass effect resulting in hyperprolactinemia. Nonsecreting pituitary adenomas, including craniopharyngiomas, sometimes cause mild hyperprolactinemia by compression of dopamine-rich blood supply or interruption of local autocrine control of prolactin secretion.

A variety of pharmacologic agents cause hyperprolactinemia. The antipsychotic drugs are notorious in this respect and exert their effect by binding to the dopamine receptor. Certain antihypertensives, such as clonidine, reserpine, and the ACE inhibitors, can increase prolactin by acting as false neurotransmitters, thereby interfering with dopamine action. Antihistamines work by interfering with the inhibitory effect of histamine on prolactin secretion. By contrast, certain antidepressants facilitate the stimulatory action of serotonin on prolactin release. The calcium channel blockers increase prolactin by an unknown mechanism. Illicit drugs can act by stimulating β-endorphins (heroin) or interfering with dopamine metabolism (cocaine).

Altered metabolism of prolactin is responsible for hyperprolactinemia in a variety of states. Hepatic failure is

TABLE 10-2. *Pathologic causes of hyperprolactinemia*

Pituitary tumors (adenomas, craniopharyngiomas)
Empty sella syndrome
Hypothalamic disorders (neoplasms, vascular disruption)
Ectopic production of prolactin (bronchogenic cancer, hypernephroma)
Pituitary or hypothalamic infiltrative disorders (e.g., sarcoidosis, granulomas)
Primary hypothyroidism
Illicit drug use
Renal failure
Hepatic failure
Chest wall lesions

commonly associated with hyperprolactinemia. This may be due to changes in the clearance of both estrogens and prolactin itself. Renal failure is also commonly associated with hyperprolactinemia. Renal transplant or dialysis are usually corrective. Hypothyroidism causes increased prolactin by decreased clearance of prolactin as well as stimulation of secretion by TRH.

Chest wall lesions can occasionally cause galactorrhea or hyperprolactinemia. Patients with herpes zoster, spinal cord disease, chest wall trauma, or surgery are included in this group. Mechanisms are poorly understood but probably involve the afferent loop that is important in lactation.

Idiopathic or functional hyperprolactinemia is a diagnosis of exclusion. Some investigators believe that these patients have microadenomas below the limits of radiographic detection. Others suggest that these patients have a functional disturbance in portal blood flow or dopamine metabolism. There is probably more than one etiology.

PHYSIOLOGIC CAUSES OF HYPERPROLACTINEMIA

Prolactin is necessary for the establishment and maintenance of lactation. Prolactin, along with insulin, estrogen, and insulin-like growth factor, prepares the breast for lactation by stimulating the proliferation of its ducts and stroma. Prolactin specifically stimulates secretion by the alveolar cells. Despite this, pregnant women do not normally lactate because high estrogen levels block lactation. After delivery, estrogen levels drop and lactation begins. Oxytocin, which allows for milk letdown by contraction of the myoepithelial cells, is released in anticipation of nursing the infant. This reflex can be triggered by hearing the infant cry. However, prolactin levels are increased only by the actual nipple stimulation of suckling. Baseline prolactin levels remain elevated and increase further within about 10 minutes of nursing. Maximum levels are attained within 10–30 minutes and levels decline by 30 minutes to 2 hours later (Fig. 10-3). In time, prolactin bursts lessen in magnitude and baseline prolactin levels gradually normalize. The speed of normalization depends largely on the frequency of lactation. In women who do not breast-feed, prolactin levels are usually normal by the end of 1–2 weeks postpartum.

Breast stimulation is another common reason for transient prolactin elevation in nonpregnant women. Sexual intercourse even without nipple stimulation increases prolactin in some women.

There is a diurnal variation in prolactin secretion. The highest levels are seen during the early morning hours (3–5 a.m.) and more modest increases are seen in the early afternoon hours. Sleep itself induces prolactin release as well.

Food, as well as hypoglycemia, can induce prolactin elevation. Because of the known prolactin-stimulating ac-

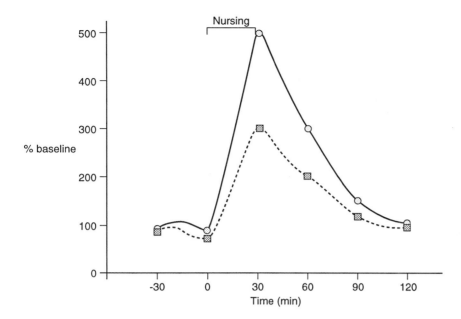

FIG. 10-3. Circulating prolactin levels in nursing women. Circles are levels in women who were 8–40 days postpartum. X represents levels in women who were 60–190 days partum. Values are expressed as a percent of baseline, the prolactin level at the time nursing began. (Data are modified from Noel et al.; see "Selected Reading.")

tivity of serotonin, foods that are rich in tryptophan are particularly apt to have this effect. Hypoglycemia causes a number of stress-related substances to be released, including prolactin.

Finally, prolactin can vary with the menstrual cycle. Both estrogen and progesterone can stimulate prolactin release. Accordingly, the periovulatory rise in estrogen and the luteal phase are both associated with increased prolactin levels.

CLINICAL PRESENTATION

The classic patient with pathologic hyperprolactinemia presents with galactorrhea and amenorrhea. Galactorrhea is the presence of a clear or white nipple discharge that occurs spontaneously or after nipple stimulation. The amount of discharge is irrelevant. Menstrual disturbances are very common in affected patients and range from luteal phase defect to amenorrhea. The higher the prolactin, the more severe the disturbance. Patients with amenorrhea and hyperprolactinemia usually have low estrogen levels, but vasomotor symptoms are not common. Hypoestrogenism can be confirmed with a negative response to progestin challenge.

Sexual dysfunction is usually not a presenting complaint, but if a careful history is taken, this symptom can frequently be elicited. Men commonly have erectile dysfunction. Loss of libido is frequently seen in both sexes. It is not clear as to whether this is a direct effect of prolactin or is caused indirectly by hypogonadism. Unfortunately, correction of hyperprolactinemia in men usually does not correct erectile dysfunction.

Certain symptoms and conditions are related to the presence of a large tumor. Macroadenomas may cause headaches, visual changes, and even seizures (neuropathy). There is no characteristic pattern to the headaches. The classic visual problem is bitemporal hemianopsia; however, diplopia and decreased visual acuity can also be seen. Seizures have been reported in cases where large tumors have invaded the medial temporal lobe. Additionally, some patients with macroadenoma have evidence of pituitary insufficiency (endocrinopathy). Dynamic testing for pituitary reserve is appropriate in these affected women.

A complete history and physical examination can target the work-up so that other conditions can be investigated as needed. Nipple discharge can be examined on a cover-slipped microscope slide. Fat globules can be seen without staining under low-power (40×) light microscopy. Laboratory studies in all patients with galactorrhea without a known cause (i.e., medication or chest wall lesion) should include a prolactin measurement obtained preferably between the hours of 9 a.m. and 11 a.m. and a TSH level (Table 10-3). If the patient has fairly regular menses, the level should be obtained in the early follicular phase of the cycle. Other laboratory stud-

TABLE 10-3. *Laboratory evaluation 11 a.m. prolactin*

Thyroid-stimulating hormone
FSH and LH—selected patients
Androgens—selected patients
Insulin tolerance test—macroadenomas

FSH, follicle-stimulating hormone; LH, luteinizing hormone.

ies that may be helpful include gonadotropin and androgen levels. These should be recommended based on specific findings in the history (amenorrhea) or physical exam (hirsutism).

Provocative tests of prolactin secretion were useful before the current era of improved pituitary imaging techniques and medical therapy. With modern imaging techniques, tumors can be identified with great accuracy and prolactin provocation tests are rarely preformed.

IMAGING STUDIES OF THE PITUITARY

It is indeed a challenge to choose which patients require imaging studies and which studies to recommend for a given patient. In making these choices, it is important to keep in mind the patient's symptoms and prolactin level. The contemporary options include coned down view of the sella, CT scan, and MRI (Table 10-4).

Coned down view of the sella is a screening test for a large pituitary/hypothalamic structural lesion that has been advocated for patients who are at low risk for macroadenoma. For example, women with modestly elevated prolactin levels (below about 60 ng/ml) and no other symptoms of endocrinopathy or neuropathy can be screened in this way.

High-detail coronal CT scan of the pituitary can detect adenomas as small as 3–5 mm. Tumors usually appear as hypodense areas and sometimes displace the infundibulum or increase the overall height of the gland. Erosion of the sellar floor is often associated with tumors and is clearly visualized. Injection of contrast material has been used to enhance the image. The images obtained may be limited in a patient with many dental fillings or with arthritis limiting the ability to hyperextend the neck.

MRI gives a more three-dimensional view and can detect tumors at least as small as the CT scan but is more sensitive in its ability to detect soft tissue lesions. If contrast material is injected, MRI is probably better able to detect optic chiasm compression, cavernous sinus compromise, and an empty sella. Both of these techniques are considerably more expensive than plain X-rays. It is therefore desirable to limit their use. Either of these high-resolution imaging studies should be used in patients where a detailed study of the pituitary is desired, such as women with significant elevations of prolactin.

TABLE 10-4. *Imaging options in patients with hyperprolactinemia*

Plain X-rays
CT scan
MRI

THERAPY

Symptomatic hyperprolactinemia or troublesome galactorrhea are common reasons for treatment. Practitioners must choose between medical therapy and, if an adenoma is present, surgery or radiation. Medical therapy is the current treatment of choice. There is also a role for observation in selected patients.

Bromocriptine is the most commonly used drug for hyperprolactinemia in the United States. It belongs to the class of drugs known as ergot alkaloids. Bromocriptine is approved by the Food and Drug Administration for hyperprolactinemia, pituitary adenoma, Parkinson's disease, and most forms of galactorrhea.

Bromocriptine acts directly on the anterior pituitary as a dopamine agonist to lower serum prolactin. In patients with tumors, bromocriptine acts directly on the lactotroph. It lowers rates of DNA proliferation and may even produce cellular necrosis within the tumor.

Bromocriptine has a fairly short half-life, about $3\frac{1}{2}$ hours. This necessitates more than once-a-day dosing; usually twice daily is sufficient. After a single dose, peak plasma levels are attained in 2–3 hours and remain detectable for 8–12 hours. The drug is metabolized in the liver and largely excreted in the feces.

Prolactin levels usually respond within hours of drug administration (Fig. 10-4). Thus, there is no reason to delay monitoring of prolactin levels. In some patients with tumors, high resolution studies document shrinkage within 4–6 weeks. However, other patients require several months to achieve tumor shrinkage. In either case, it is sufficient to follow prolactin levels and titrate medication dosage accordingly. Resumption of ovulatory cycles is likely as the prolactin normalizes. This should be monitored so that the drug can be discontinued in the event of pregnancy. Additional ovulation induction agents can be used concurrently if bromocriptine alone is not successful.

Side effects are commonly seen, occurring in up to 70% of patients. Gastrointestinal problems such as nausea, vomiting, cramping, and constipation are frequent. Central nervous system effects include dizziness, syncope, headache, nightmares, and, in rare cases, hallucinations and seizures. Gradual increases in the dose and prandial administration tend to minimize the occurrence of side effects.

There are two alternative routes of bromocriptine administration. A depot parenteral preparation of bromocriptine has been developed that would allow for monthly injections. Clinical efficacy and side effect frequency are similar to oral bromocriptine. However, this preparation should work well for patients who require long-term therapy, such as those with macroadenomas. Vaginal administration of bromocriptine is highly effective with a lower incidence of side effects. Absorption is excellent. A longer half-life is observed, which often allows for use of a lower dose of medication.

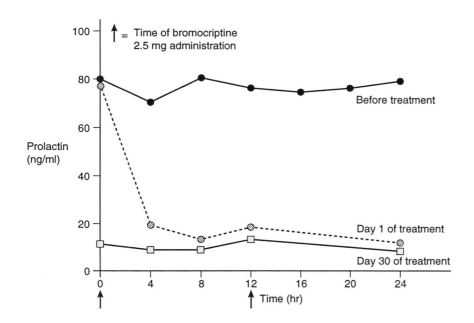

FIG. 10-4. Pharmacokinetics of prolactin secretion after bromocriptine administration. Hyperprolactinemic patients were studied before treatment *(black circles)*, on the first day of treatment *(lighter circles)*, and after 1 month of treatment *(boxes)*. The arrows on the x axis show the times of bromocriptine administration. (Modified from Moro et al.; see "Selected Reading.")

Other ergot alkaloids have been used to treat hyperprolactinemia (Table 10-2). Only pergolide is available in the United States. Side effects from pergolide are similar to bromocriptine. However, pergolide has the advantage of once daily administration. Pergolide has similar efficacy to bromocriptine, though there are few controlled trials.

Quinagolide (CV205-502) is a new, nonergot dopamine agonist. It appears to have equal efficacy with bromocriptine with fewer side effects. While it is not yet clinically available, its improved tolerability suggests promise.

SURGERY

Transsphenoidal resection of pituitary adenomas was a popular therapy because of the rapid rate of improvement. However, the high efficacy of medication coupled with poor permanent cure after surgery has reduced its popularity. Cure rates and morbidity rates are closely related to tumor size and skill of the surgeon (Fig. 10-5).

Therapeutic success after resection of microadenomas is much greater than after macroadenomas. Initial normalization of prolactin occurs in about 70% of cases. Morbidity and mortality rates are quite low, about 0.2–0.4%, in most series. Transient diabetes insipidus and CSF rhinorrhea are common. Long-term follow-up shows that about half of these patients have a recurrence of symptoms within 5 years.

Macroadenomas are a greater therapeutic challenge. Initial normalization occurs in only 20–50% of cases. Recurrence rates may be as high as 90%. Morbidity and mortality rates remain low, at 6% and 0.9%, respectively. However, the nature of complications is more often serious. Pituitary function, which is often compromised pre-operatively in these patients, frequently worsens after surgery.

Radiation is usually reserved for patients who are refractory to medical and surgical therapy. The published literature shows a cure rate of only 10% in such uncom-

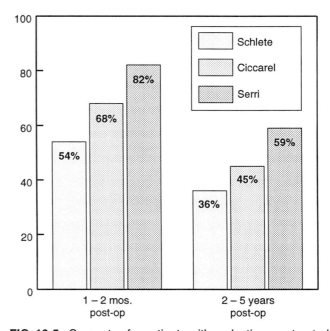

FIG. 10-5. Cure rates for patients with prolactinomas treated surgically. For each series, prolactin levels were obtained in the first 4–8 weeks after surgery and again 2–5 years after surgery. Most of the patients had microadenomas. A small number of patients with macroadenomas are included in each series. Because their numbers were so few, they are combined with data from patients with smaller tumors.

mon patients, if used as a postoperative therapy. Of patients treated with a combination of radiation and bromocriptine, about 30% are cured. Because of the poor response rate and the potential for postirradiation hypopituitarism, this therapy is not widely used.

There is also a role for "therapeutic abstinence" in selected patients. Long-term data indicate that most patients with idiopathic hyperprolactinemia or microadenomas need not be treated if the patient is asymptomatic. Risk of growth of a microadenoma is probably only about 5% and is usually accompanied by increases in prolactin or the development of symptoms. The only long-term health risk to hyperprolactinemia-induced amenorrhea is osteoporosis. Hormone replacement therapy or low-dose oral contraceptives can be given safely to affected patients.

PREGNANCY

Hyperprolactinemic patients who conceive generally do well despite the fact that pregnancy is a physiologic stimulus to lactotroph hyperplasia. Symptomatic pituitary enlargement occurs in only about 5% of cases. However, patients with untreated macroadenomas develop significant enlargement in 15–35% of cases. Bromocriptine has been used successfully in this setting.

Monitoring of most hyperprolactinemic patients who become pregnant is clinical. The variability of prolactin levels and the physiologic stimulus of high estrogen levels make this measurement useless. Patients should be questioned about headaches, visual changes, or other symptoms of pituitary enlargement. Visual field studies should be performed in symptomatic patients.

If extrasellar growth is documented, the patient should be treated with bromocriptine. Over 300 children have received this medication while in utero. No increased birth defects or ill effects have been documented. Transsphenoidal surgery is reserved for patients who remain resistant to medication.

SELECTED READING

Control of Normal Prolactin Secretion

Ben-Jonathan N. Dopamine: a prolactin inhibiting hormone. *Endocr Rev* 1985;6:564–589.

Hattori N. The frequency of macroprolactinemia in pregnant women and the hyeterogeneity of its etiologies. *J Clin Endocrinol Metab* 1996;81: 586–690.

Jones EE. Hyperprolactinemia and female infertility. *J Reprod Med* 1989; 34:117–126.

Katz E, Adashi EY. Hyperprolactinemic disorders. *Clin Obstet Gynecol* 1990;33:622–639.

Noel GL, Suh HK, Frantz AG. Prolactin release during nursing and breast stimulation in postpartum subjects. *J Clin Endocrinol Metab* 1974;38: 413.

Pathologic Causes of Hyperprolactinemia

Kletzky OA, Davajan V. Hyperprolactinemia: diagnosis and treatment. In: Mishell DR, Davajan V, Lobo RA, eds. *Infertility, Contraception and Reproductive Endocrinology*, 3rd ed. Boston: Blackwell Scientific, 1991; 356–357.

Molitch ME. Pathologic hyperprolactinemia. *Endocrinol Metab Clin North Am* 1992;21:877–901.

Yen SSC. Prolactin in human reproduction. In: Yen SSC, Jaffe RB, eds. *Reproductive Endocrinology*. 3rd ed. Philadelphia: WB Saunders, 1991; 357–388.

Clinical Management of Hyperprolactinemia

Corenblum B, Donovan L. The safety of physiological estrogen plus progestin replacement therapy and oral contraceptive therapy in women with pathological hyperprolactinemia. *Fertil Steril* 1993;59:671–673.

Kupersmith MJ, Rosenberg C, Kleinberg D. Visual loss in pregnant women with pituitary adenomas. *Ann Intern Med* 1994;121:473–477.

Lewis V, Parsons AK. Bromocriptine and related compounds for ovulation induction in hyperprolactinemia. In: Collins RL, ed. *Ovulation Induction.* New York: Springer-Verlag, 1991;124–144.

Schlechte J, Dolan K, Sherman B, Chapler F, Luciano A. The natural history of untreated hyperprolactinemia: a prospective analysis. *J Clin Endocrinol Metab* 1989;68:412–418.

Pituitary Imaging

Elster AD. Imaging of the sella: anatomy and pathology. *Semin Ultrasound, CT MRI* 1993;14:182–194.

Johnson MR, Hoare RD, Cox T, Dawson JM, Maccabe JJ, Huw Llewelyn DE, McGregor AM. The evaluation of patients with a suspected pituitary microadenoma: computer tomography compared to magnetic resonance imaging. *Clin Endocrinol* 1992;36:335–338.

Rasmussen C, Larsson SG, Bergh T. Long term follow-up of the sella trucica in hyperprolactinemic women. *Aust NZ J Obstet Gynaecol* 1990;30: 257–264.

Medical Therapy of Hyperprolactinemia

Ferrai C, Crosignani PG. Medical treatment of hyperprolactinemic disorders. *Hum Reprod* 1986;1:507–514.

Molitch ME, Elton RL, Blackwell RE, Caldwell B, Chang RJ, Jaffe R, Joplin G, Robbins RJ, Tyson J, Thorner MO. Bromocriptine as primary therapy for prolactin secreting macroadenomas: results of a prospective multicenter study. *J Clin Endocrinol Metab* 1985;60:698–705.

Moro M, Maraschini C, Toja P, Masala A, Alagna S, Rovasio PP, Ginanni A, Lancranjan I. Comparison between a slow-release oral preparation of bromocriptine and regular bromocriptine in patients with hyperprolactinemia: a double blind, double dummy study. *Horm Res* 1991;35: 137–141.

Philosophe R, Seibel MM. Novel approaches to the management of hyperprolactinemia. *Curr Opin Obstet Gynecol* 1991;3:336–342.

Vance ML, Evans WS, Thorner MO. Bromocriptine. *Ann Intern Med* 1984; 100:78–91.

Surgical Therapy of Prolactinomas

Ciccarelli E, Ghigo E, Miola C, Gandini G, Muller EE, Camanni F. Long-term follow-up of "cured" prolactinoma patients after successful adenomectomy. *Clin Endocrinol* 1990;32:583–592.

Schlechte JA, Sherman BM, Chapler FK, Van Gilder J. Long term follow-up of women with surgically treated prolactin-secreting pituitary tumors. *J Clin Endocrinol Metab* 1986;62:1296–1301.

Serri O, Rasio E, Beauregard H, Hardy J, Somma M. Recurrence of hyperprolactinemia after selective transphenoidal adenomectomy in women with prolactinoma. *N Engl J Med* 1983;309:280–283.

Pregnancy and Hyperprolactinemia

Gemzell C, Wang CF. Outcome of pregnancy in women with pituitary adenoma. *Fertil Steril* 1979;31:363–372.

Molitch ME. Pregnancy and the hyperprolactinemic woman. *N Engl J Med* 1985;312:1364–1370.

Prager D, Braunstein GD. Pituitary disorders during pregnancy. *Endocrinol Metabol Clin North Am* 1995;24:1–14.

Samaan NA, Schultz PN, Leavens TA, Leavens ME, Lee YY. Pregnancy after treatment in patients with prolactinoma: operation versus bromocriptine. *Am J Obstet Gynecol* 1986;155:1300–1305.

Clinical Reproductive Medicine,
Edited by Bryan D. Cowan and David B. Seifer
Lippincott-Raven Publishers, Philadelphia © 1997

CHAPTER 11

Androgen Excess Disorders

Stephen R. Lincoln

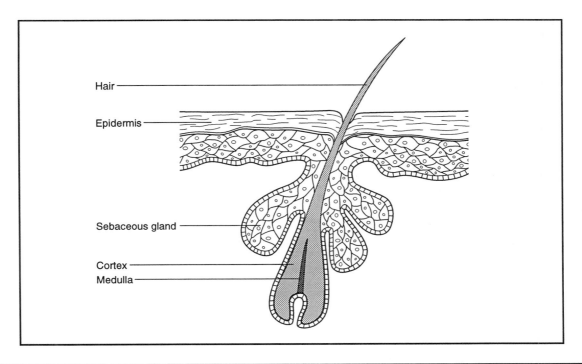

Hirsutism
Hair Follicle Growth and Development
Endocrinology of Hair Growth
Androgen Production
Evaluation of the Hirsute Patient

Differential Diagnosis of Hirsutism
Special Circumstances of Hirsutism in Pregnancy
Treatment of Hirsutism
Medical Therapy
Selected Reading

S. R. Lincoln: Department of Obstetrics and Gynecology, University of Tennessee, Memphis TN
38163

HIRSUTISM

Excessive facial and body hair in locations where hair is not commonly found in women is defined as hirsutism. Hirsutism may result from a hyperandrogenic state that signifies metabolic alterations allowing activation and stimulation of hair follicles in male pattern locations. Virilization is a more severe state of hyperandrogenism resulting in masculinization of the female (Table 11-1). Although hirsutism may reveal a cosmetic disfigurement, rarely is it associated with a life-threatening disease. Virilization, on the other hand, may represent a potentially malignant androgen-producing neoplasm and deserves an urgent evaluation.

HAIR FOLLICLE GROWTH AND DEVELOPMENT

Hair follicles develop in utero at 8–10 weeks gestation. The total endowment of hair follicles is determined at birth and can never increase. The number of follicles varies by ethnic origin (eg, Italians > Asians), but interestingly, not by gender (male = female). Hair follicles begin as nests of columnar epithelium invaginating into the underlying dermis where the hair follicle root bulb is derived. The epithelial column hollows out to form the hair canal, arrector pili attach, and sebaceous glands arrive to form the pilosebaceous apparatus (Fig. 11-1).

Hair growth occurs in cycles and is a result of three phases. The anagen phase is initiated with shedding of the old hair within the follicle, followed by stimulation and growth of the new follicle. Once the growth phase is complete, the hair follicle enters the rapid involution phase

TABLE 11-1. *Signs of androgen excess*

Hirsutism	Virilization
Facial hair	Clitoromegaly
Intermammary hair	Amenorrhea
Male escutcheon	Deepening of the voice
Abdominal hair	Decreased breast size
Hair on upper legs	Increased muscle mass
Temporal balding	

and the shaft ceases to grow, the root moves upward within the follicle, and the hair bulb shrivels. After the catagen phase, hair follicles enter the telogen or resting phase until a new cycle begins.

Hair on the head has a very long growing (anagen) phase (2–3 years) and a short resting (telogen) phase resulting in this hair constantly growing in length and shedding. However, hair on the forearm has a short anagen phase and long telogen phase resulting in short stable hair. This is important clinically as medical treatment for hirsutism may take 6–12 months before any visual effect becomes apparent.

ENDOCRINOLOGY OF HAIR GROWTH

"Sexual hair" refers to those hair follicles that respond to the sex steroids. Locations of sexual hair follicles include the pubic area, axillae, lower abdomen, thighs, legs, arms, chests, and face. Androgens predominantly initiate and stimulate hair growth, as well as increase the diameter and pigmentation of individual hairs. In contrast, the estrogens retard initiation and stimulation of hair growth. In addition, estrogens may increase the synchrony of anagen phase growth leading to periods of exclusively

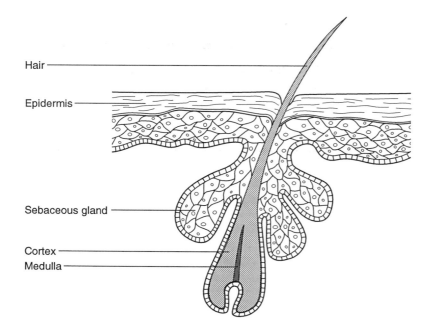

FIG. 11-1. Pilosebaceous unit.

Hair

Epidermis

Sebaceous gland

Cortex
Medulla

TABLE 11-2. *Effect of steroids on hair growth*

Androgens: Initiate and stimulate growth, pigment hair, transform vellous hair to terminal hair
Estrogens: Synchronize growth stages and possibly retard androgen effects
Progestins: Minimal

growth or shedding. This synchrony may lead to perceived increased growth or shedding in high estrogen states (ie, pregnancy). Once the high estrogen state is removed, the synchrony disappears. The effects of progestins are controversial and they probably have minimal effects on hair growth (Table 11-2).

ANDROGEN PRODUCTION

Hair follicles responsive to sex steroids remain dormant until puberty when rises in androgens begin stimulation and growth of pubertal hair. When levels reach the "adult female" range, hair growth occurs in the pubic region, axillae, and extremities in female areas. If levels rise to the "adult male" range, hair growth occurs on the face, chest, back, and male pattern escutcheon occurs. Androgen production in the female occurs from two sources: the adrenal glands and the ovaries. The most important androgens include testosterone, dihydrotestosterone (DHT), androstenedione, dehydroepiandrosterone (DHEA), and dehydroepiandrosterone sulfate (DHEAS). Figure 11-2 reviews the contributions of the androgens from the adrenal and ovarian sources.

Approximately 25% of circulating testosterone in normal women is secreted directly by the ovary and another 25% directly from the adrenal glands. The remaining 50% of testosterone arises from peripheral conversion of androstenedione which, in turn, is secreted equally from the adrenal and ovary. The adrenal glands also secrete the vast majority of the less androgenic steroids DHEA and DHEAS. At target sites for androgen activities (ie, hair follicles), testosterone is converted to DHT by the enzyme 5α-reductase. Both testosterone and DHT interact with the androgen receptor, but DHT has a higher binding affinity and hence is more potent.

Circulating testosterone is bound to protein for transport and only a small fraction is free and active (Fig. 11-3). The majority of testosterone molecules are bound to the protein sex hormone-binding globulin (SHBG) whereas the remaining molecules are bound to albumin. In normal women, only 1% of circulating testosterone is free whereas hirsute women may have higher levels of the unbound fraction. The protein SHBG is synthesized in the liver and small changes in SHBG can greatly influence free testosterone concentration. The balance of SHBG depends on levels of other steroids that have action on or are metabolized by the liver. The production of SHBG is increased in states of excessive estrogens or thyroid hormones and decreased by excessive androgens or decreased thyroid hormones. Hypothyroidism, for example, can result in hirsutism due to decreased SHBG where the total concentration of testosterone remains constant.

EVALUATION OF THE HIRSUTE PATIENT

Only a limited number of disorders result in hirsutism. Hirsutism in pregnancy will be considered separately at the conclusion of the chapter. Intersex disorders (undermasculinized XY patient or virilized XX patient) are an extremely rare form and are discussed in Chapter 5. If a female patient has normal pelvic anatomy exam, is not pregnant, and is not taking androgen medications (ie, danazol, anabolic steroids), the differential diagnosis of hirsutism can be summarized in Table 11-3.

Evaluation of the hirsute patient focuses on excluding the rare but serious pathologic conditions that produce androgen excess. Testosterone or DHEAS will be elevated in neoplasms of the ovary or adrenal, respectively. Elevations of 17α-hydroprogesterone (17-OHP) will be found in congenital adrenal hyperplasia. If menstrual irregularities are present, thyroid and pituitary evaluations are indicated. When Cushing's syndrome is suspected, a screening test (ie, dexamethasone suppression) is indi-

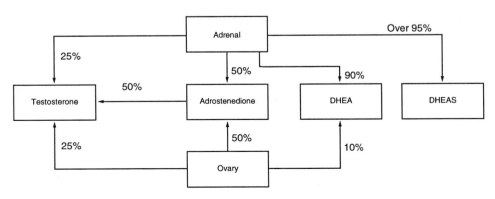

FIG. 11-2. Androgen production.

FREE AND PROTEIN-ASSOCIATED TESTOSTERONE

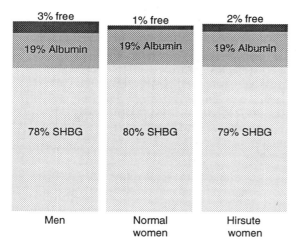

FIG. 11-3. Free and protein-associated testosterone.

cated. Table 11-4 summarizes the initial laboratory assessment of the hirsute patient.

The initial history and physical examination will often lead to the cause of hirsutism. The onset of hirsutism in association with puberty that is not progressive is the hallmark of idiopathic hirsutism or estrogenized/androgenized polycystic ovarian syndrome (PCOS). Particularly important is the presence of hirsutism that occurs remote from puberty and progresses rapidly. This later scenario is associated with neoplasia. Assessment of the quantity of hirsutism can include the use of the Ferriman–Gallwey system to document the location and extent of disease. Photographs can also be used to record data for future comparison after treatment. Microscopic measurement of hair follicle diameter is another method to observe progression or regression of hirsutism.

DIFFERENTIAL DIAGNOSIS OF HIRSUTISM

Idiopathic hirsutism (also labeled constitution or familial) is the most common nonpathologic cause of hirsutism and may represent over 50% of patients. It is characterized by normal laboratory evaluations, regular menstrual cycles, and an absence of virilization. Idiopathic hirsutism is frequently familial and found more

commonly in women of Mediterranean ancestry. The hirsutism is slow growing (years) and may be viewed as an increased tissue sensitivity to normal levels of androgen. Increased 5α-reductase activity has been found in this group of women. Idiopathic hirsutism is a diagnosis of exclusion and pathologic causes must be excluded.

Polycystic ovarian syndrome (PCOS) is the most common pathologic cause of hirsutism. The triad of obesity, hirsutism, and oligo-ovulation is the hallmark of PCOS but it is important to remember that not all three signs are always present. The unifying features of this group includes mild androgen excess and an increased luteinizing hormone (LH) to follicle-stimulating hormone (FSH) ratio. The etiology of PCOS continues to be an enigma. It is helpful to consider PCOS as an endpoint of several mechanisms that cause a steady state of estrogenization and androgenization with anovulation.

Menstrual irregularities in hirsute patients with PCOS often begin soon after menarche. Virilization is rarely present and basic laboratory evaluation is essentially normal. However, slight elevations of T (100–150 ng/dl) or DHEAS (400–600 ml/dl) may occur and the LH/FSH ratio is usually >2:1 (normal 1:1). Not all patients need gonadotropins measured, but sometimes levels are helpful to confirm the diagnosis.

Stromal hyperthecosis can be viewed as a severe form of PCOS but different characteristics exist. The history is consistent with PCOS including menstrual irregularities and androgen excess, but progressive signs of virilization may begin to occur with stromal hyperthecosis. Mild degrees of temporal balding, decreased breast size, and clitoromegaly may develop as well as weight gain and increased muscle mass. Virilization should alert the physician to the possibility of a neoplasm, but stromal hyperthecosis has a slow progression whereas neoplasms present with a rapid progression to virilization.

Laboratory values reveal testosterone approaching tumor levels (200 ng/dl) with minimal elevation of DHEAS. Retrograde ovarian vein catheterization has shown that the elevated testosterone arises from the ovary. Ovarian biopsy will reveal nests of luteinized theca cells. In contrast to PCOS, the gonadotropin ratio is frequently close to 1.

Late onset (also known as nonclassical or adult onset) congenital adrenal hyperplasia (CAH) may be present in

---

TABLE 11-3. *Diagnosis of hirsutism*

%	Cause	T	DS	17-OHP	Virilized	Comments
50	Idiopathic	NL	NL	NL	No	↑ Tissue sensitivity
40	PCOS	NL-SL ↑	NL-SL	NL	No	↑ LH/FSH
5	Stromal hyperthecosis	SL ↑	NL-SL	NL	Occasionally	NL LH/FSH
1–4	CAH	NL	NL-SL −	>200 mg/dl	No	ACTH test
<1	Cushing	NL	NL	NL	No	Dex screen
<1	Ovarian tumor	>200 ng/dl	NL	NL	Yes	Rapid progression
<1	Adrenal tumor	NL	>700 mg/dl	NL	Yes	Rapid progression

PCOS, polycystic ovarian syndrome; CAH, congenital adrenal hyperplasia; LH, luteinizing hormone; FSH, follicle-stimulating hormone; ACTH, adrenocorticotropic hormone.

TABLE 11-4. *Initial lab assessment*

Testosterone
Dehydroepiandrosterone sulfate
17-hydroxyprogesterone
Menstrual irregularities: prolactin and thyroid-stimulating hormone
Suspect Cushing's—dexamethasone suppression test

1–10% of hirsute patients. Incidence varies according to ethnic populations studied and late onset CAH is most common in Alaskan Yupik Eskimos and Ashkenazi Jews. The syndrome arises when the pituitary "recognizes" decreased cortisol production and compensates for the adrenal insufficiency by increasing ACTH production. However, precursors to cortisol increase at the site of the enzyme deficiency (see Fig. 11-4) and the excess precursors are shunted into androgen production. The excess androgens leads to hirsutism.

The most common enzyme defect in late onset CAH is 21-hydroxylase deficiency. The enzyme defects are inherited (autosomal recessive) and the gene (located on chromosome 6) responsible for 21-hydroxylase has been described including various nucleotide inversions, deletions, and mutations responsible for the deficiency. The variable defects result in a range of clinical presentations. Some hirsute women thought to have PCOS really have late onset CAH.

Diagnosis is made by finding elevated precursor levels of 17α-hydroxyprogesterone (>200 ng/dl) in a screening test. The 17α-hydroxyprogesterone (17-OHP) screen must be drawn in the follicular phase to avoid false posi-

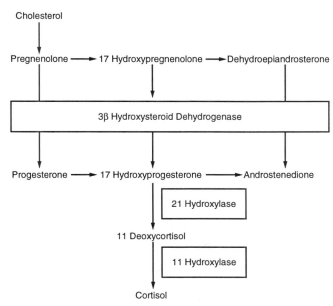

FIG. 11-4. Steroidogenesis pathway and congenital adrenal hyperplasia enzyme defects.

tives (17-OHP rises due to corpus luteum production in the secretory phase) and in the early morning to avoid false negatives (circadian decrease of 17-OHP) that parallel cortisol and ACTH. If the screening level is elevated, the ACTH stimulation (Fig. 11-5) test is performed to

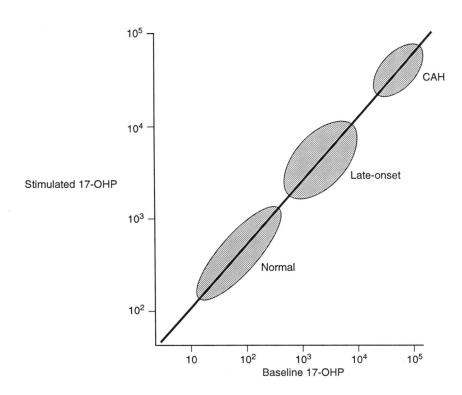

FIG. 11-5. ACTH stimulation and congenital adrenal hyperplasia

confirm the diagnosis. Synthetic ACTH (Cortrosyn 250 μg) is given intravenously and 17-OHP is measured at time zero (x axis) and 1 hour (y axis). Levels of 17-OHP >1000 ng/dl make the diagnosis. The normal post-ACTH value of 17-OHP is <320 ng/dl.

Cushing's syndrome is a rare cause of hirsutism. Cushing's syndrome is a state of excess cortisol production and can arise from several sources. Pituitary ACTH-producing adenoma (Cushing's disease), ectopic ACTH production by tumor (lung or kidney), or autonomous over-secretion of cortisol by the adrenal (tumor) can all lead to glucocorticoid excess. Characteristics include hirsutism of a fine lanugo type, centripital obesity, pigmented abdominal striae, dorsal neck fat pads, peripheral muscle wasting, weakness, moon facies, hypertension, hypokalemia, and ecchymosis.

When clinical suspension of hypercortisolism arises, the overnight dexamethasone suppression test (1 mg at 11 p.m. followed by 8 a.m. cortisol level) or a 24-hour urinary free cortisol level can be used for screening. Serum cortisol <5 mg/dl after suppression or urinary-free cortisol <100 mg (urine test) exclude Cushing's. If the screening test is abnormal, more extensive testing, including extended low- and high-dose suppression, serum ACTH levels, and possibly radiographic studies, is required to diagnose Cushing's and define the etiology of cortisol excess.

Androgen-producing tumors are the most uncommon but potentially lethal causes of hirsutism. The clinical history of rapidly progressing hirsutism followed by virilization can take place in only a few months. Baseline measurements of testosterone (<200 ng/dl) and DHEAS (<700 mg/dl) effectively exclude an androgen-producing tumor as a cause of hirsutism. Androgen-secreting ovarian tumors are usually palpable (80%) on bimanual exam and include Sertoli–Leydig cell tumors, granulosa cell tumors, gynandroblastomas, and Brenner tumors. Adenomas and carcinomas of the adrenal gland can secrete large amounts of DHEAS and other androgens. Metastasis of both ovarian and adrenal tumors can frequently occur before detection.

SPECIAL CIRCUMSTANCES OF HIRSUTISM IN PREGNANCY

When virilization occurs with pregnancy, clinical suspicion for a luteoma of pregnancy should arise. A luteoma is not a true ovarian neoplasm but represents an exaggerated response of ovarian stroma to human chorionic gonadotropin (hCG). Solid luteomas (unilateral in approximately 45% of cases) are associated with normal pregnancy and androgen excess. Luteomas may rarely cause virilization of a female fetus. True androgen-secreting tumors of the ovary are rare since these neoplasms inhibit ovulation. Theca luteal cysts may arise in pregnancy and the condition is referred to as Hyper Reactio Luteinalis. Multiple theca luteal cysts arise usually due to high levels of hCG, are almost always bilateral, and may be associated with trophoblastic disease. Virilized female fetuses have not been reported with theca luteal cysts and the cysts regress postpartum. Surgery is rarely required except in extreme cases of rupture or torsion.

TREATMENT OF HIRSUTISM

Hirsutism is not a specific disease but a sign of a spectrum of conditions. The etiology of hirsutism should be ascertained and treatment should focus on the condition that results in hirsutism. Serious pathologic causes of hirsutism are rare but require specialized care. Androgen-producing neoplasms of the adrenal or ovary require surgical exploration and often adjuvant chemotherapy. Cushing's syndrome require precise localization of the lesion and treatment involves removal of the source. Late onset congenital adrenal hyperplasia requires replacement doses of the delinquent corticosteroids.

Treatment of the remaining causes of hirsutism (idiopathic, PCOS, and stromal hyperthecosis) can be considered together. Medical treatment is aimed at reducing the amount of androgens produced (usually at the ovary) and decreasing the synthesis and actions of androgens at their peripheral sites. It is important to remember new hair follicles will no longer be stimulated with medical therapy, but previously established hair follicles remain. Only mechanical removal of established terminal hair will show visible improvement. It often requires 6–12 months before medical and depilatory therapy show visible results. Mechanical therapies include shaving, tweezing, waxing, or depilatory pads. Permanent removal can only be accomplished with electrolysis.

MEDICAL THERAPY

Estrogen- and progestin-containing oral contraceptives (OCPs) have been a mainstay in the treatment of hirsutism. They function to suppress ovarian steroidogenesis. Patients with PCOS also benefit from the induction of regular menses and protection from continuous estrogen on the uterine endometrium. There is no clinically apparent distinction between low-dose, high-dose, or multiphasic combination of OCPs and the treatment of hirsutism. New formulations of OCPs include less androgenic progestins (gestodene, norgestimate, and desogestrel). All OCPs are associated with increases in SHBG and decreases in free testosterone levels in laboratory studies.

Spironolactone is a diuretic found to have three significant antiandrogen actions. It competes with androgens at the androgen receptor in the hair follicle, reduces 5α-reductase activity, and inhibits ovarian androgen biosynthesis. Spironolactone is most effective at doses of 200 mg daily in divided doses (100 mg bid) but may be reduced after 3–6 months of therapy. Side effects can occur and include diuresis in the beginning stages of treatment, fatigue, and occasionally dysfunctional bleeding. Spironolactone is a potassium-sparing diuretic and hyperkalemia may also occur. A newer 5α-reductase inhibitor (finasteride) has been reported to achieve the clinical responses at 5 mg/day.

Flutamide is a new nonsteroidal antiandrogen that has shown promising results in the treatment of hirsutism. Flutamide directly inhibits hair growth and may have fewer side effects than spironolactone. Doses of 250 mg tid have been shown to be effective and further clinical trials are underway. Neither flutamide nor spironolactone has been approved for use in pregnancy, and if not on OCPs, other methods of contraception should be employed.

Long-acting gonadotropin-releasing hormone analogs (GnRH-a) also show promise as a treatment of hirsutism. The reversible "medical menopause" effectively inhibits pituitary LH secretion and may be extremely effective in the treatment of hirsutism. However, long-term treatment (>6 months) is not recommended due to adverse bone demineralization and lipid profiles in the estrogen-deprived patient on GnRH-a. Current trials are investigating its use with estrogen and progesterone.

SUGGESTED READING

American College of Obstetricians and Gynecologists. Evaluation and treatment of hirsute women. ACOG Tech Bull No. 203, 1995.

American College of Obstetricians and Gynecologists. Hyperandrogenic chronic anovulation. ACOG Tech Bull No. 202, 1995.

Azziz R, Dewakly D, Owerbach D. Nonclassic adrenal hyperplasia: current concepts. *J Clin Endocrinol Metab* 1994;78:810–815.

Heiner JS, Greendale GA, Kawakami AK, Papolt PS, Fisher M, Young D, Judd HL. Comparison of a gonadotropin-releasing hormone agonist and a low dose oral contraceptive given alone or together in the treatment of hirsutism. *J Clin Endocrinol Metab* 1995;80:3412.

Marcondes J, Minnani S, Luthold W, Wajchenberg B, Samojlik E, Kirschner M. Treatment of hirsutism in women with flutamide. *Fertil Steril* 1992;57:543.

Pittaway D, Maxson N, Wentz A. Spironolactone in combination drug therapy for unresponsive hirsutism. *Fertil Steril* 1985;43:878.

Speroff L, Glass R, Kase N. *Hirsutism in Clinical Gynecologic Endocrinology and Infertility*, 5th ed. Baltimore: Williams and Wilkins, 1994;483–513.

Clinical Reproductive Medicine,
Edited by Bryan D. Cowan and David B. Seifer
Lippincott-Raven Publishers, Philadelphia © 1997

CHAPTER 12

Menopause

Delbert L. Booher

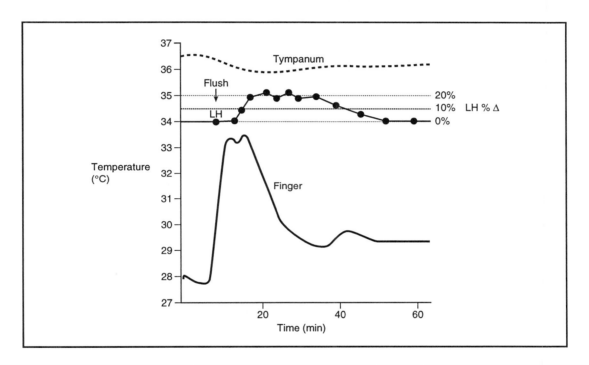

Definition
Endocrinology
Climacteric "Syndrome"
Major Areas of Menopausal Change

Menopausal Hormone Replacement Therapy
Clinical Tips in Menopausal Management
Cost and Benefit
Suggested Reading

D. L. Booher: Program for Mature Women, Department of Gynecology and Obstetrics, The Cleveland Clinic Foundation; Department of Reproductive Biology, Case Western Reserve University; Department of Obstetrics and Gynecology, The Cleveland Clinic Foundation Health Sciences Center, Cleveland, OH 44195

Contemporary management of menopause addresses the continuum of events associated with the effects of estrogen deprivation on quality and duration of life for mature women. Although life expectancy for women has increased by 30 years since the turn of the century, to 78.2 years, the average age of onset of menopause, 51, has not changed significantly. Consequently, the average woman can now expect to live one third of her life in the postmenopausal period. One sixth of the U.S. population consists of postmenopausal women, and the number of women age 65 and older will increase.

DEFINITION

The classic definition of menopause was the final menstrual period. The contemporary approach to menopause is evaluation and management of all events related to lack of adequate estrogen that occur after the last menstrual period. The definition established by the International Menopause Society is that menopause begins rather than ends with the last menstrual period.

ENDOCRINOLOGY

Menopause is the endocrine deficiency disorder of adult onset hypogonadism. The postmenopausal hormonal profile is elevated gonadotropic hormones due to low estradiol and possibly to low levels or decreased effectiveness of ovarian inhibin. Total ovarian estrogen production is low, there is an increased conversion of androstenedione to estrone and reversal of the premenopausal estrone/estradiol ratio. Additionally, elevated luteinizing hormone (LH) may increase testosterone production by ovarian stroma in some women. There is an estrogen-dependent decrease in sex hormone-binding globulin (Chapter 9). This increases the bioactivity of androgens and augments skin and hair changes related to androgens.

CLIMACTERIC "SYNDROME"

Major menopausal changes can be categorized into subgroups, including neuroendocrine changes, urogenital atrophy, androgen-dependent skin and hair disorders, osteoporosis, and cardiovascular disease. The antiquated concept that menopause is nothing more than hot flushes, psychosocial adjustment, and vaginal dryness that will resolve is no longer an acceptable approach to evaluation and management of the menopause.

MAJOR AREAS OF MENOPAUSAL CHANGE

Vasomotor Instability

Hot flushes and night sweats occur in 85% of women undergoing natural or surgical menopause and continue for 3–5 years in 45%. Nearly 15% experience hot flushes near the time of menstruation as they approach meno-

pause. Vasomotor instability appears to arise from estrogen *withdrawal* which affects the central α-adrenergic system, and not from low estrogen *per se*. Luteinizing hormone (LH) is released coincident to hot flushes but is not the cause of the hot flush. For example, patients with pituitary insufficiency have hot flushes but cannot release LH. In addition, injection of gonadotropins does not induce flushes. Finally, administration of GnRH agonists to inhibit LH release has no effect on hot flushes. Adrenergic agents and prostaglandins have been shown to release GnRH and affect thermo-regulatory function. Thus, it is hypothesized that estrogen withdrawal in the central nervous system induces changes in catecholamines and prostaglandins that produce the hot flushes.

Objective findings at the time of the hot flush include increased rate of skin electrical conductants, increased skin temperature, and decreased internal body (core) temperature (Fig. 12-1). Events that trigger hot flushes include cigarette smoking, alcohol, caffeine, stress, and heat. The patient may experience an aura, then a focus of flushing on the upper trunk which spreads upward to the shoulders, neck, and face. This may be associated with palpitations, headaches, and dizziness. The mean duration of flushing is 3.3 minutes; then it may conclude with perspiration. Insomnia frequently ensues when episodes occur at night. Nonspecific treatment can be directed at control of environment, lifestyle, clothing, and stress management.

Hot flushes respond well to supplemental estrogen therapy in most women. For those women unable to use estrogen, progestins have been shown to be helpful. Oral medroxyprogesterone acetate (MPA), 10-20 mg daily, or Depo MPA, 150–300 mg intramuscularly every 1–3 months, will modify hot flush frequency and intensity. Caution is advised with this management in that androgenicity of long-term progestin therapy may increase cardiovascular risk. Other agents suggested for treatment of vasomotor instability include clonidine, methyldopa, antiprostaglandins, and a mixture of phenobarbital and belladonna (Bellergal). Clonidine, an α-adrenergic agonist, transdermal therapeutic system in dosages of 100–200 μg/day, has been shown to be effective in 50–60% of patients, although 40% discontinue usage due to norepinephrine-like side effects. Naprosyn, an antiprostaglandin, in doses of 250 mg bid has been shown to be approximately 50% effective and generally well tolerated. Methyldopa, in the range of 750 mg/day, has some value with mode of action related to reduction in tissue concentration of serotonin, dopamine, norepinephrine, and epinephrine. Bellergal-S every 12 hours PRN has been our traditional therapy, although recent double-blind studies indicate little more than a placebo effect.

Psychological Changes

Subtle changes in psychological function exist due to estrogen deficiency. These include nonspecific com-

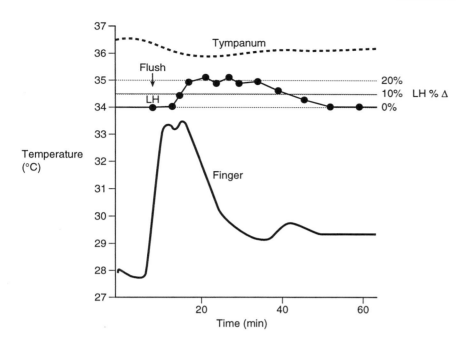

FIG. 12-1. Association of hot flushes with serum LH rises and peripheral and core temperature changes.

plaints such as irritability, anxiety, nervousness, depression, fatigue, forgetfulness, loss of memory, and inability to concentrate. Such complaints are characteristic of sleep deprivation and can be explained partially on the basis of interrupted sleep. However, neuropeptide changes suggest the existence of a complex communication system within the central nervous system needed for maintenance of psychological homeostasis. Neuropeptides related to ACTH, β-endorphin, and neurohypophyseal hormones modulate many central nervous system functions (Table 12-1). These comprise motivation, attention, concentration, arousal, learning and memory processes, pain, mood, aggression, and social, sexual, and maternal behavior. In addition, these neuropeptides are also involved in the regulation of body temperature, blood pressure, sleep, respiration, central blood flow, and brain metabolism. Several neuropeptides posses neurotropic opiate-like, neuroleptic-like, psychostimulant, and analeptic effects.

Some releasing hormones also possess central nervous system effects. For example, thyrotropin-releasing hormone functions as an endogenous arousal agent and has analeptic-like properties, corticotropin-like-releasing hormone, and somatostatin enhance sympathetic activity and induce behavioral activation, and luteinizing hormone-releasing hormone is involved in sexual behavior.

Thus, climacteric complaints may be related to neuropeptide alterations resulting from decreased levels of sex steroids. In evaluation of psychiatric dysfunction, other sources of depression must also be considered. A therapeutic trial of supplemental estrogen therapy can be prescribed, but if depressive symptoms persist, psychiatric evaluation should be pursued.

Urogenital Atrophy

Urogenital tissues become atrophic in specific response to lack of adequate estrogen. The labia majora flatten and wrinkle and the clitoris decreases in size. The Bartholin glands produce less secretions, and pubic hair becomes sparse but more coarse.

Vaginal atrophy results in a loss of elasticity associated with shortening and narrowing of the vagina. The vaginal epithelium becomes thin, sensitive, friable, and less resistant to infection. There is decreased glycogen in the vaginal epithelial tissue, decreased Döderlein bacteria, and increased vaginal pH. Maturation index shows primarily basal cells. Decreased vaginal secretions may lead to dyspareunia.

Tissues of the uterine cervix, uterine fundus, and fallopian tubes undergo involutional atrophy that is generally asymptomatic. Atrophic endometrium can cause postmenopausal bleeding. The base of the urinary bladder and urethra are also derived from Mullerian tissue and are estrogen-sensitive. Epithelial changes in the lining of the urethra and trigone of the bladder after menopause are similar to those of the vagina and may result in atrophic cystitis, atrophic urethritis, urethral caruncles, urethral shortening, and urinary incontinence. The urethral syndrome associated with loss of

TABLE 12-1. *CNS releasing hormones involved in sexual behavior*

ACTH
Thyrotropin-releasing hormone
Corticotropin-like-releasing hormone
Luteinizing hormone

bladder sphincter tone is characterized by recurrent bacterial urethritis with dysuria, frequency, urgency, nocturia, and postvoiding dribbling. Local or systemic supplemental estrogen therapy is helpful in treating all of these symptoms.

Urinary incontinence develops in approximately 40% of postmenopausal women. Evaluation of incontinence is by history, physical examination, and selective urodynamic studies. Urgency incontinence due to bladder irritability is frequently associated with atrophic changes of the urinary bladder, although possible urinary tract infection must be excluded.

Sexual Function

Sexual function can be altered by a combination of psychological changes and urogenital atrophy. Multiple environmental factors can be involved including marital disharmony, lifestyle stresses, and illness. Local genital factors leading to dyspareunia include atrophy of the vulva, vagina, and pelvic supportive structures. Libido may be altered in postmenopausal women associated with serum levels of estrogen, progesterone, and testosterone. Approximately half of testosterone in women is derived from ovarian sources. Thus, testosterone therapy may be appropriate in the younger, ovariectomized patient. However, caution should be exercised in the use of testosterone supplements in other women. The postmenopausal patient is already subjected to a testosterone-dominated hormonal milieu due to lack of adequate estrogen. Additional testosterone may significantly increase some menopausal changes associated with excessive testosterone, including skin and hair changes, and increased cardiovascular risk. Furthermore, there is little evidence that androgens enhance libido in postmenopausal women. Psychological evaluation is frequently needed in conjunction with hormonal therapy to satisfactorily improve sexual dysfunction. Vaginal moisturizing lotions and personal vaginal lubricants can be helpful adjuncts to decrease dyspareunia.

Skin and Hair Changes

Skin and hair changes are due to a combination of lack of adequate estrogen plus relative dominance of testosterone. Hypoestrogenism results in decreased anagen phase hair growth, decreased skin collagen, and loss of skin elasticity with skin wrinkling. The epidermis becomes thin and fragile with blending of epidermal pili. Reduced secretions of sweat and oil glands result in skin dryness and itching. The testosterone-dominant hormonal milieu contributes to androgen excess skin and hair disorders, including male pattern baldness, thinning of hair, receding hairline, hirsutism, and adult onset acne. Other androgen effects include redistribution of body fat, tendency to gain weight, and deepening of voice.

Androgen excess skin and hair disorders in postmenopausal women can be significantly modified with supplemental estrogen therapy. Systemic hormone therapy reduces pituitary LH release and thus decreases ovarian stromal production of androstenedione and testosterone. Oral estrogen therapy will also elevate serum sex hormone binding globulin and thus decrease free serum testosterone (Chapter 9). Adjuncts to estrogen therapy include spironolactone (antitestosterone effect) and minoxidil topical solution to reduce male pattern balding.

Osteoporosis

Osteoporosis is epidemic in the United States today. Nearly half of the 41.5 million women in the United States over age 50 have some degree of osteopenia and suffer 1.4 million fractures per year at a cost of 9–10 billion dollars. Postmenopausal (type I) osteoporosis causes 80% of all fractures and nearly all hip fractures in postmenopausal women. Approximately 25% of white women will have vertebral compression fractures by age 60 and 50% by age 75. Approximately one third of white women will experience hip fracture by age 85 and 20–25% of all women will sustain such a fracture by age 90. Hip fracture is by far the most serious consequence of osteoporosis with mortality exceeding 50,000 deaths in postmenopausal women in the United States per year. Of women experiencing hip fracture, 15% will die within 3 months due to complications of fracture including pulmonary edema, myocardial infarction, and pulmonary embolus. Another 25% of these women will suffer significant morbidity and nearly half of survivors remain invalid in chronic care facilities.

The clinical profile of women at risk for osteoporosis includes white race, family history of osteoporosis, phenotypically short and petite, light skeleton, blond with fair complexion, and early age of menopause (Table 12-2). Avoidable factors related to lifestyle include smoking, physical inactivity, and nutritional factors. Secondary causes of osteoporosis include chronic renal failure, gastrectomy, intestinal bypass, and malabsorption syndromes. Associated endocrinopathies include hyperparathyroidism, hyperadrenalism, and diabetes. Associated medications include steroids, anticonvulsants, heparin, aluminum antacids, methotrexate, and excessive supplemental thyroid replacement therapy. Using these criteria, approximately 30% of all postmenopausal women will be identified as being high risk for osteoporosis and justify further evaluation and management.

A variety of radiographic methods have been developed to assess bone mineralization including plain radiography, single-photon absorptiometry, dual-photon ab-

TABLE 12-2. *Clinical profile of women at risk for osteoporosis*

Indigenous
    White race
    Family history of osteoporosis
    Phenotypically short and petite
    Light skeleton
    Blond with fair complexion
    Early age of menopause
Lifestyle
    Smoking
    Physical inactivity
Nutritional
    Inadequate calcium
    Inadequate vitamin D
    Excessive alcohol
    Excessive caffeine
Secondary causes
    Chronic renal disease
    Gastrectomy
    Intestinal bypass
    Malabsorption syndromes
Associated endocrinopathies
    Hyperparathyroidism
    Hyperadrenalism
    Diabetes mellitus
Associated Medications
    Steroids
    Anticonvulsants
    Heparin
    Aluminum antacid
    Methotrexate
    Excessive supplemental thyroid replacement therapy

sorptiometry, quantitative digital radiography, computed tomography, quantitative computerized tomography, dual-electron X-ray absorptiometry (DEXA), and neutron activation analysis. Plain radiography is the most readily available but is the least sensitive of all methods in that 25–30% of bone mineral content must be lost before osteopenia can be diagnosed by routine X-ray. DEXA is a newer technique offering high sensitivity and specificity, very low radiation exposure, reduced cost, brief time for evaluation, and excellent precision. Indirect measurements of bone metabolism can be obtained through measurement of serum alkaline phosphatase that reflects osteoblastic activity, and urinary calcium and hydroxyproline that reflect osteoclastic activity. A single determination of body fat mass, urinary calcium and hydroxyproline, and serum alkaline phosphatase has been shown to identify 79% of fast bone losers (bone loss >3% per year) and 78% of slow bone losers. Fast losers have higher urinary hydroxyproline and calcium levels and lower body weight.

Drugs currently approved by the Food and Drug Administration for the treatment of osteoporosis include estrogen, calcium, biphosphates (alendronate), and calcitonin, all of which decrease bone resorption. Supplemental estrogen therapy combined with calcium and exercise will prevent development of osteoporosis in most women. Bone demineralization accelerates when estrogen therapy is discontinued.

Low-risk women do well with calcium and exercise alone. Exercise equivalent to one-half hour of walking every other day is encouraged for all women. Calcium absorption decreases with age, so that oral intake must increase as women grow older. A total dietary calcium intake of 1200 mg/day is recommended before age 55 and 1500 mg per day thereafter.

Alternative antiresorptive therapy for osteoporosis prevention in women who cannot use estrogen includes tamoxifen and biphosphonates. Tamoxifen (20 mg/day) is as effective as estrogen in maintaining bone mineral density. However, data are limited and fracture risk has yet to be determined. Other biphosphonates and estrogen antagonists are currently under investigation with optimistic initial reports.

Cardiovascular Disease

Cardiovascular disease is by far the leading cause of mortality in women in the United States. Mortality figures combining heart attack and stroke approach 500,000 deaths per year. It has been known since the 1930s that the incidence of cardiovascular disease in women before menopause is approximately one fourth that of men. Cardiovascular mortality in women age 40–44 is 1.3 per 1000 per year but increases 17-fold to 22.1 by age 65–69. Cardiovascular disease in men during those same years increases less than fivefold from 5.7 to 26.7 per 1000 per year. It is evident that cardiovascular disease in women increases dramatically within 10–15 years after menopause, although it never quite reaches the same incidence as that seen in men.

Cardiovascular disease is a multifactorial disease involving blood pressure, total cholesterol, high-density lipoproteins, low-density lipoprotein, diabetes, hematocrit, blood viscosity, endothelial factors, vasoactive peptides, and blood clotting factors.

One probable mechanism for cardiovascular protection of premenopausal women is estrogen-induced alterations in serum cholesterol and lipoproteins. Epidemiologic data have linked lipoproteins to cardiovascular risk. High-density lipoproteins (HDLs) remove excess cholesterol from the tissues and return it to the liver for metabolism and excretion, whereas low-density lipoproteins (LDLs) transport cholesterol to peripheral tissues for deposition and steroid synthesis. Higher levels of HDL and lower levels of LDL and cholesterol are cardioprotective. Estrogens decrease total cholesterol and LDL and increase HDL. The lower HDL levels found in men compared to women may be associated with testosterone and could explain differences in risks for cardiovascular disease. Coincident with the perimenopausal increase in cardiovascular disease, most women experience a rise in serum cholesterol.

The relative increased incidence of cardiovascular disease seen in menopause may be due to a loss of estrogen's protective impact on cholesterol and lipoproteins. Most prospective cohort studies report reduced relative risks for cardiovascular disease in women who used supplemental estrogen. The Boston Nurses Healthy Study provided over 100,000 person-years of observation among 32,317 postmenopausal women initially free of coronary disease and reported "ever use" of menopausal estrogen led to a 50% reduction in fatal and nonfatal coronary disease. Current users had a 70% reduction in risk. The only major descent study came from the Framingham Study. Here a significant increase in cardiovascular mortality among ever-users of estrogen replacement was observed. However, this study included women using high-dose estrogen in the form of oral contraceptives. This study is considered flawed for that reason. The majority of epidemiologic evidence supports the position that modern estrogen replacement therapy provides protection against cardiovascular disease in menopausal women.

Hypertension is another important factor in cardiovascular disease. There is a slight but occasionally significant elevation in renin substrate associated with hepatic first-pass effect of oral estrogen. There is also a 5–7% incidence of idiosyncratic hypertensive reaction associated with the use of oral estrogen therapy. However, diastolic and systolic blood pressures are reduced in most normotensive and hypertensive patients placed on estrogen therapy. Hypertension alone is not a contraindication to hormone replacement therapy. In addition, adverse blood pressure reactions can be averted by avoiding hepatic first-pass effect with the use of non-oral estrogen when needed.

Diabetes is also related to cardiovascular disease. Menopause, as such, is not diabetogenic and surgical removal of the ovaries does not affect the results of the glucose tolerance test. Oral contraceptives frequently produce reversible diabetogenic effects related to dose and type of estrogen and progestin and the duration of administration. Estrogen replacement therapy can produce a reversible alteration in glucose metabolism that is not associated with hyperinsulinism. Progestins affect carbohydrate metabolism and can induce hyperinsulinemia and vascular changes if therapy is prolonged. Patients on hormone replacement therapy including a progestin should thus have regular blood glucose evaluations. Diabetes, especially mature onset, is not felt to be a contraindication to hormone replacement therapy.

Thrombogenic complications related to cardiovascular disease require three obligatory conditions. Damage to vascular intima, impaired blood flow, and hypercoagulability are required for thrombosis formation. The literature regarding coagulation in relation to hormone replacement therapy is often confusing because it is based on oral contraceptives. There is a slight, but generally insignificant, reduction in antithrombin III related to the first-pass hepatic effect of oral estrogen. Progestins do not affect various clotting factors and may increase fibrinolytic activity. Recent research has indicated that hormone replacement therapy affects vasoactive proteins (thromboxane A_2, prostacyclin I_2, and vasoactive peptides). Estrogen alters prostaglandin synthesis in favor of prostacyclin activity which causes vasodilatation and decreased platelet adhesiveness. Estrogen also decreases smooth muscle vascular tone. It is concluded that there is no causal relation between menopausal doses of hormone replacement therapy and deep vein thrombosis, stroke, and myocardial infarction. Superficial thrombophlebitis and varicose veins are not a contraindication to hormone replacement therapy. In addition, a single remote episode of deep vein thrombosis related to a single specific event, such as a surgical procedure, is not an absolute contraindication to hormone replacement therapy. Furthermore, nonoral estrogen has essentially no effect on liver-mediated blood clotting factors.

MENOPAUSAL HORMONE REPLACEMENT THERAPY

Indications

The estrogen deprivation of menopause impairs both quality and duration of life, and improvement of both is the goal of management. Estrogen should be recommended to all women who do not have a significant contraindication to use of this therapy. The major indications for menopausal hormone replacement therapy are risk of cardiovascular disease and osteoporosis. Secondary indications include neuroendocrine changes, which encompass vasomotor instability, psychological problems, urogenital atrophy with associated sexual function, and androgen-excess skin and hair disorders.

Evaluation

Menopause is an ideal time to reinvolve women in a health care maintenance program. Early diagnosis and management of major medical problems can significantly improve the quality and duration of life in menopausal women. Major areas for screening and annual evaluation include cardiovascular disease, osteoporosis, and cancer.

Prior to initiation of menopausal hormone replacement therapy, a complete history and physical examination should be performed (Table 12-3). Significant laboratory studies include Pap smear, baseline mammogram, stool guaiac, serum cholesterol, and serum glucose concentration. Liver function studies should be done in women with a past history of liver disease. Bone densitometry (DEXA) is done selectively and is not recommended routinely prior to or during therapy. Pretreatment endometrial biopsy is not recommended for all women. Endome-

TABLE 12-3. *Requirements prior to hormone replacement therapy*

Complete history and physical exam
Laboratory studies
  Pap smear
  Baseline mammogram
  Stool guaiac
  Lipid profile
  Serum glucose
Discretionary studies
  Liver function studies
  Bone densitometry
  Endometrial biopsy

TABLE 12-4. *Contraindications to hormone replacement therapy*

Traditional contraindications
  Estrogen-dependent malignancy
    Breast
    Endometrium
  Acute liver disease
  Acute vascular thrombosis
  Chronic impaired liver function
  Unexplained abnormal uterine bleeding
  Possibility of pregnancy
Modifiers to be monitored
  Migraine headaches
  Seizure disorders
  Thrombophlebitis
  Strong family history of breast cancer
  Leiomyomata
  Endometriosis
  Familial hyperlipidemia
  Gallbladder disease
  Pancreatitis
  Diabetes mellitus

trial biopsy should be performed in women with a history of irregular bleeding and women at increased risk for endometrial cancer.

Once therapy is initiated, women should be reevaluated in approximately 3 months to determine response to therapy, appropriateness of bleeding pattern, and significant side effects. Blood pressure should be determined with breast and pelvic examinations done selectively in relation to symptoms. Endometrial biopsy may be indicated if any bleeding pattern is inappropriate. Following the initial 3-month evaluation, patients should be seen at 6- to 12-month intervals.

Contraindications to Estrogen Therapy

There are few absolute contraindications to estrogen therapy (Table 12-4). Traditional contraindications include estrogen-dependent malignancy of breast or endometrial tissue, acute liver disease, acute vascular thrombosis, chronic impaired liver function, unexplained abnormal uterine bleeding, and possibility of pregnancy. However, the use of estrogen therapy after treatment of endometrial cancer can be considered on an individual basis related to stage and grade of malignancy and time period since treatment. Breast cancer was generally considered a life-long contraindication to estrogen. However, recent evidence recommends that individualization should occur based on stage and grade of malignancy, duration of time since therapy, and significance of the problem for which estrogen is being considered.

Estrogen is inadvisable in the presence of an active source of embolization but can be considered in a patient who had a single embolic episode previously when the source of embolization is no longer present. These women are particularly good candidates for transdermal estrogen administration, which has essentially no effect on clotting factors.

Other conditions that can be modified by estrogen therapy but are not contraindications to therapy include migraine headaches, seizure disorders, thrombophlebitis, strong family history of breast cancer, leiomyomata, endometriosis, familial hyperlipidemia, gallbladder disease, pancreatitis, and diabetes. These conditions need to be monitored during estrogen therapy.

Compliance

Only 34% of women who could benefit from hormone replacement therapy are receiving these benefits. The major reason for not initiating hormone replacement therapy is fear of cancer. The major reason for discontinuation of therapy is the return of menstrual bleeding. In first-time users, 20% stopped taking medication within 9 months, 10% used it on an intermittent basis, and 20–30% never had their prescriptions filled because they were not fully convinced of the benefits and safety of therapy.

Unopposed estrogen will lead to a 5- to 7-times increased incidence of endometrial cancer. However, multiple studies have reported that the addition of a progestin to a menopausal hormone replacement program will decrease the endometrial cancer incidence below the control population and actually reduce endometrial cancer.

Breast cancer risk is the other malignancy of concern of menopausal estrogen users. A recent meta-analysis screened 556 articles published in the last 18 years and summarized data from 35 of these articles. The combined results provided strong evidence that menopausal therapy consisting of 0.625 mg/day or less of conjugated estrogens does not increase breast cancer risk. The overall relative risk of breast cancer associated with hormone replacement therapy revealed a 7% increase related to the type, duration, and dosage of therapy. The overall insignificance of this number must be kept in mind when counseling patients regarding hormone replacement therapy.

Regarding menstrual bleeding, newer treatment schedules with daily progestin will induce endometrial atrophy and amenorrhea in the majority of women within 12–15 months. These newer treatment schedules are being studied extensively at the present time. Initial reports are optimistic regarding safety in relation to endometrial cancer and cardiovascular risks. Patients seem happy with these replacement schedules and rarely discontinue therapy

TABLE 12-5. *Different classes of estrogens*

Naturally occurring estrogens
  Estrone
  Estradiol
  Conjugated estrogens
Synthetic estrogens
  Ethinyl estradiol
  Mestranol
  Quinestrol
Nonsteroidal estrogens
  Diethylstilbestrol
  Chlorotrianisene

when patient education is carried out regarding the safety and cancer risks.

Estrogen

There are several classes of estrogens (Table 12-5). Naturally occurring estrogens include estrone, estradiol, and conjugated estrogens. Synthetic estrogens include ethinyl estradiol, mestranol, and quinestrol. Nonsteroidal estrogens include diethylstilbestrol and chlorotrianisene. Natural estrogens are preferred in menopausal hormone replacement therapy.

Estrogen can be administered orally, transdermally, vaginally, and by injection. Estrogen delivered orally is transported by enterohepatic circulation to the liver where it undergoes first-pass hepatic metabolism before being transported to peripheral tissues. First-pass liver metabolism is beneficial on lipids but detrimental on factors regulating blood pressure, blood clotting, and triglycerides.

Transdermal administration has the advantage that estrogen is delivered through the skin directly into the peripheral circulation. Estrogen is carried to target tissue without first passing through the liver, thus precluding negative influences on coagulation factors or triglycerides.

Both transdermal and oral estrogen administration are effective in treating major changes associated with estrogen deprivation. Transdermal estrogen and oral estrogen have equal effects on osteoporosis and cardiovascular disease. However, transdermal estrogen requires more time to achieve a similar impact on the lipid profile. Transdermal estrogen has been found to have an additional benefit of reducing rather than elevating the triglyceride level. Oral estrogen may be more effective in treating androgen-excess skin and hair disorders in that transdermal estrogen has less effect on liver production of sex hormone-binding globulin resulting in relatively more free circulating testosterone.

Vaginal estrogen is recommended primarily for local treatment of urogenital atrophy. With atrophic vaginal mucosa, there is initial absorption of vaginal estrogen with measurable increased estrogen in peripheral circulation. However, with recornification of vaginal epithe-

lium, absorption decreases and significant elevation of estrogen in peripheral circulation is difficult to maintain. Vaginal estrogen administration offers the same advantage as transdermal estrogen administration in avoiding first-pass liver metabolism effects.

Injectable estrogen is not recommended for routine menopausal management. Initial serum estrogen levels during the first 10–12 days following administration are higher than needed; then estrogen drops to below ideal therapeutic range. It is also inconvenient and expensive for the patient to return at scheduled intervals for reinjection. Injectable estrogen avoids first-pass liver effects.

Progestins

The use of progestins in menopausal hormone replacement therapy is controversial. The need for a progestin to prevent endometrial hyperplasia and cancer is well established if the uterus is present. However, progestins can be associated with premenstrual syndrome symptoms and have a detrimental effect on cardiovascular risk. Progestational agents exhibit androgenic effects that vary depending on the agent, dose, and route of administration. Progestins are not recommended after hysterectomy. Earlier studies suggesting that breast cancer decreased with the use of progestins have not been confirmed.

At the present time, progestin is primarily administered orally (Table 12-6). Synthetic progestins in the United States include medroxyprogesterone acetate (MAP), norethindrone (NET), norethindrone acetate (NET-A), and norgestrel (NGE). MAP is a 21-carbon compound derived from progesterone, is minimally androgenic, and is the most commonly prescribed progestin in the United States. However, approximately 10–15% of women complain of premenstrual syndrome-like symptoms associated with this medication.

Natural progesterone may also be used but is not yet generally available. Commercial development of natural progesterone has been impaired by problems with absorption. Absorption is related to particle size and suspension vehicle. Micronized native progesterone is well absorbed, producing adequate serum levels, secretory endometrial effect, little impact on lipid profile, and few premenstrual syndrome-like symptoms.

Treatment Regimens

Hormone replacement schedules are compared in Fig. 12-2. The older schedules of cyclic estrogen with or without cyclic progestin are discouraged and the European schedule of continuous estrogen is now being recommended. Progestin for 12 days is indicated if the uterus is present to prevent endometrial hyperplasia. Recent stud-

TABLE 12-6. *Different therapeutic options of progestins*

Medroxyprogesterone acetate (MPA)
Norethindrone (NET)
Norethindrone acetate (NETA-A)
Natural progesterone (NP)

ies indicate progestin may be used at only 2- to 3-month intervals without significant increased risk of endometrial hyperplasia.

Another approach to menopausal hormone replacement therapy is continuous daily administration of both estrogen and progestin. This schedule is intended to induce endometrial atrophy and amenorrhea, and avoid the side effect of menstrual bleeding. Unfortunately, endometrial involution may be slow, and bothersome bleeding may occur and require endometrial evaluation.

Selected Estrogens

Selected estrogens and starting dosages are noted in Table 12-7. Estrace is micronized 17β-estradiol, which is the principal estrogen secreted by the premenopausal ovary. When administered orally, estradiol is conjugated and degraded by the liver to estrone. Estrace has a short half-life and dosage must frequently be given on a BID schedule to maintain adequate serum levels and control of symptoms.

Estraderm Climara and Vivelle are 17β-estradiol administered transdermally. Estraderm is specifically recommended for patients with remote history of thrombophlebitis, hypertension developing on oral estrogen, migraine headaches, hyperglycemia, immediate postoperative period, whenever bypass of the digestive system is de-

HORMONE REPLACEMENT SCHEDULES

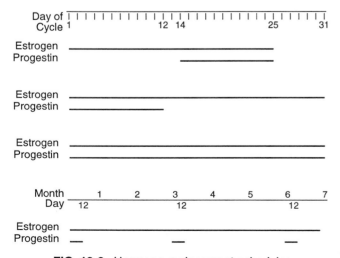

FIG. 12-2. Hormone replacement schedules.

TABLE 12-7. *Selected estrogens and starting dosages*

Name	Ingredients	Recommended starting dose (mg/day)
Oral Estrogens		
Estrace	Micronized estradiol	1.0
Estratab/Menest	Esterified estrogen	0.625
Estratest HS	Esterified estrogen plus methyltestosterone 1.25 mg	0.625
Ogen/Ortho Est	Estrone	0.625
Premarin	Conjugated estrogens	0.625
Premphase	Conjugated estrogens plus medroxyprogesterone acetate 5 mg 14 of 28 days	0.625
Prempro	Conjugated estrogens plus medroxyprogesterone acetate	0.625
Nonoral Estrogen (transdermal)		
Estraderm	17β-Estradiol	0.05
Vivelle	17b-Estradiol	0.05
Climara	17b-Estradiol	0.05

sirable, and for women who smoke. The clinical disadvantage of Estraderm is skin irritation in approximately 17% of patients, which can usually be managed by placing the patch on the back below the belt line area and the use of local cortisone cream after patch removal. The newer matrix systems used in Climara and Vivelle are better tolerated.

Estratab is esterified estrogen, which is a combination of estrogenic substances, principally estrone sulfate, with a small amount of equilin sulfate. Estratest is the same as Estratab plus methyltestosterone. Estratest half-strength contains 0.625 mg of Estratab with 1.25 mg methyltestosterone. Estratest full-strength is double the amount of Estratest HS. Clinically, Estratest is used in young, ovariectomized women with sexual dysfunction.

Ogen and Ortho Est are estropipate, which is purified estrone with no equine estrogens. It is preferred by some because of its purity. Clinically, estropipate is slightly weaker than esterified or conjugated estrogens of comparable milligram dosage because it is pure estrone.

Premarin is conjugated estrogen containing a mixture of estrogenic substances including estrone sulfate, equilin, equilenin, estradiol, and trace amounts of other equine estrogens. Premarin is our oldest estrogen and consequently has the largest clinical base. The antioxidant activity of equine estrogens is greater than that of human estrogens, which may be clinically relevant in prevention of cardiovascular disease and some types of cancer.

The initial starting estrogen dosages are noted in Table 12-7. Estrogen dosage may be increased if needed to control neuroendocrine symptoms but should not be decreased below the recommended starting dosage if decreased cardiovascular risk and osteoporosis prevention are intended treatment goals.

TABLE 12-8. *Selected progestins and starting dosages*

Name	Ingredients	Recommended starting dose (mg/day)
Cyclic Progestins		
Amen	Medroxyprogesterone acetate	5.0
Cycrin	Medroxyprogesterone acetate~	5.0
Micronor	Norethindrone	0.35
Nor QD	Norethindrone	0.35
Provera	Medroxyprogesterone acetate	5.0
Natural micronized progesterone	Progesterone	200
Premphase	Medroxyprogesterone acetate 14 of 28 days plus conjugated estrogens 0.625 mg daily	5.0
Daily Progestins		
Provera	Medroxyprogesterone acetate	2.5
Cycrin	Medroxyprogesterone acetate	2.5
Natural micronized progesterone	Progesterone	100
Prempro	Medroxyprogesterone acetate plus conjugated estrogens 0.625 mg daily	2.5

Selected Progestins

Selected progestins and starting dosages are noted in Table 12-8. Amen, Cycrin, and Provera are all medroxyprogesterone acetate, which is the favored starting synthetic progestin. Provera and Cycrin are available in 2.5-mg, 5-mg, and 10-mg dosages. Amen is a scored 10-mg tablet that can be conveniently broken in two.

Micronor and Nor QD are low-dose progestin-only oral contraceptives containing norethindrone 0.35 mg, which is slightly less potent than 5 mg of medroxyprogesterone acetate. Norethindrone is recommended as the first option for patients with significant premenstrual syndrome-like side effects with medroxyprogesterone acetate.

The progestin dosage in the continuous combined estrogen/progestin replacement program calls for progestin dosage approximately one half that of the conventional 12-day progestin schedule. Norethindrone is not available in the required dosage. Higher progestin dosage in the continuous combined replacement schedule will induce endometrial atrophy more quickly. However, long-term, high-dose daily progestin may increase cardiovascular risk and is not recommended.

CLINICAL TIPS IN MENOPAUSAL MANAGEMENT

Initiation of Therapy

Symptoms of premenstrual syndrome can blend with those of early menopause. Estrogen deficiency can usually be diagnosed on the basis of the patient's age, bleeding pattern, and symptomatology. When question persists, elevated serum FSH and low serum 17β-estradiol (approaching or below 40 pg/ml) is diagnostic of estrogen deficiency. In perimenopausal patients ovulatory with hot flushes near menses, supplemental estrogen consisting of conjugated estrogens 0.3 mg daily will provide significant relief of hot flushes. When patients become anovulatory for 6 months, a progestin is added to the treatment regimen and the estrogen dose is increased as needed to control symptoms. Another option in this perimenopausal time is a low-dose combination oral contraceptive that does not contain norgestrel. This choice is particularly indicated in women still needing contraception and can be used in nonsmokers until age 55. Initiation of conventional menopausal hormone replacement therapy is ideally begun within 1 year of the final spontaneous menstrual period, although significant benefits can still be achieved starting therapy years later.

Duration of Therapy

Duration of therapy is dictated by the indication for which therapy was originally initiated. Cardiovascular indications may require life-long therapy. Osteoporosis prevention indicates 10–15 years or more of hormonal therapy related to age at menopausal onset. Neuroendocrine changes involving vasomotor instability and psychological changes are generally self-limiting problems in which therapy can be tapered or discontinued within 3–5 years. Urogenital atrophy will continue for the remainder of life, although changes may become asymptomatic with time. Changes associated with sexual function and skin may also become asymptomatic with time.

Discontinuation of Therapy

Menopausal hormone replacement therapy is discontinued when maximal benefit of therapy has been accomplished, when previous indications for therapy are no longer a problem, or when potential risk of therapy exceeds potential benefit. Dosage of estrogen therapy should generally be stepped down gradually; otherwise hot flushes may recur. When a progestational agent is administered cyclically, both estrogen and progestin should be discontinued following the final day of progestin administration. Hormone replacement therapy may need to be discontinued abruptly if the patient develops a contraindication to the use of therapy.

Inappropriate Uterine Bleeding

Uterine bleeding usually occurs on day 9–10 or beyond of cyclic progestin. Bleeding will usually last no more than 5-7 days then stop with no more bleeding until day 9-10 or beyond of the following progestin cycle. Bleeding at other times is considered inappropriate and endometrial evaluation is indicated. Following a negative endometrial evaluation, continued inappropriate bleeding should be evaluated by hysteroscopy, transvaginal ultrasound, saline infusion uterine sonography, and/or dilatation and curettage.

Uterine bleeding on the continuous combined estrogen-progestin therapy regimen is variable during the first 9-15 months of therapy but should not occur more than every 25-30 days with flow not longer than 7-10 days or heavier than a usual menstrual period. Bleeding outside these parameters requires endometrial evaluation. Hysteroscopy, sonography, and/or dilatation and curettage procedures may be selectively indicated. Following evaluation, patients can be observed with reassurance. If bleeding is an excessive nuisance, daily progestin dosage can be doubled for three months to induce earlier endometrial atrophy, then return to the conventional dosage schedule. Another clinical option at initiation of a continuous combined therapy regimen is to begin with a higher dosage progestin during the first three months to induce earlier endometrial atrophy, then begin conventional low-dose daily continuous combined estrogen-progestin therapy.

Testosterone

Testosterone is recommended in women below age 50 who have undergone bilateral ovariectomy who complain of decreased sexual function not responding to conventional estrogen replacement therapy. Testosterone may also be indicated in other selected problems with sexual dysfunction relative to loss of libido.

Breast Tenderness

Breast tenderness is commonly associated with estrogen therapy. Tenderness will resolve over time in most patients. Caffeine restriction and weight loss help reduce tenderness. Cycling off estrogen for 5 days following completion of the progestin phase of the cycle can be recommended if the problem persists.

Smoke Cessation

All people should be encouraged to stop smoking and referred to a smoke cessation program when needed. Smoking women enter menopause $1\frac{1}{2}$ to 2 years earlier than nonsmokers. Smokers have significantly increased cardiovascular disease; osteoporosis; lung cancer; urogenital malignancies including bladder, vulvar, and cervical cancer; and premature senile skin changes. Nonoral estrogen administration is recommended in smokers to avoid first-pass liver metabolism effect.

Contraception

Contraception should be maintained for at least a year following the patient's last spontaneous menstrual period. Menopausal doses of hormone replacement therapy will not suppress spontaneous ovulation. Natural family planning is unreliable due to irregular ovulation. Intrauterine contraceptives are an option. Low-dose oral contraceptives that do not contain norgestrel can be used until age 55 in women who do not smoke. Injectable contraceptives, including the subcutaneous norgestrel implant and Depo MPA, are also viable options.

Therapeutic Alternatives

Women who cannot or will not use conventional menopausal hormone replacement therapy can be offered other options therapy. Patients with breast cancer can be offered tamoxifen (10 mg BID), which has approximately the same effect as conjugated estrogen 0.625 mg daily in reducing most menopausal changes except hot flushes. Periodic endometrial evaluation is indicated on the same schedule as if unopposed estrogen were being used. Therapy should otherwise be directed at specific areas of menopausal changes. Cardiovascular risk can be decreased with lifestyle modifications related to diet, smoking, and exercise and the use of blood pressure- and cholesterol-modulating medications when indicated. Osteoporosis risk can be reduced with calcium, exercise, calcitonin, and biphosphates. Urogenital atrophy can be reduced with a vaginal moisturizing lotion and dyspareunia reduced with personal lubricants during intercourse. Androgen-excess hair disorders can be reduced with spironolactone and minoxidil. Hot flushes can be reduced by avoiding triggering events including heat, alcohol, caffeine, cigarette smoke, and stress. Hot flush frequency and intensity can also be reduced with clonidine, antiprostaglandins, and synthetic progestins. Natural progesterone should not be used in patients with breast cancer (it can be converted to estrone and estradiol). Stress management may be indicated for psychologic support.

COST AND BENEFIT

The beneficial impact of menopausal hormone replacement therapy on the care of mature women is significant. Decreased mortality in the United States with use of this therapy includes 250,000 fewer heart attacks and strokes and 30,000 fewer hip fractures. Endometrial cancer mortality is also decreased slightly. The cost side of the equation relates to increased breast cancer risk. The projected breast cancer mortality for 1996 is 44,300. Recent studies have indicated no increased breast cancer risk at lower estrogen doses and only a 7% overall increased risk for all dosages. Thus, increased breast cancer mortality of zero to 3101 lives per year is balanced by a savings of 280,000 lives per year from cardiovascular disease and osteoporosis. In addition, with total cost of cardiovascular disease in men and women projected to exceed $100 billion in 1995, a 50% reduction of this disease in women would save billions in health care expenditures. The cost–benefit ratio relating to lives and dollars is by far in favor of menopausal hormone replacement therapy.

Quality of life cannot be measured in terms of lives or dollars, but involves sense of well being, cognitive function, day-to-day coping, functioning at home and on the job, self-perception, and perception by others. Providing increased quality and duration of life for the increasing population of postmenopausal women justifies our concern for and involvement with this group of women.

SELECTED READING

Andrews WC. Menopause and hormone replacement. *Obstet Gynecol* 1996;87:S1–S53.

Grady D, Petitti D, Rubin SM, Audet A-M. Guidelines for counseling postmenopausal women about preventive hormone therapy. *Ann Intern Med* 1992;117:1038–1041.

Grady D, Rubin SM, Petitti DB, Fox CS, Black D, Ettinger B, Ernester VL, Cummings SR. Hormone therapy to prevent disease and prolong life in postmenopausal women. *Ann Intern Med* 1992;117:1016–1037.

Lobo RA. Estrogen replacement: the evolving role of alternative delivery systems. *Am J Obstet Gynecol* 1995;175:981–1006.

Mishell DR, ed. Interdisciplinary review of estrogen replacement therapy. *Am J Obstet Gynecol* 1989;161:1825–1868.

New concepts in menopausal management. *Comtemp Ob/Gyn Supplement* (Editorial), November 1995.

Post Graduate Medicine: A Special Report. Proceedings of the Second Annual Symposium on the Long-Term Effects of Estrogen Deprivation. New York: McGraw-Hill, April 1989.

Utain WH, et al. Current perspectives in the management of the menopausal and postmenopausal patient. *Obstet Gynecol* 1990;75:1S–81S.

Writing Group for the PEPI Trial. Effects of estrogen or estrogen/progestin regimen on heart disease risk factors in postmenopausal women. *JAMA* 1995;273:199–208.

Clinical Reproductive Medicine,
Edited by Bryan D. Cowan and David B. Seifer
Lippincott-Raven Publishers, Philadelphia © 1997

CHAPTER 13

Dynamic Testing of Glandular Reserve

Lisa Barrie Schwartz and David B. Seifer

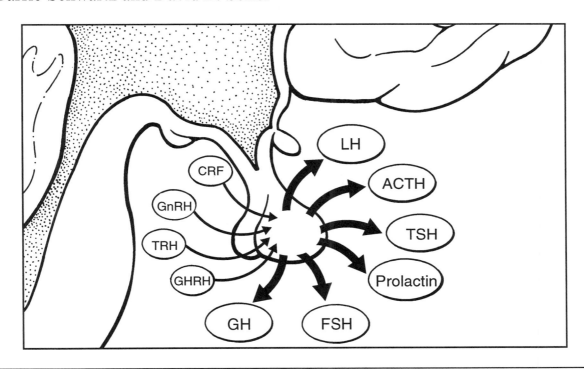

Definitions of Dynamic Testing
**Basic Principles of Suppression and
    Stimulation Tests**
Hormonal Deficiencies
  Gonadotropin Deficiency
  Thyroid Deficiency
  Prolactin Deficiency
  Growth Hormone Deficiency
  ACTH Deficiency

Hormonal Overproduction
  Thyroid Excess
  Prolactin Excess
  Growth Hormone Excess
  ACTH Excess
  Androgen Excess
  Combined Testing
Summary and Future Direction
Suggested Reading

   L. B. Schwartz: Department of Obstetrics and Gynecology, New York University Medical Center,
New York, NY 10016; and D. B. Seifer: Department of Obstetrics and Gynecology, The Ohio State
University Medical Center, Columbus, OH 43210

DEFINITIONS OF DYNAMIC TESTING

Dynamic testing refers to suppression and stimulation tests. Suppression tests assess hormonal overproduction, and stimulation tests evaluate diminished glandular reserve or function.

Stimulation tests are informative when patients have normal baseline values but diminished hormonal reserve, and provide information regarding the integrity of the system under stress. A substance that normally stimulates the primary target organ is infused and hormone levels are measured before and after stimulation. Pathologic conditions such as tumor, infection, hemorrhage, or immunologic disease can result in diminished reserve. Prolonged absence of stimulation can cause an attenuated response to an acute stimulus. Stimulation testing is useful in evaluating the following conditions: precocious puberty, hypothyroidism, short stature, Addison's disease, and hyperandrogenism.

Suppression testing evaluates hormonal overproduction in elevated baseline hormone conditions and assesses autonomous hormonal secretion. A substance known to suppress the system is administered, before and after which hormone levels are obtained. Suppressibility indicates that hormone overproduction is not autonomous. Hyperthyroidism, hyperprolactinemia, acromegaly, Cushing's syndrome, and hyperandrogenism can be evaluated with specific suppression tests.

BASIC PRINCIPLES OF SUPPRESSION AND STIMULATION TESTS

Tables 13-1 and 13-2 review the clinical relevance, guidelines for interpretation, side effects, and contraindications of the more commonly used suppression and stimulation tests.

Suppression and stimulation tests (SSTs) have unique value in evaluating the integrity of the endocrine system under dynamic conditions. They are usually safely and easily performed under proper medical surveillance. The wide array of normal variation between and within individuals (such as circadian rhythms and pulsatility) can be more carefully evaluated with dynamic testing. Subtle degrees of dysfunction that single-hormone assays may not detect can be revealed in the context of challenge tests. Many functional glandular responses become abnormal only after pituitary reserve has become greatly compromised. Suppression and stimulation tests can evaluate the feedback control and the location of the abnormality (ie, hypothalamus, pituitary, or end-organ). Dynamic testing may also determine the etiology of various syndromes (ie, Cushing's syndrome, hyperandrogenism, and hyperprolactinemia).

Some difficulties in interpreting suppression and stimulation tests stem from lack of standardization of dosage, administration, and variations of timing of hormone measurements. Lack of consideration of the altered response with age can also make reliable interpretation more difficult. In addition, responses to SST may vary within an individual menstrual cycle and between individuals because of differences in sex, stage of puberty, or age. The coexistence of medical ailments, depression, obesity, anorexia, drug use, and/or disturbed sleep patterns represent additional confounding factors that prevent simple interpretation of suppression and stimulation tests.

Any situation that affects the specificity of a radioimmunoassay (RIA) will affect the specificity of a suppression and stimulation test. Specific examples include the presence of hormone fragments, prohormones, glycosylated glycoproteins, binding proteins, γ-globulins, ectopic hormonal secretion, and cross-reactions between subunits of different glycopeptides. Sensitivity can be altered by storage methods or transport delay.

Suppression and stimulation tests must be interpreted within the appropriate clinical context with regard to the objective of the test. Recognizing the trend or alteration is often more informative than the absolute hormone levels themselves.

HORMONAL DEFICIENCIES

Gonadotropin Deficiency

Gonadotropin-releasing hormone (GnRH) is a hypothalamic decapeptide secreted in a pulsatile fashion that stimulates secretion of pituitary luteinizing hormone (LH) and follicle-stimulating hormone (FSH). Disrupted pulsatile release of GnRH leads to interrupted episodic gonadotropin secretion resulting in amenorrhea or oligomenorrhea. The GnRH test is one of the more frequently used stimulation tests by both gynecologists and pediatricians because of its broad clinical relevance in evaluating patients with syndromes such as amenorrhea or oligomenorrhea, precocious puberty, and anorexia nervosa. The test can also be used to assess serially pituitary reserve following transsphenoidal surgery and pituitary irradiation, and to monitor response to treatment of various syndromes.

The GnRH stimulation test was initially proposed to distinguish pituitary from hypothalamic dysfunction. Following measurement of baseline LH and FSH, 2.5 µg/kg up to 100 µg maximum of GnRH is infused and LH and FSH measured at 0, 30, 60, 90, and 120 minutes. The response is influenced by the menstrual cycle, with greater stimulation of LH seen in the luteal phase. During the proliferative phase, the normal response is a doubling of LH from baseline and a 1.5 times increase in FSH. In the luteal phase, LH increases to four to eight times baseline and FSH increases to two times baseline. After GnRH administration, peak levels of LH and FSH occur at 30 and 60 minutes, respectively.

Classically, patients with pituitary failure do not respond, and a blunted response is seen in hypothalamic failure. In reality, the GnRH test has not proven reliable as a test to discriminate hypothalamic versus pituitary causes of hypogonadotropic hypogonadism as originally anticipated. The overlap in responses is too large. Clinically, it has been more useful to demonstrate that the pituitary is capable of gonadotropin release when stimulated.

Another useful test for evaluating amenorrhea is the clomiphene stimulation test. Clomiphene citrate (100 mg orally daily for 7 days) is given after measurement of baseline gonadotropins. Normally, both LH and FSH should double on day 8. A subnormal response suggests hypothalamic-pituitary disease.

In general, the response to exogenous GnRH in children reflects the presence of endogenous GnRH "priming" of the pituitary. In prepubertal children, the hypothalamus is extremely sensitive to negative feedback by very low levels of gonadal steroids. As puberty is approached, hypothalamic sensitivity gradually lessens leading to increased GnRH secretion. With continued GnRH exposure, the pituitary becomes more responsive and secretes more gonadotropins, especially LH. With endogenous GnRH as a primer, pituitary sensitivity to exogenous GnRH is enhanced as children approach puberty. The GnRH test in normal prepubertal children produces an absent or diminished response (with the magnitude of the FSH rise greater than that of LH). With the onset of puberty the LH response to the GnRH test rises briskly. LH values may rise to four to six times baseline, and there is usually little or no change in FSH. The GnRH test can be used to monitor treatment of sexual precocity with GnRH analogs by documenting prepubertal gonadotropin responses.

Low-weight anorectics have consistently displayed low and nonpulsatile basal LH and FSH levels with reduced 24-hour LH secretion. Their LH response to GnRH has been reported to be both blunted and normal, with a normal or exaggerated FSH response. Although normal-weight bulimics also have low basal gonadotropin levels, they have been found to have a hyperresponse of LH to exogenous GnRH. This response has been even more exaggerated during hospitalization, resembling the heightened LH response to exogenous LRH reported in anorectics after weight recovery. Higher LH response to GnRH at the onset of treatment has been shown to be related to restoration of the menstrual cycle during successful treatment, which suggests that its use has a predictive value. GnRH testing has been used to follow the course of the disease process. Increased LH secretion after GnRH during treatment suggests that the patient is recovering, whereas decreased LH response indicates progressive disease.

Thyroid Deficiency

Thyroid gland (primary), pituitary (secondary), and hypothalamic (tertiary) dysfunction can all lead to the hypothyroid state. TSH is elevated in primary but decreased in secondary and tertiary disease. The thyrotropin-releasing hormone (TRH) stimulation test is a useful method to evaluate subtle subclinical thyroid disorders that single hormonal assays may not detect (ie, TSH and T_4 may be in the normal range). To evaluate TSH reserve, 200–500 μg of TRH is infused and TSH measured at 0, 30, 60, 90, 120, and 180 minutes. Normally, TSH rises from 5 to 30 μU/ml above baseline by 30 minutes. Absence of such a response is seen with pituitary failure (secondary). Delayed response (45–90 minutes) with slow return to baseline suggests hypothalamic disease (tertiary). An exaggerated TSH response to TRH may be diagnostic of equivocal or mild primary hypothyroidism.

The TRH stimulation test can also indirectly evaluate euthyroid patients with other forms of hypothalamic-pituitary diseases. Acromegalic euthyroid patients have diminished TSH response to TRH and dramatic increases in growth hormone following exogenous TRH. TRH stimulates secretion of prolactin, and therefore an inadequate response suggests lactotrope failure. Blunted TSH response to exogenous TRH can occur in euthyroid patients with other disorders such as depression, critical illness, and anorexia/bulimia.

Initiation of thyroid replacement therapy depends on the free T_4 and not the results of the TRH stimulation test. Patients with abnormal responses to TRH stimulation should have their thyroid indexes monitored clinically.

Prolactin Deficiency

Prolactin secretion is absent only when there is complete failure or destruction of the pituitary gland. As the principle hormone involved in milk biosynthesis, failure of lactation is usually the only presenting symptom of hypoprolactinemia. In fact, the failure to lactate within the first 7 postpartum days may be the first symptom of Sheehan's syndrome (hypopituitarism following intrapartum infarction of the pituitary gland). Inability of the pituitary to secrete prolactin in response to stimulation (ie, with TRH, metoclopramide, chlorpromazine, or insulin-induced hypoglycemia) is diagnostic of diminished prolactin reserve.

Growth Hormone Deficiency

In general, short stature in children is the only symptom of growth hormone (GH) deficiency. Identification of GH deficiency in children is usually required to justify GH replacement therapy. Psychosocial factors such as behavioral disturbances, neglect, and malnutrition can result in short stature and biochemically resemble GH

TABLE 13-1. *Stimulation testing of the*

Hormone-deficient	Clinical gynecologic syndrome	History	Physical examination	Screening tests
1. LH/FSH	Amenorrhea, oligomenorrhea, infertility, hypoestrogenic symptoms	Weight changes, stress, drugs, psychiatric problems, neurologic complaints, postmenopausal, delayed puberty	Neurologic examination, inspect vaginal mucosa	Pregnancy test, prolactin, FSH/LH, TSH, progestin challenge
2. TSH (hypothyroidism)	Menstrual disorders, hypothyroidism, infertility, galactorrhea	Fatigue, dry coarse skin, reduced body/scalp hair, swelling, cold intolerance, decreased sweating, husky voice, weight gain despite anorexia, decreased memory, hearing impairment, constipation, muscle cramps, arthralgias, paresthesias	Bradycardia, nonpitting edema, yellow complexion, large thyroid, ataxia, peripheral neuropathy	TFTs, TSH, prolactin
3. Prolactin	Failure of lactation	Inability to breast-feed	Neurologic examination, breast examination	Prolactin
4. GH	Adults—none, children—growth disorders	Symptoms of other pituitary diseases; rule out behavioral disturbances, neglect, and malnutrition in children	Neurologic examination, short stature	GH

pituitary (evaluation of hypopituitarism)

Stimulation tests	Normal response	Interpretation of results	Side effects	Contraindications
a. GnRH 100 μg IV	LH 2 × BL at 30 min and FSH 1.5 × BL at 60 min (proliferative phase); LH 4–8 × BL (luteal phase)	No response with pituitary failure, blunted response with hypothalamic failure	Transient thirst	None described
b. Clomiphene citrate 100 mg/d × 7 d PO	LH 2 × BL and FSH 2 × BL on day 8	Subnormal response suggests hypothalamic or pituitary disease	Visual symptoms, headache, dryness or hair loss, nausea, vomiting, vasomotor flushes, bloating, soreness, breast discomfort	Liver disease, abnormal uterine bleeding
a. TRH 200–500 μg IV	Increased TSH 5–30 μU/ml in 30 min	Exaggerated response (1°) or no response (2°) suggests pituitary failure, delayed response with slow return to BL suggest hypothalamic disease (3°) (Diminished TSH response also occurs in euthyroid patients with pituitary lesions, especially acromegaly)	Transient high blood pressure, an urge to void, fascial flushing	None described
a. TRH 200–500 μg IV	Prolactin 2 × BL in 15–30 min	Inadequate response suggests failure of lactotropes	Transient high blood pressure, an urge to void	None described
b. Chlorpromazine 25 mg IM/PO	Prolactin 2–3 × BL in 60–90 min	No response with pituitary or hypothalamic failure	Hypotension, dizziness, extra-pyramidal reactions	Cannot use in combination with CNS depressants
c. Metoclopramide 10 mg IV	Prolactin 6 × BL	Blunted response with hypothalamic or pituitary disease	Extrapyramidal symptoms	Gastrointestinal hemorrhage, obstruction, or perforation; pheochromocytoma; epilepsy
d. Insulin-induced hypoglycemia	Not standardized	Not standardized	See 4a	See 4a
a. Insulin IV 0.05–0.15 U/kg BW	Glucose <40 mg/dl or <50% BL, GH >7 ng/ml at 60 min	Subnormal response on two tests suggests pituitary insufficiency	Provokes adrenal crisis in patients with adrenal or pituitary insufficiency, produces adrenergic stimulatory hypoglycemia symptoms, angina	Adrenal or pituitary failure, diabetes, cardiac or cerebrovascular disease, pheochromocytoma or insulinoma, epilepsy
b. GHRH (no established protocol) 1 μg/kg IV bolus	No established protocol	No established protocol	Facial flushing	None described
c. Exercise × 20 min	GH >7 ng/ml	Subnormal response with GH deficiency	None described	None described
d. Arginine 30 g IV over 30 min	GH >7 ng/ml at 60 min	Subnormal response with GH deficiency	None described	Liver or renal disease
e. L-dopa 500 mg PO	GH >7 ng/ml at 90 min	Subnormal response with GH deficiency	Orthostatic symptoms, nausea	Narrow angle glaucoma, malignant melanoma, patients on MAOIs
f. Vasopressin 10 U IM	GH >5 ng/ml at 60 min	Subnormal response with GH deficiency	Transient warmth, abdominal cramps, false defecation urge, ECG changes	Elderly, cardiovascular disease
g. Glucagon 1 mg IM	GH >5 ng/ml at 150 min	Subnormal response with GH deficiency	Nausea, vomiting, hypoglycemia	Pheochromocytoma, insulinoma, diabetes, elderly, cardiovascular disease

TABLE 13-1.

Hormone-deficient	Clinical gynecologic syndrome	History	Physical examination	Screening tests
5. Corticotropin	Amenorrhea	Fatigue, weight loss, anorexia, loss of axillary hair, skin pigmentation	Hypotension, unexplained hypovolemic shock (with acute insufficiency)	Low morning serum cortisol

LH, Luteinizing hormone; FSH, follicle-stimulating hormone; TSH, thyroid-stimulating hormone; GnRH, gonadotropin-releasing hormone; BL, baseline; TFT, thyroid function test; CNS, central nervous system; GH, growth hormone; BW, body weight; GHRH, growth hormone–releasing hormone; MAOI, monoamine oxidase inhibitor; OHCS, hydroxycorticosteroids.

(Continued.)

Stimulation tests	Normal response	Interpretation of results	Side effects	Contraindications
a. Insulin IV 0.05–0.15 U/kg	Glucose <40 mg/dl or 50% BL, cortisol increased by 10 mg/dl with peak ≥20 μg/dl in 60 min	Inadequate response suggests failure in hypothalamic pituitary adrenal axis	See 4a	See 4a
b. Metyrapone 750 mg PO every 4 h × 24 h	Cortisol <7 μg/dl, 17-OHCS 2 × BL and increased 10–40 mg/24 h Deoxycortisol >10 μg/dl at 8:00 am 24 h after dose	Subnormal response suggests either primary or secondary adrenal insufficiency	Adrenal crisis in patients with adrenal or pituitary failure	Known adrenal or pituitary failure
c. Synthetic corticotropin (Cortrosyn 250 μg IV)	Cortisol increased by ≥7 μg/dl to values >18 μg/dl by 1 h	Subnormal response suggests either primary or secondary adrenal insufficiency	Allergic reaction, facial flushing	Asthma
d. Prolonged corticotropin stimulation 250 μg IV Cortrosyn every d × 3d	Cortisol 15–40 μg/dl on day 1, and 30–60 μg/dl on days 2, 3; 17-OHCS 15–40 mg/24 h day 1 and 30–40 mg/24 h days 2,3	In secondary, but not primary, adrenal insufficiency cortisol secretion will increase after 3 days of priming	Allergic reaction, facial flushing	Asthma
e. CRF 100–500 μg IV (no well-established protocol)	Corticotropin 3.6 × BL at 30–60 min, cortisol 2.3 × BL at 60–90 min, aldosterone 1.6 × BL at 60 min	Blunted or no response with pituitary disease, exaggerated response with hypothalamic disease	Cold/warm sensation, slight increase in BP	None described
f. Glucagon 1 mg IM	Cortisol >18 μg/dl or ≥μg/dl above BL	Blunted response with failure in the pituitary adrenal axis	See 4g	See 4g

TABLE 13-2. *Suppression*

Hormone overproduced	Clinical gynecologic syndrome	History	PE	Screening test
1. Hyperthyroidism	Amenorrhea/ oligomenorrhea	Nervousness, tremor, weight loss, increased appetite, palpitations, heat intolerance, emotional lability, muscle weakness, neck swelling, hyperdefecation, rapid speech, fidgety	Exophthalmos, tachycardia, enlarged thyroid, warm smooth skin, tremor, proximal muscle weakness	TFTs, TSH
2. Prolactin (hyperprolactin)	Oligomenorrhea/ amenorrhea, galactorrhea, hypoestrogenic symptoms, infertility	Stress, hypothyroidism, drug use, chest trauma, breast stimulation, pregnancy, suckling, estrogen therapy, chronic renal failure, hypoglycemia	Bitemporal hemianopsia, breast discharge, confirm presence of fat globules under low-power light microscopy	Prolactin ≥25 ng/ml, TFTs/TSH, CT scan
3. GH (acromegaly)	Age-dependent increased skeletal growth causing "giantism" (before epiphyseal fusion); during adult life; soft tissue swelling, hypertrophied extremities and face, thick leathery skin, increased hair growth and pigmentation, increased sweating, prognathism, deepened voice, visceromegaly, peripheral neuropathy	During childhood— gigantism; during adult life—slow development of signs and symptoms of "tissue overgrowth"	Stimata of acromegaly	GH, somatomedin C, CT/MRI of the brain

testing of the pituitary

Suppression test	Normal response	Interpretation of results	Side effects	Contraindications
a. T$_3$ suppression test 75 – 100 µg T$_3$ (Cytomel) every day for 1 wk or 3 mg T$_4$	24-h RIA uptake <50% BL	In patients with hyperthyroidism or autonomous thyroid function, there is no RIA suppression	None described	Cardiovascular disease
b. (TRH stimulation)	See Table 13-1	Suppressed TSH response to TRH is consistent with the diagnosis of hyperthyroidism (also have blunted prolactin response)	See Table 13-1	See Table 13-1
a. L-dopa 500 mg PO	Prolactin < 150 µg/L	Suppression indicative of functional hyperprolactinemia rather than microadenoma	See Table 13-1, 4e	See Table 13-1, 4e
b. Bromocriptine 2.5 mg PO	Prolactin < 58–83% BL	Suppresses both functional and tumorous hyperprolactinemia	Hypotension, dizziness, headache	Sensitivity to any ergot alkaloids, patients on antihypertension medication
c. Nomifensine 200 mg PO	Prolactin <65% BL	Nonsuppression with prolactinomas	None described	None described
d. (TRH stimulation)	See Table 13-1	Diminished response indicative of prolactinomas	See Table 13-1	See Table 13-1
e. (Insulin-induced hypoglycemia)	See Table 13-1, 4a	Subnormal response with tumor patients, and excessive response with nontumor patients	See Table 13-1, 4a	See Table 13-1, 4a
f. (Chlorpromazine 25 mg IM)	See Table 13-1, 3b	Flat response with prolactinomas (increased prolactin response with higher doses)	See Table 13-1, 3b	See Table 13-1, 3c
g. (Metoclopramide 10 mg PO)	See Table 13-1, 3c	Impaired response with prolactinoma	See Table 13-1, 3c	Diabetes
a. Glucose suppression test 2 g/kg BWPO or 0.5 g/kg BW IV	GH <5 ng/ml	Paradoxical response to hyperglycemia	None described	Diabetes
b. (TRH stimulation)	Paradoxical growth hormone response to TRH (sharp increase in GH after TRH administration)	TRH also increases growth hormone secretion in advanced renal failure, anorexia nervosa, and severe malnutrition	See Table 13-1	See Table 13-1

TABLE 13-2.

Hormone overproduced	Clinical gynecologic syndrome	History	PE	Screening test
4. Corticotropin (Cushing's syndrome)	Signs of cortisol excess, hirsutism, oligomenorrhea	Proximal muscle weakness, depression, osteoporosis, spontaneous ecchymoses, petechiae, inability to concentrate	Hirsutism, striae, acne, central obesity with round face and truncal fat accumulation, hypertension, hyperpigmentation	Androgens, electrolytes, 24-h urine cortisol >100 µg/24 h, CT scan, plasma corticotropin
5. Androgens (Hyperandrogenism)	Hirsutism, androgenization, PCOD, oligomenorrhea, infertility, virilization	Clitoromegaly, male hair pattern, temporal balding, voice change, drug intake	Elevated BP, hirsutism, clitoromegaly, male hair distribution	DHEA/DHEAS, androstenedione, testosterone, 24-h urine steroids (17-OHCS, 17-KS, 17-KGS), 17-OHP, 24-h urine free cortisol

RIA, Radioimmunassay; TRH, thyrotropin-releasing hormone; 17-OHCS, 17-hydroxycorticosteroid; PCOD, polycystic ovarian disease; DHEA, dehydroepiandrosterone; DHEAS, dehydroepiandrosterone sulfate; KS, potassium sulfate; KGS, 17-ketogenic steroid; OHP, hydroxyprogesterone; ACTH, adrenocorticotropic hormone; hCG, human chorionic gonadotropin; OC, oral contraceptive. All other abbreviations as in Table 13-1.

(Continued).

Suppression test	Normal response	Interpretation of results	Side effects	Contraindications
a. Overnight dexamethasone 1 mg PO at 11 pm	Cortisol <6 µg/dl	If elevated, probably Cushing's syndrome (in the absence of obesity, estrogen, depression, phenytoin, stress, alcoholism)	None described	None described
b. Low-dose dexamethasone 0.5 mg PO every 6 h × 2 d	17-OHCS <4 mg/24 h, urinary free cortisol <20 µg/24 h on D#2, serum cortisol <5 µg/dl on D#2	If elevated, probably Cushing's syndrome (in the absence of obesity, estrogen, depression, phenytoin, stress, alcoholism)	None described	None described
c. High-dose dexamethasone 2 mg PO q 6 h × 2 d	Urinary 17-PHCS ≤4% day 2, serum cortisol <10 µg/dl on day 2	Suppression of corticotropin and cortisol in Cushing's disease; no suppression with autonomous adrenal function or ectopic corticotropin production	None described	None described
d. CRF 100–500 µg IV	See Table 13-1, 5e	Exaggerated response in Cushing's disease, and flat response with ectopic corticotropin production	See Table 13-1, 5e	See Table 13-1, 5e
a. (ACTH stimulation) Cortrosyn 250 µg IV	Not standardized	Elevated precursor hormones with adrenal enzyme defects	See Table 13-1	See Table 13-1
b. Prolonged dexamethasone 2 mg PO q d × 2 wk	DHEAS <400 ng/ml, cortisol <40 ng/ml	Suppression of androgens to normal indicates adrenal origin of androgens	None described	None described
c. (HCG 5000 U qOD × 3 d)	Not standardized	Rise in androgens indicates ovarian etiology	Ovarian hyperstimulation	Ovarian cysts
d. OC 50 µg mestranol and 1 mg norethindrone daily × 3 wk PO	Testosterone and androstenedione reduced by half	Reduced androgens if of ovarian etiology (cannot rule out tumors)	Thromboembolic disease	Cerebrovascular or coronary disease, hepatitis, breast and endometrial cancer, pregnancy, smokers, congenital hyperlipidemia

deficiency. Random basal GH levels may be low but are not reliable for distinguishing between normal patients and those with deficient GH.

Evaluation of GH deficiency has been most commonly and reliably performed with the indirect insulin challenge test (ICT), although other methods have been described, such as GH-releasing hormone (GHRH), sleep, exercise, arginine, L-dopa, vasopressin, corticotropin, and glucagon (see Table 13-1). Normally, GH is suppressed by hyperglycemia and stimulated by other factors including hypoglycemia, arginine, and sleep. The ICT creates a hypoglycemic state after insulin (0.05–0.15 U/kg not to exceed 10 U) is infused to the fasted patient. Glucose and GH are measured at 0, 30, 45, 60, 90, and 120 minutes. Glucose must decrease by 50% or to <40 mg/dl, following which GH normally increases to >7 ng/ml, peaking at 60 minutes. Contraindications to the ICT include suspected panhypopituitarism (because of possible profound hypoglycemia) and cardiac or cerebrovascular disease (because of reflex sympathetic discharge). Intravenous glucose and hydrocortisone should be available for emergent use. Hypothyroidism or obesity impair the GH response.

L-dopa and insulin-induced hypoglycemia are reportedly the most reliable stimuli. However, growth hormone responses to L-dopa are often reduced in depressed patients. More variable results are obtained from arginine, vasopressin, and glucagon. Glucagon has been found to be a reliable, reproducible, and safe alternative to the ICT, with response impaired by age but not sex. Due to the variable results reported with the array of GH stimulation tests, it is generally believed that GH deficiency should be diagnosed only after inadequate responses to two different types of GH stimulation tests.

Both basal and provoked GH levels have been shown to depend on pubertal stage. An increase in GH secretion has been reported with increasing sexual maturation. Thus, in evaluating children with this testing, only those in the same pubertal stages should be compared.

ACTH Deficiency

ACTH is normally secreted in a pulsatile fashion with greater frequency and amplitude in the early morning, shortly before awakening. A nadir is reached in the evening to about half the morning value. Thus, there is a diurnal pattern with ACTH and cortisol levels highest in the early morning and lowest in the evening. Either the loss of diurnal variation or abnormal secretion can result in various syndromes (see Tables 13-1 and 13-2).

Indirect stimulation testing has traditionally been applied to evaluate the integrity of the hypothalamic-pituitary-adrenocortical axis. Most commonly used has been insulin-induced hypoglycemia, also referred to as the ICT. Insulin (0.05–0.15 U/kg) is infused, and both glucose and cortisol are measured at 0, 30, 45, 60, 90, and 120 minutes. With induced hypoglycemia, cortisol increases by 10 μg/dl with peak value >20 μg/dl within 60 minutes. Hypoglycemia followed by an inadequate cortisol response reflects insufficient corticotropin reserve and indicates failure in the hypothalamic-pituitary-adrenal axis.

The metyrapone test has been the next most commonly used indirect test. Metyrapone interferes with the 11-hydroxylation step in cortisol synthesis by blocking 11b-hydroxylase enzyme activity. By limiting cortisol synthesis, the negative feedback action of cortisol is prevented and ACTH secretion normally increases and drives the overproduction of cortisol precursors more proximal to the block (11-deoxycortisol, urinary 17-hydroxycorticosteroids [17-OHCS]). Baseline 24-hour urine for 17-OHCS is collected for 2 days. On day three, 750 mg of metyrapone (300 mg/m^2 in children) is administered orally every 4 hours for 24 hours. On day 4, 8 a.m. cortisol and 11-deoxycortisol are obtained and 24-hour urine for 17-OHCS is collected. Cortisol <7 mg/dl indicates adequate blockade, and 11-deoxycortisol >10 mg/dl represents a normal response. 17-OHCS should be twice baseline and increase to 10–20 mg/24 hours.

To stimulate the adrenal cortex, 250 mg synthetic ACTH (Cortrosyn) is given either intramuscularly or intravenously to the fasted patient. Cortisol is measured at 0, 30, and 60 minutes, and normally increased by >7 mg/dl to 18 mg/dl in 1 hour. Subnormal response is diagnostic of adrenal insufficiency but does not distinguish primary (end-organ) from secondary dysfunction. In adrenal insufficiency due to hypothalamic or pituitary dysfunction (secondary Addison's disease), cortisol secretion will increase after priming of the adrenal cortex. This is accomplished by the prolonged 3-day ACTH stimulation test. Twenty-four hour urine 17-OHCS is collected for 2 days, following which 250 mg Cortrosyn is infused daily for 3 days. Normally, cortisol increases by 15–40 mg/dl on day 1 reaching 30–60 mg/dl the following day, and 17-OHCS increases by 15–40 mg/24 hours on day 1 to ultimately 30–40 mg/24 hours. Lack of response suggests end-organ failure. Although more useful in the past, these tests have recently been surpassed by the ACTH RIA and aldosterone measurements.

The new direct synthetic corticotropin-releasing factor (CRF) stimulation test may replace indirect testing. The CRF test involves infusing 100–500 mg CRF and collecting blood samples at 0, 15, 30, 45, 60, 90, and 120 minutes after measuring baseline corticotropin and cortisol. A blunted or absent response suggests pituitary disease. An exaggerated response is consistent with hypothalamic dysfunction.

Glucagon has been reported to be safe, reliable, and reproducible for the assessment of anterior pituitary secretion of both ACTH (as measured by cortisol) and GH. Cortisol responses are decreased in men and in subjects with basal hypercortisolism but are not influenced by age.

HORMONAL OVERPRODUCTION

Thyroid Excess

Patients with elevated thyroid hormone (hyperthyroidism) due to either endogenous secretions or exogenous intake have suppressed TSH secretion following TRH administration. This consistent finding of suppressed TSH response to exogenous TRH in hyperthyroidism has enabled the TRH stimulation test to replace the older more cumbersome triiodothyronine (T$_3$) suppression test in evaluating subclinical or equivocal hyperthyroidism.

Prolactin Excess

The clinical syndrome and etiologies of hyperprolactinemia are summarized in Table 13-2. Increased prolactin levels are associated with a spectrum of ovulatory dysfunction including luteal phase defects, anovulation, and amenorrhea. Unlike the other pituitary hormones, prolactin is under chronic inhibitory control by hypothalamic dopamine. Reduced or absent dopamine leads to elevated prolactin levels. Many of the causes of hyperprolactinemia involve aberrant hypothalamic production of this prolactin-inhibiting factor (PIF). Agents that inhibit hypothalamic PIF include pharmacologic substances (ie, phenothiazine, reserpine, amphetamines, opiates, diazepam, α-methyldopa, and tricyclic antidepressants), physiologic factors (ie, prolonged intensive suckling), and pathologic states (ie, elevated estrogen states as in polycystic ovarian disease (PCOD); stresses such as trauma, surgery, and anesthesia; and hypothalamic lesions). Pituitary tumors can secrete prolactin independently, and the elevated TRH in patients with hypothyroidism can act as a prolactin-releasing factor.

Patients with prolactin levels >30 ng/ml should undergo a hyperprolactinemia workup. Many suppression (L-dopa, bromocriptine, nomifensine) and stimulation (TRH, metoclopramide, chlorpromazine, insulin-induced hypoglycemia) tests (see Table 13-2) have been evaluated for their ability to determine the etiology of hyperprolactinemia. Most of these tests produced conflicting results.

The TRH stimulation test has been most widely used. Normally, prolactin doubles 15–20 minutes after TRH administration. Patients with prolactinomas have blunted and delayed response to TRH. Although useful in differentiating normal patients from those with hyperprolactinemia, the TRH stimulation test has not been demonstrated to be diagnostic of prolactinomas.

Hyperprolactinemic patients with coexisting hypothyroidism or pregnancy reportedly have normal prolactin response to exogenous TRH. Patients with hyperthyroidism or hypothalamic/pituitary deficiencies without coexisting hyperprolactinemia have blunted prolactin response to exogenous TRH.

Growth Hormone Excess

GH measurements can confirm the diagnosis of acromegaly, but early detection is dependent on recognizing clinical symptoms (see Table 13-2). Repetitive GH sampling is necessary because GH is secreted episodically. The mean of hourly GH levels (from 8 a.m. to 4 p.m.) is calculated. In persons with acromegaly, if the mean GH is >2.5 μg/L, then somatomedin C will be elevated. The glucose suppression test and paradoxical GH response to exogenous TRH are classic diagnostic tools. Nonsuppression or paradoxical rise of GH in response to hyperglycemia has been reported in active acromegaly as opposed to suppression in quiescent acromegaly. Paradoxical GH response to several provocative tests reportedly suggests that normal endogenous regulation of GH secretion by stimulatory GHRH and inhibitory somatomedin is disordered in persons with acromegaly.

ACTH Excess

The clinical symptoms and diagnostic evaluation of Cushing's syndrome are summarized in Table 13-2. The 24-hour urine free cortisol and 1-mg overnight dexamethasone suppression test (DST) are initial screening tests. The overnight test involves administering 1 mg of dexamethasone orally at 11 p.m. and measuring an 8 a.m. cortisol. Normally, cortisol will suppress to <5 μg/dl. Patients who suppress do not have Cushing's syndrome. However, lack of suppression is not sufficient for the diagnosis of hypercortisolism, and additional studies are required.

When the overnight 1-mg DST is abnormal, the next step in the evaluation of Cushing's syndrome is the more cumbersome low-dose 2-mg DST. After two 24-hour urine collections for cortisol and 17-OHCS, 0.5 mg dexamethasone is given orally every 6 hours for 2 days. Daily 24-hour urine and 4 p.m. cortisol on day 2 are obtained. Normally, 17-OHCS is <4 mg/24 hr, urine free cortisol is <20 μg/24 hr, and serum cortisol is <5 μg/dl on day 2. Nonsuppression of 17-OHCS and cortisol is diagnostic of Cushing's syndrome. Obesity, exogenous estrogen, depression, phenytoin, and stress are confounding factors. Patients with Cushing's syndrome also lack cortisol response to the ICT due to their suppressed endogenous CRH secretion.

Once the diagnosis of Cushing's syndrome is established, the next step is to identify the underlying cause of the hypercortisolism. The differential diagnosis includes ACTH-producing pituitary tumors (Cushing's disease), adrenal adenoma/carcinoma, and ectopic ACTH production. The high-dose DST will suppress pituitary ACTH and cortisol in Cushing's disease but will not suppress the hypercortisolism from autonomous adrenal function or ectopic ACTH-producing tumors. The high-dose DST follows the same protocol as the low-dose test except that 8 mg, instead of 2 mg, of dexamethasone is used. In patients with Cushing's disease, 17-OHCS levels are <40% of baseline and cortisol is <10 μg/dl on day 2. A less expensive, less cumbersome, high-dose DST has been developed in which, after obtaining baseline cortisol levels, 8-mg oral dexamethasone is given at night and 8 a.m. cortisol is measured. Cortisol <5% of baseline indicates suppression.

The CRF stimulation test, although not yet standardized, has been useful in distinguishing pituitary from adrenal or ectopic causes. In normal patients, ACTH and cortisol increase after exogenous CRF. Patients with pituitary Cushing's have an exaggerated response (although the difference in response may not be distinct enough to differentiate the two). However, patients with ectopic and adrenal Cushing's syndrome have a flat response to CRF. The CRF stimulation test has a 91% sensitivity and 95% specificity in distinguishing pituitary from ectopic and adrenal causes. These values are similar to those of the high-dose DST. The diagnostic power of each test has been shown to be enhanced when two tests are used in combination.

A blunted or normal CRF-induced ACTH response 7–10 days after surgery for pituitary Cushing's has been reported to be predictive of remission. Most patients have suppressed responses to CRF during the early postoperative period. The CRF test has also been used to monitor the rate of recovery of normal ACTH secretion in patients who were surgically cured of adrenocortical tumors.

Differentiating autonomous adrenal function from an ectopic ACTH-producing tumor will be facilitated by ACTH measurements as these assays become more sophisticated. Patients with an adrenal source of hypercortisolism have suppressed pituitary ACTH, whereas ACTH is elevated with an ectopic source.

Hypercortisolemia has been described to occur in about 40–50% of patients with major depressive disorders ("pseudo-Cushing's state"). Failure to suppress cortisol levels with the 1-mg DST occurs in about 40–50% of patients with major depression and has even been used to diagnose depression in psychiatry. This has led to some confusion between diagnosing the pathologic glucocorticoid excess of Cushing's disease versus the hypercortisolism of depressive illness, especially in depressed patients with hirsutism, obesity, and elevated free cortisol levels. Use of the higher dose DST may help differentiate between the two. Also, because hypercortisolism seems to resolve with recovery from the depressive episode, postponing the DST until this time can alleviate diagnostic confusion. In fact, the DST can be used as an objective method to follow patients recovering from depression. The DST has also been used to differentiate depression from chronic pain syndromes.

Dynamic testing has been used to evaluate the hypercortisolism seen in patients with anorexia nervosa. The hypercortisolism can be quite pronounced, approaching levels seen in patients with Cushing's disease or severe depression. Proposed etiologies have included both peripheral (ie, decreased cortisol clearance, lower affinity for cortisol-binding globulin, and glucocorticoid receptor defects) and central (ie, a defect in the hypothalamic-pituitary regulation of the adrenal axis) mechanisms. Before correction of weight loss, anorectic patients have marked hypercortisolism but normal baseline ACTH levels. A marked reduction in ACTH response to CRH has been reported, remaining unchanged a month after body weight correction even though the hypercortisolism resolved. However, responses were to normalize 6 months after weight loss correction. This suggests that the hypercortisolism in patients with anorexia results from a defect at or above the level of the hypothalamus since the blunted ACTH response to CRH reflects an intact negative feedback effect of hypercortisolism at the pituitary level in underweight patients with anorexia, which corrects with return to normal body weight.

Androgen Excess

When androgen levels are elevated (hyperandrogenism), but not in the tumor range, suppression and stimulation testing may be utilized to differentiate an ovarian from an adrenal source. Ovarian suppression has been accomplished with oral contraceptives. With ovarian hyperandrogenism, testosterone and androstenedione should be reduced by approximately half. The DST has been used to evaluate the adrenal contribution to hyperandrogenism. For adequate adrenal androgen suppression, the prolonged DST has been described. Two milligrams or oral dexamethasone is administered daily for 2 weeks. If cortisol is <40 ng/ml and DHEAS <400 ng/ml (demonstrating adequate adrenal suppression), then the source of excess androgens is considered to be adrenal. If the hyperandrogenism is not suppressed, then the source of excess androgens is considered to be of ovarian or mixed origin, respectively.

Ovarian stimulation testing with human chorionic gonadotropin (hCG) is not standardized, results are variable, and it is not commonly used clinically. A rise in androgens occurs if hyperandrogenism is of ovarian etiology. Adrenal stimulation testing with Cortrosyn (1 mg intravenously), although also not yet standardized, is clinically relevant and frequently used to diagnose adrenal enzyme defects such as 21-hydroxylase, 11β-hydroxylase, and 3b-hydroxysteroid dehydrogenase deficiencies. Precursor hormones are elevated after stimulation in affected patients.

Approximately 1–6% of hyperandrogenic women have late onset adrenal hyperplasia (LOAH). The characteristic clinical presentation is peri- or postpubertal onset of hirsutism, acne, or oligomenorrhea and other signs of virilization. Most commonly used clinically for detection of LOAH in the workup of hyperandrogenic women, 17-hydroxyprogesterone (17-OHP) is measured after adrenal stimulation with exogenous ACTH and compared to the normal response. Basal 17-OHP levels >200 ng/dl predict that stimulated 17-OHP levels at 30 minutes will be consistent with LOAH (>1200 ng/dl). Therefore, adrenal stimulation testing to exclude LOAH is recommended when follicular unsuppressed morning 17-OHP levels are >200 ng/dl. A 17-OHP level 30 minutes after 250 µg Cortrosyn >1200 ng/dl is diagnostic of the 21-hydroxylase deficiency type of LOAH. It is important that measurement of *basal* 17-OHP be performed in the morning during the follicular phase of the menstrual cycle because luteal 17-OHP may confuse the diagnosis. However, the ACTH stimulation test can be done at any time during the menstrual cycle.

Combined Testing

Multiple simultaneous testing, also called combined testing, of the hypothalamic-pituitary axis with several agents allows efficient testing of multiple pituitary functions. TRH (500 mg), GnRH (100 µg), and insulin (0.10 U/kg not to exceed 10 U) are simultaneously infused to the fasted patient, and glucose, GH, cortisol, prolactin, TSH, LH, and FSH are measured every 15 minutes for 180 minutes. Results are interpreted in a similar manner as described for each individual test (see Table 13-1). Combined testing of normal subjects is reliable, safe, efficient, and cost-effective. Equivalent results and similar side effects occur as with single testing.

SUMMARY AND FUTURE DIRECTION

In summary, suppression and stimulation tests are used clinically in many circumstances to diagnose endocrinopathy, formulate treatment decisions, and follow therapeutic responses in various conditions. They are, however, limited by lack of standardization, specificity and sensitivity problems, and confounding factors. Direct suppression and stimulation tests, such as CRF, may render indirect testing with agents such as ICT or metyrapone obsolete. Structurally modified releasing hormones have provided more sensitive testing. For example, structural modification of TRH by substituting a methyl group of the three position of the histidine moiety (methyl TRH) has been described. This molecule has eightfold greater bioassay activity and fivefold greater activity than TRH. Naltrexone, an opioid antagonist, induces secretion of LH, prolactin, ACTH, and cortisol. Naltrexone could serve as a provocative multiple stimulus.

More sophisticated RIAs, such as ACTH, may eliminate the need for some suppression and stimulation tests, and make others more accurate and informative. Baseline hormone levels do not always reflect subtle or mild endocrine dysfunction. Such disorders may only manifest themselves with dynamic testing.

Other diagnostic tests can be used in combination with or in lieu of SSTs. Examples of such tests include magnetic resonance imaging, computed tomography, adrenal and ovarian vein catheterization, iodomethylcholesterol scanning, and inferior petrosal venous sampling.

ACKNOWLEDGMENT

This chapter has been adapted and modified from an article by Schwartz LB, Seifer DB: The role of stimulation and suppression testing of the endocrine system. *Clinical Consultations in Obstetrics and Gynecology* 3:174-189, 1991.

SUGGESTED READING

Definitions of Dynamic Testing

Schlaff WD. Dynamic testing in reproductive endocrinology. *Fertil Steril* 1986;45:589–606.

Basic Principles of SSTs

Donald RA. The assessment of pituitary function. *Clin Biochem* 1990;23: 23–30.
Faber J, Kirkegaard C, Rasmussen B, et al. Pituitary-thyroid axis in critical illness. *J Clin Endocrinol Metab* 1987;65:315–320.
Schwartz LB, Seifer DB. The role of stimulation and suppression testing of the endocrine system. *Clin Consult Ob/Gyn* 1991;3:174–189.

Gonadotropin Deficiency

Guisti M, Torre R, Traverso L, et al. Endogenous opioid blockade and gonadotropin secretion: role of pulsatile luteinizing hormone–releasing hormone administration in anorexia nervosa and weight loss amenorrhea. *Fertil Steril* 1988;49:797–801.
Kaplan LS, Grumback MM. Clinical review 14: Pathophysiology and treatment of sexual precocity. *J Clin Endocrinol Metab* 1989;69:1087–1089.
van Binsbergen CJM, Coelingh Bennink HJT, Odink J, et al. A comparative and longitudinal study on endocrine changes related to ovarian function in patients with anorexia nervosa. *J Clin Endocrinol Metab* 1990;71: 705–710.

Thyroid Deficiency/Excess

Hershmon JM. Use of thyrotropin-releasing hormone in clinical medicine. *Med Clin North Am* 1978:62:313–325.

Growth Hormone Deficiency

Dierich JR. Serum growth hormone levels in provocation tests and during nocturnal spontaneous secretion: a comparative study. *Acta Paediatr Scand* 1987;337:48–59.
Gelato MC, Malozowski S, Caruso-Nicoletti M, et al. Growth hormone (GH) responses to GH-releasing hormone during pubertal development in normal boys and girls: comparison to idiopathic short stature and GH deficiency. *J Clin Endocrinol Metab* 1986;63:174–179.
Rao RH, Spathis GS. Intramuscular glucagon as a provocative stimulus for the assessment of pituitary function: growth hormone and cortisol responses. *Metabolism* 1987;36:658–663.

ACTH Deficiency

Kaye TB, Crapo L. The Cushing syndrome: an update on diagnostic tests. *Ann Intern Med* 1990;112:434.

Prolactin Excess

Archer DF, Harger JM, Moore EE, et al. Validity of hypothalamic-pituitary testing in hyperprolactinemia: prolactin response to insulin hypoglycemia and arginine. *Am J Obstet Gynecol* 1981;141:556–561.

Ayalan D, Persitz E, Ravid R, et al. The diagnostic value of pharmacodynamic tests in the hyperprolactinaemic syndrome. *Clin Endocrinol* 1979; 11:201–215.

Barbieri RL, Cooper DS, Daniels GH, et al. Prolactin response to thyrotropin-releasing hormone (TRH) in patients with hypothalamic-pituitary disease. *Fertil Steril* 1985;43:66–73.

Growth Hormone Excess

Shibasaki T, Hotta M, Masudo A, et al. Studies on the response of growth hormone (GH) secretion to GH-releasing hormone, thyrotropin-releasing hormone, gonadotropin-releasing hormone, and somatostatin in acromegaly. *J Clin Endocrinol Metab* 1986;63:167–173.

ACTH Excess

Avgerinos PC, Chrousos GP, Nieman LK, et al. The corticotropin-releasing hormone test in the postoperative evaluation of patients with Cushing's syndrome. *J Clin Endocrinol Metab* 1987;65:906–913.

Boyar RM, Hellman LD, Roffwarg H, et al. Cortisol secretion and metabolism in anorexia nervosa. *N Engl J Med* 1977;296:190–193.

France RD, Krishnan KRR. The dexamethasone suppression test as a biologic marker of depression in chronic pain. *Pain* 1985;21:49–55.

Gold PW, Loriaux DL, Roy H, et al. Responses to corticotropin-releasing hormone in the hypercortisolism of depression and Cushing's disease. Pathophysiology and diagnostic implications. *N Engl J Med* 1986;314: 1329–1335.

Nieman LK, Chrousos GP, Oldfield EH, et al. The ovine corticotropin-releasing hormone stimulation test and the dexamethasone suppression test in the differential diagnosis of Cushing's syndrome. *Ann Intern Med* 1986;105:862–867.

Schrell U, Fahlbuschr, Buchfelder M, et al. Corticotropin-releasing hormone stimulation test before and after transsphenoidal selective microadenomectomy in 30 patients with Cushing's disease. *J Clin Endocrinol Metab* 1987;64:115–119.

Androgen Excess

Abraham GE, Maroulis GB, Boyers SP, et al. Dexamethasone suppression test in the management of hyperandrogenized patients. *Obstet Gynecol* 1981;57:158–164.

Azziz R, Rafi A, Smith BR, et al. On the origin of the elevated 17-hydroxyprogesterone levels after adrenal stimulation in hyperandrogenism. *J Clin Endocrinol Metab* 1990;70:431–436.

Azziz R, Zacur HA. 21-Hydroxylase deficiency in female hyperandrogenism: screening and diagnosis. *J Clin Endocrinol Metab* 1989;69: 577–584.

New MI, Speiser PW. Genetics of adrenal steroid 21-hydroxylase deficiency. *Endocr Rev* 1986;7:331–349.

Taylor L, Ayers JST, Gross MD, et al. Diagnostic considerations in virilization: iodomethylnorcholesterol scanning in the localization of androgen secreting tumors. *Fertil Steril* 1986;46:1005–1010.

Combined Testing

Cohen R, Bouquier D, Biot-Laporte S, et al. Pituitary stimulation by combined administration of four hypothalamic releasing hormones in normal men and patients. *J Clin Endocrinol Metab* 1986;62:892–898.

Summary and Future Direction

Mendelson JH, Mello NK, Cristofaro P, et al. Use of naltrexone as a provocative test for hypothalamic-pituitary hormone function. *Pharm Biochem Behav* 1986;24:309–313.

Clinical Reproductive Medicine,
Edited by Bryan D. Cowan and David B. Seifer
Lippincott-Raven Publishers, Philadelphia © 1997

CHAPTER 14

Oral Contraceptives

Michael D. Fox

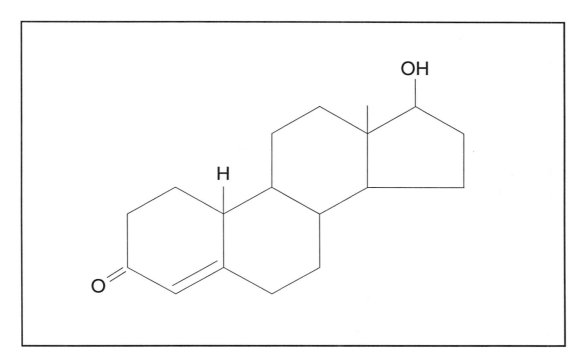

Pharmacology and Formulation
  The Estrogen Component
  Progestins
  Formulations
  Mechanism of Action
  Metabolic Effects
  Cardiovascular Effects
  Endocrine Effects
  Gastrointestinal Effects
  Oral Contraceptives and Neoplasia
  Other Effects Related to Oral Contraceptive Use
Clinical Usage
  Starting Oral Contraceptives
  Side Effects of Oral Contraceptive Use
  Postcoital Contraception ("Interception")
  Other Methods of Oral Contraception
Summary
Suggested Reading

M. D. Fox: Division of Reproductive Endocrinology, Department of Obstetrics and Gynecology,
St. Vincent's Hospital, Jacksonville, FL 32216

In the last 30 years, hormonal contraception has become the most used reversible contraceptive measure worldwide. Since the introduction of oral contraceptives (OCs) in 1960, we have seen dramatic alterations in their formulation and usage resulting in substantial decreases in adverse effects. The goal of research and development has been to optimize contraceptive efficacy while minimizing the overall side effect profile. There are three developmental milestones in the evolution of OC usage: (a) reduction of component steroids; (b) development of "phasic" formulations to further reduce dosage and prevent breakthrough bleeding; and (c) introduction of the "new generation" progestins, which are highly selective and have an improved side-effect profile compared to traditional progestins. These three changes taken together have dramatically reduced the incidence of serious complications associated with OC use, such as thromboembolism and coronary heart disease. Additionally, metabolic effects such as changes in the lipoprotein profile and coagulation factors have been substantially reduced and for the most part are now considered of no clinical consequence. As a direct result, many women who were once ineligible for OC use are now able to safely utilize this extremely effective method of contraception. This has been especially beneficial to women aged 35 through menopause.

Early formulations contained high doses of estrogen and progestin that were responsible for an increased incidence of untoward side effects. Many recommendations made by the Food and Drug Administration (FDA) are based largely on studies of patients taking these early preparations. These now outdated recommendations unfortunately continue to be perpetuated by patients, media reports, and physicians alike. Since more than 10 million women in the United States are using this form of birth control annually, we should dispel common misconceptions regarding OCs.

In general, the term oral contraception is applied to estrogen–progestin combinations or progestin-only formulations (so-called minipill). Another use of OCs is as a post-coital contraceptive (so-called interception). The contraceptive steroids used in OCs are synthetic and the hormonal state produced is pharmacologic. An understanding of currently used hormonal components of OCs and their particular side-effect profiles will afford the practitioner the chance of choosing the combination best suited for individual patient needs. The OC chosen should provide maximum protection against pregnancy while using the lowest dose of steroid possible to secure maximum safety to the patient.

PHARMACOLOGY AND FORMULATION

The Estrogen Component

Estrogens can be classified according to occurrence (natural versus synthetic) or by structure (steroidal versus

TABLE 14-1. *Component steroids of current oral contraceptive preparations*

Estrogens
Ethinyl estradiol
Mestranol
Progestins
Estranes
Norethindrone
Norethindrone acetate
Ethynodiol diacetate
Gonanes
Norgestrel (dextro/levo)
Desogestrel[a]
Norgestimate[a]
Gestodene[b]

[a]New progestins.
[b]Not currently available in the United States.

non-steroidal). Naturally occurring steroidal estrogens include estradiol-17β (E_2), estrone (E_1), and estriol (E_3) as well as equine or conjugated estrogens (equilin, equilenin, 17α-dihydroequilin, etc.). Ethinyl estradiol and mestranol are both synthetic, steroidal estrogens (Table 14-1). Diethylstilbestrol (synthetic) and plant or phytoestrogens (natural) are nonsteroidal in structure.

Prior to 1930, initial work with estrogens found that excessive oral amounts of the naturally occurring estrogens would be required to inhibit ovulation. Later, it was found that the addition of an ethinyl (-C≡CH) group at the 17 position inhibited hepatic degradation and made the compound much more active orally. This compound, ethinyl estradiol (EE), is the most potent oral estrogen in use in the United States and is used in the majority of OCs on the market today. A less commonly used estrogen is the 3-methyl ether of EE, mestranol. Mestranol must be first converted to EE by cleavage of the methyl group in the liver prior to becoming biologically active, and this occurs with 60% efficiency. Thus, a 50-μg dose of mestranol is roughly equivalent to 35 μg of EE. Ethinyl estradiol and mestranol are the only two synthetic estrogens currently used as components of OCs.

Most studies looking at the pharmacokinetics of OC steroids have demonstrated a large interindividual and intraindividual variation in response to oral dosing. Serum levels of EE peak at 1–2 hours after an oral dose and decline rapidly until 6–8 hours after dosing, at which time a more gradual decline occurs. The second phase of the elimination period is slowed by the enterohepatic circulation whereby EE is secreted into the bile, deconjugated in the gastrointestinal tract, and reabsorbed into the bloodstream. EE administered orally is at least 200 times more potent than estradiol. Thus, 5 μg of EE is the equivalent of 1 mg of micronized estradiol.

Progestins (syn: progestagens, progestogens, gestagens)

Synthetic progestins are derivatives of either progesterone or testosterone. All progestins used in OCs are derivatives of testosterone but lack the 19 carbon; hence the name 19-nortestosterones. They are further subdivided into estranes and gonanes (Table 14-1). Until recently, there were only four progestins used in OCs: norethindrone, norethindrone acetate, ethynodiol diacetate (estranes), and norgestrel (gonane). Norethindrone acetate and ethynodiol diacetate are structurally related to norethindrone and undergo rapid hydrolysis and subsequent conversion to norethindrone and its metabolites. Norgestrel is a racemic mixture of dextro- and levonorgestrel although only levonorgestrel has any biological activity. Compared to the estranes, levonorgestrel has more progestational and androgenic effects and possesses no estrogenic activity.

Concerns over the intrinsic androgenicity of OC progestins prompted research directed at the development of more selective progestins for use in combination OCs. Recently, two new gonane progestins, desogestrel and norgestimate, have been approved for use in the United States. Used for many years in Europe, these two agents are characterized by the potent progestational effect of levonorgestrel but have lower androgenic tendencies than any of the older agents. Together with a third progestin, gestodene (used outside the United States), these agents have been referred to as the "new generation" progestins. Large efficacy studies utilizing low-dose combinations of these progestins show an equal or better rate of ovulation suppression and pregnancy prevention when compared to existing formulations.

After an oral dose, desogestrel is rapidly converted to its active metabolite, 3-ketodesogestrel, by the gut and the liver. Norgestimate undergoes multiple degradative steps in the liver resulting in several products. Only one of the products, 17-deacetyl norgestimate, in addition to the parent compound is felt to contribute significantly to the clinical response. All the new progestins have similar pharmacokinetic properties as the traditional compounds.

The new progestins are highly selective, which refers to the ability of the drug to produce desired pharmacologic outcomes while avoiding the undesired, other receptor-mediated effects ("side effects"). For example, 3-ketodesogestrel binds 100% more effectively to the progesterone receptor than levonorgestrel and 400% more effectively than norethindrone. In the case of the androgen receptor, 3-ketodesogestrel binds 50% less than levonorgestrel. The selectivity index for a particular progestin is the ratio of its affinity for the progesterone receptor to its affinity for the androgen receptor. Using this measure, 3-ketodesogestrel is 3.5 times and norgestimate and its metabolite are 4–20 times more selective than either levonorgestrel or norethindrone. This is based primarily on animal data but has been supported by observed clinical response to the newer progestins.

The androgenic influence of progestins has the broadest spectrum of adverse effects, influencing most organ systems of the body. One antiandrogen effect of the new progestin combination OCs results from their ability to increase steroid hormone-binding globulin (SHBG) significantly more than older pill combinations. Increased SHBG binds more free androgen, preventing it from binding to its receptor. This results in less androgen effect. Some authors feel this to be the primary mechanism for the antiandrogen effect of OCs. Progestins also directly bind to SHBG and displace androgens, which can result in undesirable androgenic side effects. The new progestins minimize this displacement effect representing yet another mechanism for a lower androgenic profile for the new progestins. Because of the stronger progestational effect of this group of progestins, ovarian androgen production is suppressed to a greater degree. All of these effects make combination OCs containing the new progestins the first choice in hyperandrogenic patients.

Formulations

Estrogen alone can provide effective contraception by inhibiting ovulation but prolonged use results in irregular bleeding, endometrial hyperplasia, and/or carcinoma. Likewise, progestin-only agents are effective as contraceptive agents but are associated with annoying side effects such as abnormal bleeding. Combination OCs were developed to provide a stable endometrial environment, which results in more predictable and tolerable bleeding patterns. OCs contain an estrogen and progestin in either fixed dose (monophasic) or varied dose (biphasic, triphasic). The efficacy of lower dose (<50 μg of EE) is no less than higher dose preparations. However, the incidence of breakthrough bleeding is higher. Because significant side effects associated with OC use are dose-dependent, the multiphasic pills were conceived to lower the total steroid dose without amplifying breakthrough bleeding. Currently there are one "biphasic" and four "triphasic" formulations in use. In all but one instance the EE dose is constant at 35 μg and the progestin component is varied, but the cumulative monthly dose is less than that of monophasic formulations. In one pill (Triphasil) the estradiol is increased from 30 to 40 μg for 5 days during the midcycle (Table 14-2).

OCs are dispensed in packages of either 21 or 28 days of pills. Twenty-eight-day packages contain 21 days of "active" steroid tablets and 7 days of "inactive" tablets. The use of a continuous pill cycle with a pill-free interval built in to the cycle has been shown to improve compliance by maintaining a regular pill administration routine. The 21-day packages are now reserved for therapeutic usage of OCs in which continuous usage is preferred to cyclic therapy.

Mechanism of Action

Oral contraceptives achieve the prevention of pregnancy through a variety of mechanisms. The primary

TABLE 14-2. *Currently available oral contraceptive formulations*

Name (manufacturer)	Estrogen	Dose	Progestin	Dose	Androgen bioactive equivalent[a]
Brevicon (Syntex)	ethinyl estradiol	35μg	norethindrone	0.5mg	0.17
Demulen 1/35 (Searle)	ethinyl estradiol	35μg	ethynodiol diacetate	1mg	0.21
Demulen 1/50 (Searle)	ethinyl estradiol	50μg	ethynodiol diacetate	1mg	0.21
Desogen (Organon)	ethinyl estradiol	30μg	desogestrel	0.15mg	‡
Levlen (Berlex)	ethinyl estradiol	30μg	levonorgestrel	0.15mg	0.46
Loestrin 1/20 (Park-Davis)	ethinyl estradiol	20μg	norethindrone	1mg	0.53
Loestrin 1.5/30 (Park-Davis)	ethinyl estradiol	30μg	norethindrone	1.5mg	0.80
Lo-Ovral tablets (Wyeth-Ayerst)	ethinyl estradiol	30μg	norgestrel	0.3mg	0.46
Modicon (Ortho)	ethinyl estradiol	35μg	norethindrone	0.5mg	0.17
Nelova 1/35E (Warner Chilcott)	ethinyl estradiol	35μg	norethindrone	1mg	0.34
Nelova 0.5/35E (Warner Chilcott)	ethinyl estradiol	35μg	norethindrone	0.5mg	0.17
Nelova 1+50M (Warner Chilcott)	mestranol	50μg	norethindrone	1mg	0.34
Nordette (Wyeth-Ayerst)	ethinyl estradiol	30μg	levonorgestrel	0.15mg	0.46
Norinyl 1/35 (Syntex)	ethinyl estradiol	35μg	norethindrone	1mg	0.34
Norinyl 1/50 (Syntex)	mestranol	50μg	norethindrone	1mg	1.30
Ortho-Cept (Ortho)	ethinyl estradiol	30μg	desogestrel	0.15mg	‡
Ortho-Cyclen (Ortho)	ethinyl estradiol	35μg	norgestimate	0.250mg	‡
Ortho-Novum 1/50 (Ortho)	mestranol	50μg	norethindrone	1mg	0.34
Ortho-Novum 1/35 (Ortho)	ethinyl estradiol	35μg	norethindrone	1mg	0.34
Ortho-Novum 7/7/7 (Ortho)	ethinyl estradiol	35μg	norethindrone	0.5mg	0.25
			35μg	0.75mg	
			35μg	1mg	
Ortho-Novum 10/11 (Ortho)	ethinyl estradiol	35μg	norethindrone	0.5mg	0.25
			35μg	1mg	
Ortho Tri-Cyclen (Ortho)	ethinyl estradiol	35μg	norgestimate	0.180mg	
			35μg	0.215mg	
			35μg	0.250mg	‡
Ovcon 35 (Bristol-Myers)	ethinyl estradiol	35μg	norethindrone	0.4mg	0.46
Ovcon 50 (Bristol-Myers)	ethinyl estradiol	50μg	norethindrone	1mg	0.30
Ovral (Wyeth-Ayerst)	ethinyl estradiol	50μg	norgestrel	0.5mg	0.80
Tri-Levlen (Berlex)	ethinyl estradiol	30μg	levonorgestrel	0.05mg	0.29
			40μg	0.075mg	
			30μg	0.125mg	
Tri-Norinyl (Syntex)	ethinyl estradiol	35μg	norethindrone	0.5mg	0.29
			35μg	1.0mg	
			35μg	0.5mg	
Triphasil (Wyeth-Ayerst)	ethinyl estradiol	30μg	levonorgestrel	0.050mg	0.29
			40μg	0.075mg	
			30μg	0.125mg	
Progestin Only ("Mini-Pill"):					
Micronor (Ortho)	none		norethindrone	0.35mg	0.13
Nor-Q-D (Syntex)	none		norethindrone	0.35mg	0.13
Ovrette (Wyeth Ayerst)	none		norgestrel	0.075mg	0.13

[a]Adapted from Dickey RP. *Managing Contraceptive Pill Patients.* 6th ed. CIP, Inc, 1991:144–145. These data come from the rat ventral prostate assay and compares the oral contraceptive (OC) steroid response to a fixed dose of methyltestosterone. This represents older thinking on the clinical correlation between animal bioassays and response in humans. These numbers give practitioners a guide with some scientific basis with which to predict the relative response between various OC preparations.

‡According to current clinical data regarding metabolic effects of new progestins, we can speculate with some degree of certainty that their values in this assay would be less than existing OC preparations.

mechanism is through disruption of the normal hypothalamic-pituitary axis. Ovulation is inhibited by interfering with the secretion of gonadotropin-releasing hormone (GnRH), resulting in decreased production of the gonadotropins FSH and LH. It has been shown that the inhibition of ovulation is a synergistic effect between estrogen and progestin but is primarily a progestin effect. In fact, the progestin-only pills, which contain nearly the same dosage of progestin as the low-dose combination, fail to suppress ovulation in 30–50% of cycles. Furthermore, LH is not completely suppressed with newer low-dose preparations and small peaks may be demonstrated throughout the cycle. Despite the suppression of gonadotropins, ovarian steroidogenesis is not completely absent during the 21-day contraceptive portion of the cycle. Estradiol levels have been measured and range from 20 to 80 pg/ml.

The endometrium is altered by the contraceptive steroids. The histologic appearance has been described as "inactive" or "irregular secretory." It is theorized that tubal physiology is also altered. The cervical mucus, dominated by a progesterone effect, is characterized by decreased production but increased cellularity and thickness. This presumably prevents the passage of sperm through the cervix and may hinder the passage of bacterial pathogens. The latter effect may contribute to the reduction in upper genital tract infections in patients using OCs.

The estrogen component of OCs is involved in the contraceptive action by its suppressive effects on FSH secretion from the pituitary. In addition, it stabilizes the endometrium in the face of a progestational effect and reduces the incidence of breakthrough bleeding.

Metabolic Effects

There are several long-term prospective trials that have added greatly to our understanding of adverse effects associated with OC use. The U.S. groups include the Walnut Creek study, consisting of 16,638 patients enrolled between 1968 and 1972, and the Centers for Disease Control (CDC) Cancer and Steroid Hormone Study (CASH), which is multicenter and includes eight separate geographic areas of the country. British trials include the Royal College of General Practitioners (RCGP) involving more than 20,000 users matched with a similar number of controls and the Oxford Family Planning Association (OFPA) study of 17,032 women matched with the same number of controls. As stated earlier, much of this information involves the use of higher dose formulations (50–150 μg) of estrogen. Unfortunately, most of our information on lower dose preparations is based on small groups.

Cardiovascular Effects

The majority of serious side effects associated with OC use are related to cardiovascular disease. Myocardial infarction, cerebrovascular disease, and thromboembolic disease have all been associated with OC use. Estrogens generally increase hepatic protein synthesis including fibrinogen and factors II, VIII, and X. These are atherogenic but are balanced by increases in plasminogen and tissue plasminogen activator (tPA), both components of the fibrinolytic system. HDL cholesterol is increased whereas LDL is decreased. In contrast, the progestin component has been linked to cardiovascular disease by promoting a decrease in HDL and an increase in LDL, which may offset the positive effects afforded by estrogen on blood lipids. The new progestins have a favorable effect on baseline lipoprotein levels. A number of studies have confirmed a significant decrease of LDL and a concomitant increase in HDL and the HDL/LDL ratio. It will be a while before long-term data is available.

According to the results of the Lipid Research Clinics published in 1984, small changes in HDL resulted in significant alterations in cardiovascular risk whereas the association with LDL changes was less clear. Combining a low HDL with other cardiovascular risk factors such as hypertension, diabetes, obesity, etc., markedly increased risk. However, these risk associations were demonstrated in groups other than reproductive age women. If atherogenesis due to OC alterations in the lipoprotein profile

was significant, one would expect that past users would have a sustained cardiovascular risk. Interestingly, there is no evidence for an increased risk of cardiovascular disease in women who are past users of OCs. Similarly, there is no correlation with duration of OC use to cardiovascular disease, and the risk of myocardial infarction rapidly decreases to the level of nonusers with discontinuation.

The earlier RCGP study correlated OC use and an increased relative risk (4.2; 95% confidence interval, 2.3–7.7) of cardiovascular mortality, but this was not borne out in other contemporary studies such as OFPA and the Walnut Creek contraceptive studies. More recent data and updates of older data would confine statistically significant increases in risk to patients over 35 years of age who smoke. According to a recent update of RCGP, OC users who smoke more than 15 cigarettes a day may increase the risk of myocardial infarction by 3- to 4-fold over those who smoke less than 15 cigarettes per day and 5- to 10-fold over nonsmokers. Smoking clearly exerts a synergistic effect on the risk of death from myocardial infarction in OC users. For nonsmokers aged 35–44 there was a slight increase in risk. The benefits of contraception may outweigh the small risk in this group. (The overall risk of myocardial infarction due to OC use has been estimated to be 4 in 100,000, which is half of the reported risk of mortality due to vaginal birth, 9 per 100,000). In summary, the existing long-term data based on older studies suggests that there is no increased risk of mortality from OC use in women under 35. For nonsmokers over age 35 there may be a slight increase in risk, but less risk than the risk of pregnancy in this age group. Smokers above age 35 are at increased mortality from OC use. The overall risk is dose-related. Since cardiovascular disease risk has been linked to abnormal lipoprotein profiles, OCs should be chosen that provide the lowest effective dose and minimize lipid changes whenever possible.

The risk of hemorrhagic and thrombotic stroke were increased two- and threefold, respectively, in early reports. Recent data utilizing low-dose formulations do not support this association. Patients suffering from migraine headaches have varying responses to the use of OCs. Some patients observe improvement whereas others note worsening of symptoms. Because migraine headache symptoms are similar to those of an impending cerebrovascular accident, patients with severe migraines (visual changes, nausea) should probably avoid OCs in lieu of other methods of contraception.

Venous thromboembolism, a result of estrogen changes in the fibrinolytic system and the smooth muscle relaxing effect of progesterone, is more common in current users than in nonusers. This effect is dose-related and is much less significant in new low-dose formulations. Changes in coagulation factors such as decreased prothrombin, increased factors VII and VIII, fibrinogen, and plasminogen are all of small magnitude and essentially independent of the type of progestin used (including the new generation progestins). This would support the fact that this is an estrogen-mediated phenomenon. The relative risk of deep venous thrombosis and pulmonary embolism is reported to be from 4 to 11 for current users. However, the effect does not linger after discontinuation. Most of the venous thromboembolic events in patients using low-dose preparations are associated with other risk factors such as trauma or immobilization. In patients undergoing elective surgery, OCs should be discontinued for 4 weeks preoperatively and at least 2 weeks postoperatively. Some have recommended prophylactic heparin treatment when emergency surgery is necessary in a patient on OCs.

Women started on older high-dose OCs had a 5% incidence of hypertension. In an older study based on high-dose OCs, the average increase was 4.1 mm Hg systolic and 1 mm Hg diastolic immediately after initiation of OC use and it continued to increase modestly with use. These changes quickly reversed with discontinuation of treatment. The mechanism of OC-associated hypertension is thought to be an estrogen-induced increase in plasma angiotensinogen, the renin substrate. A compensatory decrease in plasma renin may negate the effect in most patients. Several studies of patients on a desogestrel 150 µg and EE 30 µg combination OC revealed minimal (<1 mm Hg) changes in systolic or diastolic pressures. In one study the only women who became hypertensive after institution of the new OC (0.07%) had risk factors for the development of hypertension. Some authors have postulated that OC use unmasks latent hypertensives and that no real increase in hypertension exists for users of OCs. In healthy patients, annual monitoring of blood pressure is all that is recommended.

Although OCs seldom produce hypertension, their use is not routinely recommended for patients with existing hypertension. In fact, hypertension continues to be listed as an absolute contraindication for OC use. However, in well-controlled hypertensive patients without other risk factors for heart disease in whom highly effective birth control is of primary importance, OCs can be used with caution. Informed consent should be obtained in these cases. Due to reported changes in blood pressure with OC use, patients with hypertension prior to onset of therapy need close monitoring of blood pressure. Adjustment of antihypertensive medications may be necessary during the course of therapy. Morbidity of hypertensive OC users is less than morbidity associated with pregnancy in these patients.

Endocrine Effects

Oral contraceptive use is associated with alterations in carbohydrate metabolism, but an increase incidence of diabetes mellitus has not been observed. Decreased insulin receptors, compensatory increase in insulin levels, delayed gastrointestinal absorption of glucose, and elevated blood sugar in response to carbohydrate ingestion are all observed effects in OC users. In the vast majority of healthy patients this effect is negligible and serum glucose levels are unchanged. These effects are primarily due to the progestin component of the pill. These effects are dose-related and most data concerning low-dose formulations support only minimal changes in glucose and insulin metabolism.

It is questionable as to whether patients who were gestational diabetics are at increased risk of developing frank diabetes mellitus while taking OCs. For women with pre-existing diabetes mellitus, the use of OCs has unpredictable effects. Many authors feel that the risk of pregnancy in this group far outweighs any increased risk from OC use. There have, however, been reports of thrombosis in diabetics on OCs. Diabetes is a significant heart disease risk factor and certainly if other risk factors are present another form of contraception should be used.

Estrogen increases cortisol-binding globulin (CBG) with a resultant increase in cortisol level. Progesterone competitively displaces cortisol from its binding protein causing an increase in free bioactive hormone. The long-term consequences of elevated cortisol levels are unknown but the reported magnitude of change in cortisol is small. The cortisol response to stress is not affected by pill use.

Likewise, thyroid-binding globulin is increased by estrogen and metabolic alterations are similar to those of pregnancy. The total thyroxine is elevated and resin uptake is decreased due to increased binding globulin. Measurement of TSH and free thyroxine remain accurate in the assessment of the patient's thyroid status.

Other metabolic effects include mild weight gain, breast engorgement, and tenderness. Cholasma has been reported in some patients and to a large extent is irreversible. These tend to be estrogen effects and for certain patients can be very problematic. Significant weight gain is unusual but when present would appear to be an anabolic effect of sex steroids. In most patients, dietary restriction is helpful but in a small subgroup of patients who seem to be extremely sensitive to the anabolic effects, discontinuation of OCs is eventually the only method of resolution. Weight gain was reported to be the primary reason for discontinuation in 25% of patients who stop using OCs due to intolerable side effects.

Gastrointestinal Effects

Estrogen increases hepatocellular enzyme activity and protein synthesis. A decrease in transport of bile acids has been described with estrogen and some progestins, rarely resulting in cholestatic jaundice. This condition is rapidly reversible with discontinuation of OCs. Due to this effect, OCs are strictly contraindicated in patients with chronic cholestatic liver disease. OCs are, however, safe for patients with cirrhosis or a history of hepatitis as long as the active phase of the disease has ceased.

Hepatocellular adenomas are rare liver lesions characterized by an abnormal dilatation of vascular spaces in the liver. Development of adenomas is stimulated by high-dose androgens and estrogens. Hepatic adenomas have been virtually nonexistent in users of low-dose contraceptives (<35 g EE). Patients may be asymptomatic, have epigastric or right upper quadrant pain, or present with rupture and hemoperitoneum.

Estrogen causes an increase in biliary cholesterol and early on reports linked OCs to an increase in gallstones. Today most authors believe that OCs merely accelerate stone formation in patients destined for gallbladder disease. Thus, the true incidence of gallstones is not increased when compared to controls over time.

Oral Contraceptives and Neoplasia

The CASH study demonstrated that OC use is associated with a reduced risk of endometrial (all three tissue subtypes) and ovarian epithelial carcinoma. They estimate that 2000 cases of endometrial cancer and 1700 cases of ovarian cancer annually are prevented by OC use.

A 50% reduction in the risk of endometrial cancer was seen after 12 months of OC use. This protective effect was maximized after 3 years of use and persisted for 15 or more years after discontinuation of the medication. A 40% reduction in incidence has been reported for ovarian cancer. This effect also increases with duration of use and is persistent for 10–15 years after the discontinuation of OCs.

In contrast to endometrial cancer, early studies have suggested a causal relationship between long-term OC use (>5 years) and cervical dysplasia, carcinoma in situ, and invasive cancer. Many have criticized these data with concerns that confounding risk factors such as multiple sexual partners, use of barrier contraception, and improved compliance with Pap smear screening for OC users were not properly controlled. The CASH study did not identify an association between pill use and invasive cervical carcinoma. It did conclude that the apparent increase in carcinoma in situ of the cervix was due to improved surveillance.

The RCGP, OFPA, and the Walnut Creek study have failed to demonstrate a relationship between every use of OCs and the later development of breast cancer in women aged 20–54. A recent meta-analysis of 34 studies confirmed the findings of the older studies. Although these reports are reassuring, several studies have identified subgroups of patients at risk. Some have suggested an increase in risk for early use (<25 years) and another study suggested increases with longer duration of use (>12 years). The most consistent association has been found in OC users and the development of breast cancer at a young age (<45 years). The magnitude of increase is small and breast cancer is extremely unusual in this age group. Since the numbers of patients used for comparison were very small, caution should be applied when interpreting these results.

These reports and other prompted the Centers for Disease Control to reexamine the data from CASH which were collected from 1980 to 1982 and were derived from >5000 cases of breast cancer. For women aged 20–34, the relative risk (RR) for development of breast cancer with ever use of OCs was 1.4 (1.0–2.1; 95% confidence interval), for ages 35–44 the RR was 1.1 (0.9–1.3; 95% CI), and for ages 45–54 the RR was 0.9 (0.8–1.0; 95% CI). The RRs of various subgroups in this analysis were very similar to the aggregate numbers. Overall it was concluded that OC use had no impact on the development of breast cancer.

Other Effects Related to Oral Contraceptive Use

"Postpill amenorrhea" has been variously defined as the failure to resume menses in 3, 6, or 12 months after OC discontinuation. The incidence of postpill amenorrhea is quoted as 0.7–0.8%. There is no evidence to support a role for OCs and the incidence of secondary amenorrhea. If no menses has occurred by 12 months after discontinuation of OCs a routine evaluation of amenorrhea should be undertaken.

Galactorrhea has been associated with pill use and may be aggravated by the estrogen component of the OC. In general, this effect is minimal and is reversible with discontinuation. There is no contraindication to pill use in patients with documented prolactin microadenomas. Vitamin A is increased slightly and vitamins C, B_6, and folic acid have been shown to decrease with OC use. Changes are minimal and supplemental vitamins are not required.

A great deal of emphasis has been placed on the noncontraceptive benefits of OCs (Table 14-3). These bene-

TABLE 14-3. *Noncontraceptive benefits of oral contraceptives*

Decreases in	Number of hospitalizations prevented
Endometrial cancer	2,000
Ovarian cancer	1,700
Ectopic pregnancy	9,900
Iron deficiency anemia	27,200
Dysmenorrhea	3,000
Ovarian cysts	
Leiomyoma uteri	
Pelvic inflammatory disease	
Total cases	51,000
Hospitalizations	13,300
Benign breast disease (fibrocystic, fibroadenoma)	20,000

Adapted from Ory HW. The noncontraceptive health benefits from oral contraceptive use. *Fam Plann Persp* 1982;14:182; and Peterson HB, Lee NC. The health effects of oral contraceptives: Misperceptions, controversies, and continuing good news. *Clin Obstet Gynecol* 1989;32:339–355.

fits on the whole combined with the absence of morbidity and mortality associated with unwanted pregnancy is the basis for the outstanding risk–benefit ratio associated with OC use.

CLINICAL USAGE

Starting Oral Contraceptives

A complete history and physical exam including but not limited to a risk factor analysis, blood pressure, breast exam, liver palpation, and cervical cytology should be performed on all patients considering using OC agents. The history should specifically contain inquiries to identify the presence of absolute and relative contraindications to OC use (Table 14-4). All women should have a screening cholesterol determination and consideration of a fasting glucose to rule out diabetes. Patients should be counseled about minor side effects, which will be more noticeable during the first three cycles. These include breakthrough bleeding, spotting, nausea, breast tenderness or enlargement, weight gain, and fluid retention. These symptoms are common but are largely resolved by the third cycle. Patients should be encouraged to continue a particular pill for at least 3 months before a change is considered.

OCs should be started by menstrual day 5 to provide protection during the first cycle of use. The usual recommendation for patient compliance is to have the patient begin a pack on the Sunday after the first day of menses because the packages are arranged in calendar format with Sunday as the start day. If the period begins on Sunday the patient should start that same day.

During the 7-day drug-free interval, the inhibition of the hypothalamic-pituitary axis is lifted and FSH levels

TABLE 14-4. *Risk factors for oral contraceptive use*

Absolute Contraindications:
  Thrombophlebitis or thromboembolic disorders
  History of deep vein thrombosis or thromboembolic disorders
  Cerebrovascular or coronary artery disease
  Known or suspected carcinoma of the breast
  Estrogen-dependent neoplasia
  Undiagnosed abnormal genital bleeding
  Antithrombin III deficiency
  Severe liver diseases; cholestatic jaundice of pregnancy or previous pill use, adenomas, hyperplasia, or carcinoma
  Elective surgery
  Hypercoagulable state due to inherited coagulation defect
  Known or suspected pregnancy
Relative Contraindications:
  Migraine headaches
  Diabetes mellitus
  Hypertension
  Epilepsy
  Sickle cell disease
  Crohn's disease

From FDA package insert.

TABLE 14-5. *Clinical management of missed oral contraceptive (OC) tablets*

Consecutive tablets omitted	Instruction to the patient
1	Take missed tablet immediately and the next pill at the regularly scheduled time.[a]
2	Take two tablets immediately and the next pill at the regularly scheduled time.[a]
3	Before the 10th cycle day: resume OCs on the regular schedule.[a]
4 or more	Stop OCs and start a new pack on the Sunday after the next cycle begins.[a]

Patients should be instructed that other forms of birth control are necessary during the incident cycle. If menstruation does not occur within 7–10 days following discontinuation of OCs a pregnancy test must be performed prior to reinstitution of therapy.

[a]After the 10th cycle day, stop OCs and start a new pack on the Sunday after the cycle begins.

begin to rise steadily causing the initiation of follicular recruitment. For this reason, the first few pills after this interval are probably the most critical in preventing ovulation from occurring. Contraceptive failures with OCs are most commonly associated with missing the first one or more "active" tablets each month. For example, if the first two active pills are missed, the first active tablet would be taken on cycle day 10 which may not be early enough to suppress ovulation that cycle. *Other forms of contraception should be recommended for that cycle.* If tablets are missed during the later part of the cycle, definite recommendations can be made (Table 14-5).

Postpartum initiation of OCs has been a subject of controversy related primarily to the increased incidence of thrombosis during this time period. Ovulation is virtually nonexistent during the first 3 postpartum weeks in term-pregnancy women in whom bromocriptine has not been used to suppress breast milk production. This is not the case, however, after terminations or in patients given bromocriptine. Ovulation can as early as the second postpartum week. Therefore, the general recommendation is to begin OCs at the third postpartum week after term pregnancies (nonnursing) and between the first and second weeks after early gestation terminations or abortions.

OCs have been shown to decrease milk production in breast-feeding mothers but no decrement in infant growth has been identified for healthy women. Contraceptive steroids cross into breast milk in small amounts but have not been associated with adverse effects. Despite this, it is recommended that other forms of birth control be considered in breast-feeding mothers. Progestin-only contraceptives have been suggested because they do not decrease milk supply and have not been associated with problems in newborns.

Pregnancies have occurred when OCs have been combined with other medications such as antibiotics and anticonvulsants. The mechanism is thought to be induction of hepatic degradative enzymes that cause an increase in metabolism and clearance of contraceptive steroids. Drugs included in these categories are rifampin, griseofulvin, Dilantin, phenobarbital, primidone, carbamazepine, and Coumadin. Patients on these medications should choose alternative forms of contraception. In contrast to early reports, more recent investigations demonstrate that ampicillin and tetracycline have no effect on the serum levels or effectiveness of OCs. Thus there is no need to recommend additional contraception with these medications.

Side Effects of Oral Contraceptive Use

As previously stated, the OC of choice for an individual patient contains the lowest effective dose of contraceptive steroids that has the fewest undesirable side effects. All pills currently marketed in the United States have comparable efficacy; thus the side-effect profile becomes the paramount issue. In this author's opinion, an OC containing 30–35 µg of EE combined with one of the new progestins, desogestrel, or norgestimate should be the first choice for most patients. Older patients or patients in whom estrogen risk factors may be in question could benefit from a lower EE dose such as a 20-µg preparation. The disadvantage to lowering the estrogen component is the resultant dominant progestin effect and increase in characteristic side effects. When patients return after a 3-month trial with complaints requiring a change to a different formulation, this change can be tailored to the symptom utilizing the differences in estrogenic, progestational, androgenic, and endometrial effects of the various formulations (see Table 14-2; relative androgenicity). These various activities of the OCs have been characterized for each preparation based on a combination of human and animal data. Although the use of animal data to produce complicated algorithms to fit first-time OC users with a particular formulation is not practical, the relative effects of the various preparations can be compared and this information can be utilized in a logical way to make rational medication changes for a particular patient. For example, if a patient is experiencing increases in acne, hirsutism, or an increase in LDL cholesterol, the logical choice would be to change to a formulation with less androgenic activity and increased "relative" estrogenic activity.

Minor side effects such as amenorrhea and breakthrough bleeding are commonly encountered and are aggravating to patients and clinicians alike. In some women, the low dose of estrogen is unable to stimulate the development of sufficient endometrium. This results in a thin atrophic layer too scant to produce withdrawal bleeding during the 7-day hormone-free period. From a medical standpoint this is not a significant problem because this process is completely reversible on discontinuation of OCs. The confusion for the physician and patient arises from the inability to exclude a pregnancy without withdrawal bleeding. For patients who are not bothered by the amenorrhea, repeated home pregnancy testing may be required to confirm the non-pregnant state and continue OCs. Patients who wish to menstruate regularly may require a therapy aimed at rejuvenating the endometrium. Conjugated estrogens (0.625–1.25 mg/day) may be added to the 21 days of active OCs for one or two cycles after the possibility of pregnancy has been eliminated. This generally provides resumption of menses for a prolonged period. Alternatively, switching to a formulation with more estrogenic activity may produce a more consistent pattern of withdrawal bleeding.

The most aggravating OC side effect is breakthrough bleeding. It is responsible for the discontinuation of OCs in the majority of women. This problem is more common with the newer pills with low estrogen and progestin doses. Oddly, in studies where blood levels of contraceptive steroids are correlated with episodes of bleeding, an association linking the two has not been found.

A progestin-dominant chronically decidualized endometrium is the usual cause of asynchronous bleeding. Bleeding usually presents after several months of normal withdrawal bleeding. The addition of estrogen (2.5 mg of conjugated estrogen or 20 µg of EE) to the OC regimen for the first 7 days of pill use will usually stabilize the endometrium. Most will have relief after a single course but this treatment can be repeated as necessary. For recurrent bleeding despite the above regimen, a thorough evaluation for organic causes of bleeding should be undertaken.

Postcoital Contraception ("Interception")

A special situation for OC use is that of the patient who presents with midcycle coital exposure asking for the "morning-after pill." Large doses of estrogen or estrogen-progestin combinations can be effective in the prevention of pregnancy if given within 72 hours of exposure. The mechanism of this effect is unknown. The risk of pregnancy in a random exposure has been estimated to be 7%. The failure rate of prophylactic treatment is <1%. Published data support that an effective dose is 100 µg of EE and 1 mg dl-norgestrel (eg, two pills containing 50 µg EE and 0.5 norgestrel each) taken within 72 hours of exposure and repeated 12 hours later.

Prior to institution of any regimen for postcoital contraception, the possibility of an existing pregnancy should be excluded. This mode of contraception should also be a routine part of counseling performed during a rape examination.

Other Methods of Oral Contraception

The progestin-only pill ("minipill") has been around for nearly as long as combination OCs and consists of continuous daily low-dose progestin. Currently, there are three progestin-only pills marketed in the United States (see Table 14-2). The lower dose of progestin is not sufficient to suppress ovulation and therefore the mechanism of action relies primarily on its ability to alter cervical mucus, endometrial receptivity, and possibly tubal motility. As a result, the failure rate is slightly higher than that of combination OCs. Because of increased failure rates and increased breakthrough bleeding (30–40%), patient acceptance of this method is low. However, there are situations where this method is ideal. Examples include older smoking women, lactating women, and in general any women in whom estrogen is contraindicated.

SUMMARY

In conclusion, the new low-dose OC agents are exceedingly safe except in women over 35 years of age who smoke. Unfortunately, a great deal of folklore surrounds the use of OCs most of which was derived from information gathered from early studies based on high-dose formulations. Recent public opinion polls found that 75% of women under age 35 felt that OC use was risky and 50% thought it to be more dangerous than pregnancy. We must dispel these myths and promote the health benefits that OCs afford.

SUGGESTED READING

General Reviews and Large Epidemiologic Works

American College of Obstetricians and Gynecologists Committee Opinion. *Hormonal Contraception.* ACOG Tech Bull No. 198, 1994.

Grimes DA. The safety of oral contraceptives: epidemiologic insights from the first 30 years. *Am J Obstet Gynecol* 1992;166:1950.

Kay C. The Royal College of Practitioner's oral contraception study: Some recent observations. *Clin Obstet Gynecol* 11:759, 1984.

Ramcharan S, et al. The Walnut Creek contraceptive drug study: an interim report. *J Reprod Med* 1980;25:346.

Speroff L, DeCherney A. Evaluation of a new generation of oral contraceptives. *Obstet Gynecol* 1993;81:1034.

Pharmacokinetics

Bergink W, et al. Serum pharmacokinetics of orally administered desogestrel and binding of contraceptive progestogens to sex hormone–binding globulin. *Am J Obstet Gynecol* 1990;163:2132.

Collins DC. Sex hormone receptor binding, progestin selectivity, and the new oral contraceptives. *Am J Obstet Gynecol* 1994;170:1508.

Goldzieher JW, Brody SA. Pharmacokinetics of ethinyl estradiol and mestranol. *Am J Obstet Gynecol* 1990;163:2114.

McGuire JL, et al. Pharmacologic and pharmacokinetic characteristics of norgestimate and its metabolites. *Am J Obstet Gynecol* 1990;163:2127.

Mishell DR, et al. Serum estradiol in women ingesting combination oral contraceptive steroids. *Am J Obstet Gynecol* 1972;114:923.

Metabolic Changes

Godsland IF, Crook D. Update on the metabolic effects of steroidal contraceptives and their relationship to cardiovascular disease risk. *Am J Obstet Gynecol* 1994;170:1528.

Godsland IF, et al. Clinical and metabolic considerations of long-term oral contraceptive use. *Am J Obstet Gynecol* 166:1955.

Lipid Research Clinics Program. The Lipid Research Clinics coronary primary prevention trial results. *JAMA* 1984;251:365.

Murphy AA. Effect of low-dose oral contraceptive on gonadotropins, androgens, and sex hormone binding globulin in nonhirsute women. *Fertil Steril* 1990;53:35.

Shoupe D. Effects of desogestrel on carbohydrate metabolism. *Am J Obstet Gynecol* 1993;168:1041.

Adverse Reactions

Cancer and Steroid Hormone Study. Oral-contraceptive use and the risk of breast cancer. *N Engl J Med* 1986;315:405.

Cancer and Steroid Hormone Study Group. Combination oral contraceptive use and the risk of endometrial cancer. *JAMA* 1985;257:796.

Goran S. Coagulation and anticoagulation effects of contraceptive steroids. *Am J Obstet Gynecol* 1994;170:1523.

Hankinson SE, et al. A quantitative assessment of oral contraceptive use and risk of ovarian cancer. *Obstet Gynecol* 1992;80:708.

Inger TG, et al. Oral contraceptive use and the incidence of cervical intraepithelial neoplasia. *Am J Obstet Gynecol* 1992;167:40.

Irwin KL, et al. Oral contraceptives and cervical cancer risk in Costa Rica: detection bias or causal association. *JAMA* 1988;259:59.

Lammer EJ, Cordero JF. Exogenous sex hormone exposure and the risk for major malformations. *JAMA* 1986;255:3128.

Luciano AA, et al. Hyperprolactinemia and contraception: a prospective study. *Obstet Gynecol* 1985;65:506.

Oxford Family Planning Study, Oral contraceptives and stroke findings in a large prospective study. *Br Med J* 1984;289:530.

Porter JB, et al. Mortality among oral contraceptive users. *Obstet Gynecol* 1987;70:29.

Romeiu I, et al. Oral contraceptives and cancer. *Cancer* 1990;66:2253.

Scott LD, et al. Oral contraceptives, pregnancy, and focal nodular hyperplasia of the liver. *JAMA* 1984;251:1461.

Tankeyoon M, et al. Effects of hormonal contraceptives on milk volume and infant growth. *Contraception* 1984;30:505.

Wingo PA, et al. Age-specific differences in the relationship between oral contraceptive use and breast cancer. *Cancer* 1993;71:1506.

Wynn V. Oral contraceptives and coronary heart disease. *J Reprod Med* 1991;36:219.

Benefits of Oral Contraceptive Use

Burkman RT. Noncontraceptive effects of hormonal contraceptives: bone mass, sexually transmitted disease and pelvic inflammatory disease, cardiovascular disease, menstrual function, and future fertility. *Am J Obstet Gynecol* 1995;170:1569.

Lanes SF, et al. Oral contraceptive type and functional ovarian cysts. *Am J Obstet Gynecol* 1992;166:956.

Other Hormonal Contraceptives

Chi IC. The safety and efficacy issues of progestin-only oral contraceptives—an epidemiological perspective. *Contraception* 1993;47:1.

Van Santen MR, Haspels AA. A comparison of high-dose ethinyl estradiol and norgestrel combination in postcoital interception: a study in 493 women. *Fertil Steril* 1985;43:206.

SECTION II

Reproduction

Clinical Reproductive Medicine,
Edited by Bryan D. Cowan and David B. Seifer
Lippincott-Raven Publishers, Philadelphia © 1997

CHAPTER 15

Gametogenesis

Victoria M. Sopelak

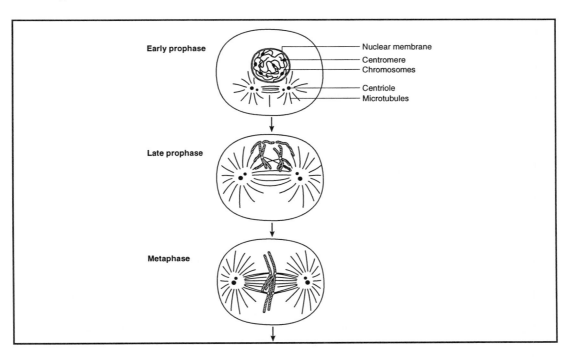

Introduction and Embryology
Ovarian Development
  Prefollicular Stage
  Development of Primordial Follicles
  Follicular Maturation
  Follicular Growth
  Resumption of Meiosis
  Fertilization

Embryogenesis
Hormonal Control of Follicular Development
Spermatogenesis
  Fetal and Postnatal Period
  Pubertal and Adult Changes
  Hormonal Control of Spermatogenesis
Suggested Reading

V. M. Sopelak: Division of Reproductive Endocrinology, Department of Obstetrics and Gynecology, University of Mississippi Medical Center, Jackson, MS 39216

INTRODUCTION AND EMBRYOLOGY

The development of male and female germ cells begins early in embryonic life and continues into adulthood. At 4–6 weeks of fetal life, 1000–2000 primordial germ cells migrate from the embryonic *yolk sac* to thickenings of mesodermal tissue known as the *urogenital ridge*. There the gonads form and incorporate the resident germ cells. The ultrastructural appearance of the primitive germ cells and the timing of migration is similar in both the male and female embryo. This early period of germ cell migration is referred to as the *indifferent stage* of sex differentiation. Irrespective of the sex of the embryo, primitive germ cells will be the only precursors of adult germ cells.

Germ cell proliferation (*mitosis*) and maturation occurs in the primitive gonad (urogenital ridge) beginning at 10 weeks of embryonic life. Mitosis involves synchronous division of localized groups of germ cells. Proliferative mitotic activity is completed in the ovary at 20–25 weeks of intrauterine life. Germ cells in the testis undergo an initial fetal stage of proliferation, a period of absent or diminished germ cell mitosis, and a second proliferative stage postnatally. Thus, the female is born with a fixed stock of oocytes but the male will continue proliferation of germ cell derivatives throughout life.

The formation of haploid gametes (*meiosis*) is a critical event during the maturation of both the sperm and the egg. The maturational changes leading to haploid gametes is referred to as *oogenesis* in the ovary and *spermatogenesis* in the testis. Oogenesis begins during prenatal development and is interrupted prior to its completion, whereas spermatogenesis is initiated at the time of sexual maturation (around the time of puberty) and continues through adulthood.

With this background, the following sections will deal with the major maturational changes that occur in the ovary and testis after these organs have formed. These changes will be correlated with chronological age and gonadal development

OVARIAN DEVELOPMENT

Prefollicular Stage

The development and maturation of a mature ovary containing competent oocytes is classified by the morphologic appearance of the germ cells. The germ cells are referred to as *oogonia* after the ninth week of embryonic life. The generation of oocytes during early embryogenesis is referred to as the *prefollicular* stage. Follicular *maturation* begins shortly after the prefollicular stage is complete but is arrested until puberty and the emergence of gonadotropic regulation of the final maturational sequences.

Mitosis regulates germ cell numbers. It is divided into distinct phases referred to as prophase, metaphase, anaphase, and telophase (Fig. 15-1). During *prophase* the chromosomes consist of two chromatids connected at the centromere. Initially, these chromosomes are surrounded by a nuclear membrane. As mitosis proceeds toward the next stage, the nuclear envelope disappears and the mitotic apparatus (microtubules and centrioles) become attached to the centromere. During *metaphase* the chromosomes line up on the equator and become attached to the polar centrioles. Paired chromatids of each chromosome separate and migrate toward opposite poles during *anaphase*. The nucleus is reformed during *telophase* resulting in two diploid cells. *Interphase* refers to the period of time between telophase of one cell division and prophase of the next. The number of germ cells increases to approximately 4–6 million by the fifth gestational month via mitosis (Fig. 15-2)

Some of the oogonia are transformed into *primary oocytes* through the process of meiosis. A peak population of approximately 7 million germ cells (comprising 2 million oogonia and 5 million primary oocytes) is reached in the two ovaries during the sixth to seventh intrauterine month (see Fig. 15-2).

Meiosis is characterized by chromosome conjugation and two successive cell divisions (first and second meiotic divisions) in which the diploid chromosome number is reduced to the haploid state (Fig. 15-3). Like mitosis, meiosis consists of four phases, referred to as prophase, metaphase, anaphase, and telophase. Unlike mitosis, meiosis is an extensive process that begins during fetal life, arrests before completion, reinitiates prior to ovulation, and concludes at the time of fertilization.

Prophase of the *first meiotic division* is highly specialized and is subdivided into five distinct substages (leptotene, zygotene, pachytene, diplotene, and diakinesis) (see Fig. 15-3). The first meiotic division extends throughout the entire intraovarian existence of the oocyte. DNA duplication ($2n$) and exchange occurs during meiosis I. With the extrusion of the first polar body, the DNA chromosome number is reduced to the haploid content (23 in the human). The *second meiotic division* is of short duration and very similar to mitosis. Normally ovulation and fertilization (restoration of the diploid state) are required to complete the second meiotic division. DNA reduction (n) occurs during the final meiotic division (see Fig. 15-3).

Leptotene is the first subdivision of prophase of the first meiotic division (prophase I). Leptotene is a presynaptic state in which the chromatin has the appearance of fine threads. The duplicated homologous chromosomes become synapsed at *zygotene*. During *pachytene*, the chromosome threads shorten and intertwine, giving the appearance of four chromatids known as *tetrads* (see Fig. 15-3). It is during pachytene that homologous chromosomes exchange reciprocal DNA in a process known as

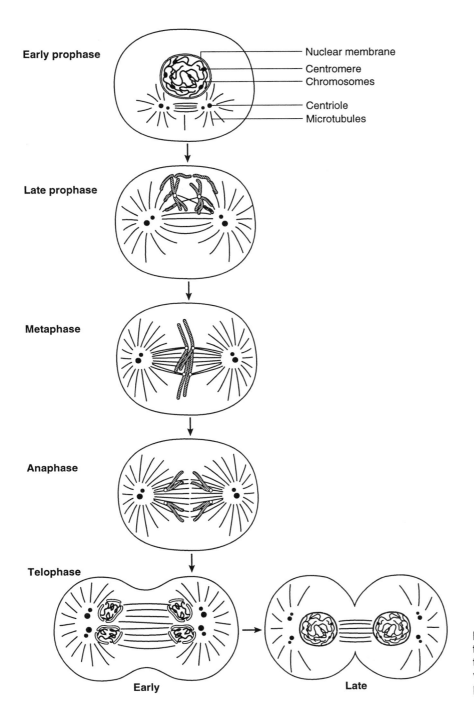

Early prophase

Nuclear membrane
Centromere
Chromosomes
Centriole
Microtubules

Late prophase

Metaphase

Anaphase

Telophase

Early

Late

FIG. 15-1. Cellular division with the formation of two daughter cells occurs through the process of mitosis. Mitosis is subdivided into prophase, metaphase, anaphase, and telophase.

chiasmata. Diplotene is the stage of meiosis whereby the paired bivalent chromosomes begin to repel each other.

During oocyte maturation, there is a prolonged resting period following diplotene. The reason for this prolonged phase of diplotene is unknown but may allow additional DNA exchange between complementary chromatids. *Diakinesis*, when the nucleolus and nuclear envelope disappear and the spindle fibers form, is delayed until shortly before ovulation. All stages up to and including diplotene are referred to as meiotic prophase I.

Development of Primordial Follicles

Primary oocytes become surrounded by a single layer of flattened granulosa cells. Cytoplasmic processes from these cells form unions with the plasma membrane of the oocyte and the oocyte–granulosa cell complex is then separated from the surrounding stroma by a basement membrane. This complex is referred to as a *primordial follicle* (Fig. 15-4). Although this process is initiated about the time of differentiation, all viable

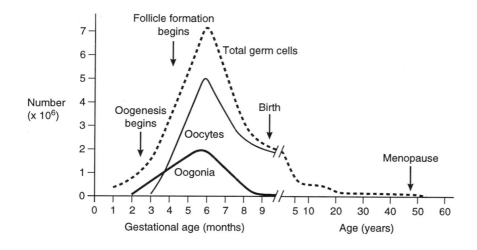

FIG. 15-2. The number of germ cells in the ovaries correlated with age. Peak numbers of germ cells are found in fetal ovaries during the sixth to seventh intrauterine month. From that time until menopause, there is a steady decline in germ cell number.

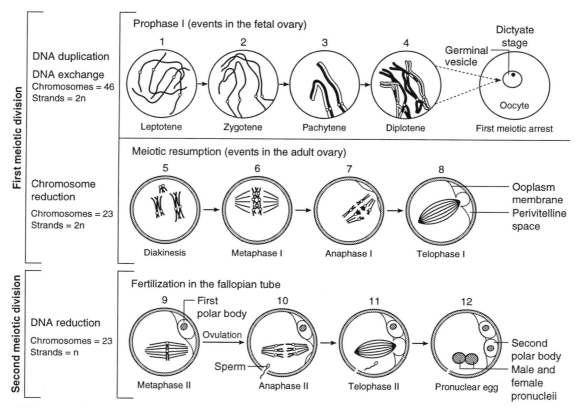

FIG. 15-3. Cellular division during meiosis reduces the chromosome complement from 46 chromosomes, 2n strands to the haploid state (23 chromosomes, n strands). For simplicity, only two pairs of chromosomes are depicted. Prophase I of the first meiotic division occurs during fetal life and is subdivided into four stages. Meiosis is arrested at the diplotene stage (first meiotic arrest) and the oocyte enters the dictyate stage. Shortly before ovulation, meiosis resumes and the oocyte proceeds through metaphase I, anaphase I, and telophase I, which completes the first maturation division. The oocyte is at the metaphase II stage when ovulation occurs. Completion of the second meiotic division (anaphase II and telophase II) takes place in the oviduct after fertilization.

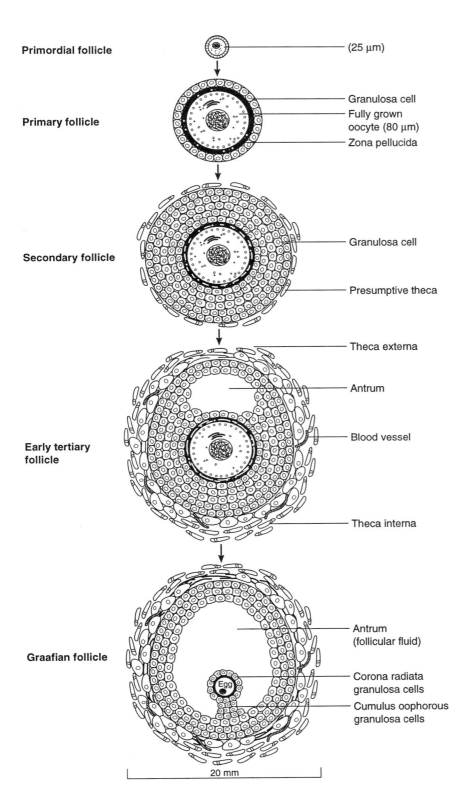

Primordial follicle — (25 μm)

Primary follicle — Granulosa cell / Fully grown oocyte (80 μm) / Zona pellucida

Secondary follicle — Granulosa cell / Presumptive theca

Early tertiary follicle — Theca externa / Antrum / Blood vessel / Theca interna

Graafian follicle — Antrum (follicular fluid) / Corona radiata granulosa cells / Cumulus oophorous granulosa cells

20 mm

FIG. 15-4. During folliculogenesis, the oocyte remains arrested at the diplotene stage but increases in size from 25 to 80 mm and becomes surrounded by granulosa cells. Follicular growth from the primary follicle to the tertiary and Graafian follicle is associated with changes in the size of the oocyte, the number of granulosa cell layers, development of the theca, formation of a fluid-filled antrum, and an overall increase in follicle size.

oocytes are not incorporated into primordial follicles until 6 months postpartum.

Some controversy surrounds the origin of the granulosa cells. It is unclear as to whether these granulosa cells are cortical (derived from somatic cells in the sex cords) or medullary in origin (arising from the ovarian stroma or rete ovarii). The cells which form the theca interna and theca externa of growing follicles are probably derived from the ovarian stroma, in common with glandular interstitial cells.

Follicular Maturation

Follicular maturation is initiated during the fifth to sixth month of gestation when the spindle-shaped granulosa cells in some of the primordial follicles differentiate into cuboidal cells. These follicles are called *primary follicles* (see Fig. 15-4). Proliferation of the granulosa cells gives rise to multiple layers of cells that contribute to follicle enlargement.

During their growth phase, the oocyte nucleus remains arrested in the diplotene stage of meiotic prophase. However, the oocyte cytoplasm undergoes extensive changes, including an increase in size (increasing from 25 to 80 μm), formation of large numbers of microvilli on the cell surface, and changes in the differentiation and distribution of cytoplasmic organelles (Fig. 15-5). The granulosa cells synthesize the *zona pellucida* that surrounds each oocyte. Cytoplasmic processes from granulosa cells traverse the zona pellucida to form gap junctions and maintain intimate contact with the plasma membrane of the oocyte (Figs. 15-4 and 15-5). Additional gap junctions are formed between adjacent granulosa cells. Because there is no direct blood supply to the growing oocyte, these gap junctions are probably responsible for transport of nutrients and other essential substances to the oocyte.

Follicular Growth

Follicular growth is associated with increases in the number of granulosa cells surrounding the oocyte, changes in the size of the oocyte itself, and formation of

a fluid-filled antrum. Follicles are classified according to these changes and include (a) *primary* or non-growing small follicles where the oocyte is enclosed by a single layer of granulosa cells; (b) *secondary* or preantral follicles where the growing oocyte is surrounded by multiple layers of proliferating granulosa and theca cells; and (c) *tertiary*, *Graafian*, or *antral* follicles in which the oocyte has terminated its growth while the surrounding cellular envelope continues to enlarge and a fluid-filled antrum is present (Fig. 15-4).

During late embryonic development theca cells differentiate from the surrounding mesenchymal cells and become incorporated into the envelope of the growing follicle. The theca interna portion of the follicle remains separated from the inner granulosa cell layers by the membrana granulosa and becomes well vascularized. Peripheral layers of these cells retain their spindle-shaped configuration, merging with the stromal cells to become known as theca externa cells.

Follicular maturation and growth begins during the seventh month of fetal life and continues until the menopause. Thus, by the fourth to sixth month postnatally, all stages of follicle development up to the point of antrum formation can be found.

Although most stages of follicle growth can be observed in the prepubertal ovary, the final maturation process culminating in ovulation does not normally occur before sexual maturity. Completion of this process requires maturation of the hypothalamic-pituitary-ovarian axis and stimulation by circulating gonadotropic hormones. Thus, before puberty follicular growth is gonadotropin-independent, whereas after puberty both go-

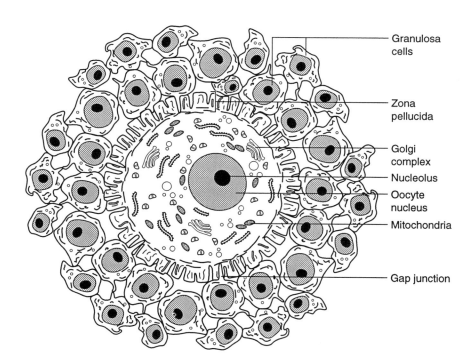

Granulosa cells

Zona pellucida

Golgi complex

Nucleolus

Oocyte nucleus

Mitochondria

Gap junction

FIG. 15-5. Oocyte growth consists of an increase in cellular size; formation of the zona pellucida, microvilli, and gap junctions; and a redistribution of cytoplasmic organelles such as mitochondria, endoplasmic reticulum, and the Golgi complex.

nadotropin-independent and dependent growth occur. Follicles that grow to a stage that require these hormones for further development undergo atresia if the appropriate gonadotropin stimulation does not occur. Ovaries from older premenarcheal girls generally have more numerous and larger follicles compared to younger females, thus accounting for the age-related increase in the weight of premenarcheal ovaries from less than 1 g at birth to 5–10 g at menarche. Even after puberty most follicles are still destined for atresia (Fig. 15-6). In part, the amount of hormone available to the follicle determines which ones successfully mature and attain ovulation.

The appearance of the follicle is changed by the formation of the fluid-filled antrum (see Fig. 15-4). During this process, the oocyte remains embedded at one side of the cavity in a mound of granulosa cells called the *cumulus oophorus*. These cumulus cells remain compact, but those nearest the zona pellucida become radially arranged and more columnar forming the *corona radiata*. The granulosa cells in other parts of the follicle wall become thinner, in contrast to the theca interna, which becomes broader with more conspicuous glandular cells.

The fluid filling the antrum (liquor folliculi) is formed from granulosa cell secretions, transudates from the blood, and numerous other products that contribute to the follicular microenvironment and influence oocyte maturation and/or ovulation. Substances derived mainly from plasma include antibodies, carbohydrates, inorganic components, lipoproteins, phospholipids, pituitary hormones, proteins, steroid-binding proteins, and nongonadal steroids such as cortisol. Substances produced mainly within the ovary include enzymes, mucopolysaccharides, nonsteroidal growth factors, and sex steroids. These products undoubtedly reach the oocyte via gap junctions be-

tween oocyte microvilli and elongated projections of the cumulus cells (see Fig. 15-5).

Resumption of Meiosis

Follicular growth to the tertiary stage is generally completed before the nucleus of the oocyte proceeds to maturation. The resumption of meiosis is dependent on previous exposure to follicle-stimulating hormone (FSH) followed by the rapid rise of circulating luteinizing hormone (LH), which occurs during the midportion of the menstrual cycle. Thus, the resting stage of meiosis (prophase I) is terminated by LH-induced resumption of meiosis about 36–48 hours prior to ovulation (Fig. 15-7).

During the first 16 hours following the onset of the midcycle LH surge the nucleolus is prominently located in the seemingly devoid nucleus (termed the *germinal vesicle* stage) (Figs. 15-3, 15-7, 15-8). Meiotic prophase I is complete when the nuclear chromatin of the oocyte passes from the diplotene stage into diakinesis (16 hours after the LH surge begins). Subsequently, the nucleolus fades and the duplicated chromosome pairs group together resulting in the formation of tetrads.

Metaphase of the first maturation division (*metaphase I*) is marked by the attachment of the chromosomes to the equator of the meiotic spindle that forms at the periphery of the cell (see Fig. 15-3). This is initiated approximately 26–30 hours after the LH surge (see Fig. 15-7). The chromosomes separate and move to opposite poles of the spindle. The spindle rotates perpendicular to the surface of the oocyte at *anaphase I*. During *telophase I*, separation of the haploid set of chromosomes is complete. The *first polar body*, consisting of one haploid set of duplicated chromosomes and a small amount of cytoplasm,

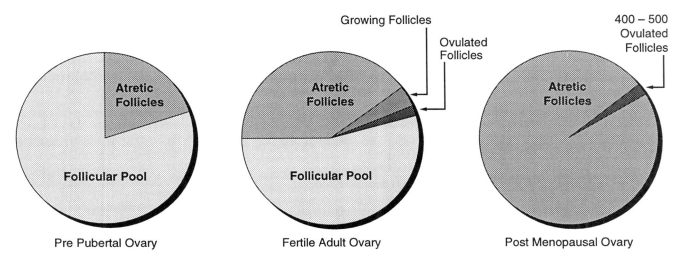

FIG. 15-6. The population of oocytes within the ovary continually changes with age. Only 400–500 oocytes will be ovulated during a woman's reproductive lifetime. Most of the oocytes in the follicular pool are lost to atresia.

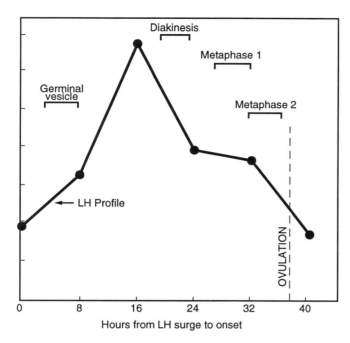

FIG. 15-7. Resumption of meiosis in tertiary follicles is triggered by the midcycle luteinizing hormone surge. The oocyte completes the first meiotic division as it proceeds through diakinesis, metaphase I, anaphase I, and telophase I. Just prior to ovulation, metaphase II of the second meiotic division is initiated. Ovulation occurs at this stage.

becomes detached from the oocyte, remains free inside the zona pellucida, and may undergo a second meiotic division (*second polar body*).

The *second meiotic division* generally begins approximately 30–34 hours after the onset of the LH surge (see Figs. 15-3 and 15-7). Since interphase and prophase of this second meiotic division are omitted, the chromosomes of the secondary oocyte remain in a condensed state and are reassembled on the equator of a second spindle formed close to the site of the first. This stage, referred to as *metaphase II*, precedes ovulation by 1 or 2 hours. It is the metaphase II oocyte that is capable of being fertilized and is ovulated (approximately 36–38 hours from the onset of the LH surge). This is the second and last interruption in oocyte meiosis.

During the 24-hour period prior to ovulation, changes occur between the oocyte and the surrounding cumulus cells. Just before ovulation, the gap junctions between the inner cumulus layer and the oocyte are almost completely lost (see Figs. 15-5 and 15-8). This breakdown in oocyte–cumulus communication may represent a mechanism that reduces or curtails the transfer of meiotic inhibitors present in the follicular fluid.

Up to this time, substances formed from granulosa cell secretions and transudates from the blood reached the oocyte via gap junctions (see Fig. 15-8). Some of these substances, such as inhibin, Mullerian-inhibiting substance (MIS), FSH-binding inhibitor, and LH receptor-binding inhibitor, affected the granulosa cells and altered their response to gonadotropins while growth factors, such as epidermal growth factor and plasma-derived growth factor, affect cell proliferation. At least three inhibitors of meiosis—cAMP, oocyte maturation inhibitor (OMI), and purine nucleosides—are produced by the granulosa cells and transmitted to the oocyte through gap junctions (see Fig. 15-8). It is only after OMI activity is either removed or rendered inactive by the preovulatory LH surge that the germinal vesicle is able to migrate to the periphery of the oocyte and meiosis resumes. This is associated with a decrease in cAMP levels within the oocyte (see Fig. 15-8).

Fertilization

In order to fertilize the oocyte, the sperm must pass through the cumulus mass, which is held together by a hyaluronic acid matrix. Hyaluronidase, an enzyme found in the acrosome of the sperm head, facilitates sperm passage through this cellular matrix. Sperm must then bind to the zona by way of both sperm receptors present at the surface of the zona and proteins present on the sperm membrane. One of the glycoproteins constituting the zona is call ZP3. It is synthesized and secreted during oocyte growth. Binding of the sperm to ZP3 on the zona is followed by release of enzymes from the head of the sperm (*acrosome reaction*). These enzymes allow the sperm to penetrate through the zona pellucida and then pass through a small space, the *perivitelline space*, prior to establishing contact with the ooplasm membrane (vitelline membrane) (see Figs. 15-3 and 15-8).

As soon as the sperm contacts the vitelline membrane, two reactions are triggered. The first is the *cortical granule reaction*. This reaction consists of fusion of the ooplasm with cortical granule membranes (Golgi-derived granules located below the ooplasm membrane) and release of the granule contents (containing hydrolytic enzymes) into the perivitelline space (see Fig. 15-8). This substance reacts with the zona to stop or prevent other sperm from entry and represents a block to polyspermy.

The second reaction triggered by contact of sperm with the vitelline membrane is resumption of meiosis in the oocyte. If the ovum is penetrated (fertilized) by a sperm cell, a process called *activation* ensues. The oocyte resumes the second meiotic division and extrudes the second polar body (containing half of the chromosomes originally present in the oocyte). The remaining chromosomes in the oocyte cytoplasm decondense and form the female pronucleus (Figs. 15-3 and 15-9). After entering the ooplasm, the sperm head decondenses and forms the male pronucleus. Thus, fertilization is demonstrated by the presence of two or more polar bodies in the perivitelline space, two pronuclei (male and female) in the

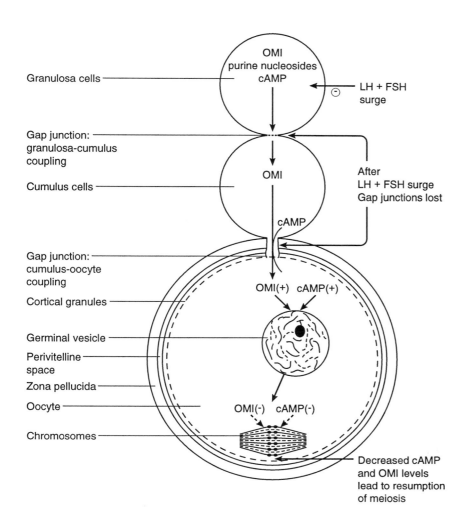

FIG. 15-8. Substances are transported to the oocyte via gap junctions. Ooctye maturation inhibitor (OMI), purine nucleosides, and cAMP are transported from the granulosa cells to the oocyte where they maintain the oocyte in meiotic arrest. It is only after the luteinizing hormone and follicle-stimulating hormone surge, when the gap junctions are lost and cAMP and OMI levels decline, that the oocyte resumes meiosis.

ooplasm, and remnants of the fertilizing sperm flagellum within the ooplasm.

Normally, pronuclei can be observed between 12 and 20 hours after fertilization. DNA replication occurs while the male and female pronuclei are in close apposition to each other in the center of the ovum (see Figs. 15-3 and 15-9). Pronuclear membranes break down after DNA replication is completed. The chromosomes from each pronuclei recondense and aggregate on an equatorial plate of the first cleavage spindle. This is the culminating point of oocyte maturation and the completion of meiosis. *Cleavage*, the initial step in *embryonic* development, is soon to follow.

Embryogenesis

Fusion of the male and female pronuclei (*syngamy*) following fertilization completes meiosis of the oocyte and returns the chromosome complement to the diploid state (46 in the human). Following fusion, activation of many pathways involved in protein and nucleic acid synthesis occurs. Approximately 27–43 hours following fer-

tilization, while still located within the fallopian tube, the unicellular fertilized oocyte (*zygote*) divides (cleaves) and forms two daughter cells, or *blastomeres* (see Fig. 15-9). Through a series of consecutive mitotic divisions, the *conceptus* is transformed into a multicellular complex. By 50 hours after fertilization, the human conceptus is still located within the fallopian tube (ampullary portion) and may contain 3–10 blastomeres still enclosed within the zona pellucida. Since cellular differentiation has not yet occurred, each of these blastomeres is theoretically *totipotent*, capable of giving rise to all of the cells needed to form an entire individual. During this period of cleavage there is no growth (enlargement) of the blastomeres. Thus, although the number of blastomeres increases, the size of the conceptus stays the same as the original oocyte due to a decrease in the size of each blastomere with each successive division.

As cleavage continues, the blastomeres form a solid ball of cells known as a *morula* (see Fig. 15-9). At 3–4 days following fertilization, fluid begins to accumulate among the cells of the morula forming a *blastocele* or blastocyst cavity. It is at this time that the cells of this *blastocyst* differentiate into lines: embryoblast and tro-

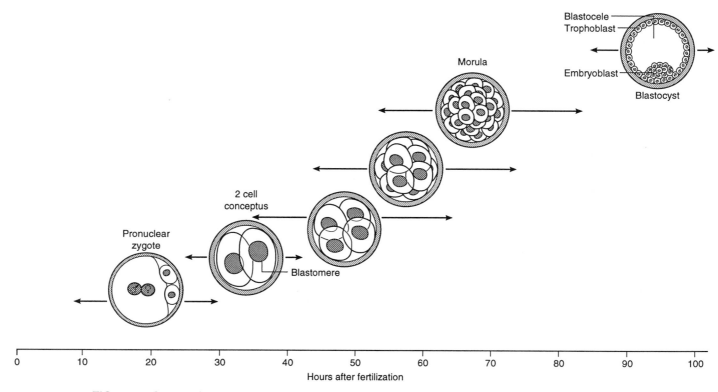

FIG. 15-9. Successful ovum penetration is evident by 20 hours after fertilization by the presence of two pronuclei (male and female) and two or more polar bodies in the perivitelline space. Following pronuclear fusion, the zygote (located within the fallopian tube) begins to divide in an organized manner, forming a conceptus with multiple blastomeres that eventually becomes a solid ball of cells (morula). By 96 hours, the cells have begun to reorganize, forming the blastocyst which now enters the uterine cavity.

phoblast. The *embryoblast* or *inner cell mass* is located at one end of the blastocele and becomes the embryo, whereas the *trophoblast*, cells enveloping the blastocele and covering the embryoblast, will form the placenta and other extraembryonic structures (see Fig. 15-9). It is at least 4 days after ovulation that this blastocyst, still encased within the zona pellucida, enters the endometrial cavity. During the fifth to sixth day following fertilization, the blastocyst lies unattached within the endometrial cavity but continues to divide and begins to lose the zona pellucida. About 6 to 6½ days following fertilization the zona pellucida is lost by "hatching" from the zona and the trophoblast nearest the embryonic pole of the blastocyst makes contact with the endometrial cells and becomes attached (*implantation*). During the subsequent week the trophoblast and blastocyst further invade the endometrium. In this fashion the *embryo*, the developing organism from the first week of development until the eighth week, becomes established.

Hormonal Control of Follicular Development

Gonadal sex is determine at the time of fertilization. The absence of a Y chromosome generally assures development of an ovary. Once ovarian differentiation has occurred, hormonal and local intraovarian factors probably regulate oogenesis. Meiosis and the formation of primary oocytes are initiated first in oogonia in the central portion of the ovary that are in contact with the rete ovarii. This finding led to the hypothesis that a *meiosis-inducing factor* was secreted by the rete ovarii that was essential for meiosis and the formation of primordial follicles. To date, however, no meiosis-inducing substance has been recognized and the role of local intraovarian factors on oogenesis remains unclear. Hormonal factors that regulate meiosis are more clearly recognized. FSH regulates the number of germ cells that undergo degeneration and controls the onset of follicular growth. However, evidence from organ cultures, maternal and fetal hypophysectomy studies, and anencephalic fetuses shows that proliferation of oogonia and the maturation of oocytes through meiotic prophase to the diplotene stage are not *totally* dependent on FSH. Germ cell differentiation and the formation of primordial follicles occur in anencephalic fetuses but development of secondary follicles is impaired when the hypothalamic-hypophyseal axis is defective. Formation of primordial follicles reaches a maximum during the 20th to 25th week of gestation. This is when fetal plasma concentrations of FSH peak and the first primary follicles are formed. In contrast, the ovaries are small and contain few primary follicles in the anencephalic female fetus. Therefore, the purported meiosis-inducing factor of the rete probably initiates meiosis and the formation of primordial follicles. However, subsequent primary oocyte maturation requires fetal pituitary gonadotropins.

The development of secondary follicles requires the presence of gonadotropins. Late in gestation placental transfer of FSH initiates secondary follicle growth, but this culminates in atresia. Although follicle growth to the antral stage occurs, the oocytes do not resume meiosis. It is thought that the meiosis-inhibiting factor, oocyte maturation inhibitor (OMI), stops meiosis in the primary oocyte. Pubertal changes that are necessary for initiation of ovulatory cycles and regulation of the ovarian menstrual cycle are described in other chapters. Once gonadotropin-dependent ovulatory menstrual cycles are initiated at 10–12 years of age, they continue until age 50–55. Thus, oocytes remain in an arrested state (prophase I) for an appreciable length of time before they undergo atresia (gonadotropin-independent) or are ovulated (gonadotropin-dependent).

SPERMATOGENESIS

Fetal and Postnatal Period

Following migration of the primordial germ cells to the urogenital ridge, the testes differentiate and the germ cells (approximately 300,000 per gonad) become distributed within the sex cords at approximately 7–8 weeks of intrauterine life. The primitive germ cells are known as *gonocytes* (Fig. 15-10). Following limited mitotic proliferation, certain gonocytes (lacking glycogen) become

arranged in pairs connected by intercellular bridges near the periphery of the sex cords, interspersed among Sertoli and Leydig cells and supporting tissues. These cells, known as *prespermatogonia*, resemble adult stem cells. In these primitive seminiferous tubules, the prespermatogonia remain relatively quiescent and do not undergo further differentiation or meiosis until late in the prepubescent period.

Pubertal and Adult Changes

During the prepubertal period, just prior to the onset of spermatogenesis, the prespermatogonia undergo nuclear condensation, nucleolar enlargement, and a cytoplasmic volume reduction. The nucleolar enlargement is most likely due to increased RNA synthesis. Spermatogenesis is not established until the time of sexual maturation and early pubertal development. Once established, continued cycles of germ cell maturation continue throughout adulthood until the time of senescence. *Spermatogenesis*, defined as the process by which a spermatogonial stem cell gives rise to a spermatozoon, can be divided into three phases: (a) a phase of *multiplication of spermatogonia* that leads to formation of spermatocytes while simultaneously maintaining their number by renewal; (b) a period during which each *spermatocyte undergoes two meiotic divisions* culminating in the formation of four haploid spermatids; and (c) a *maturation phase* during which spermatids are transformed into spermatozoa (see Fig. 15-10). In the human, the time from the beginning of the differentiation of the spermatocyte to the formation of a motile sperm takes approximately 70–75 days. In addition, 10–21 days is required for transport of the sperm through the epididymis to the ejaculatory duct.

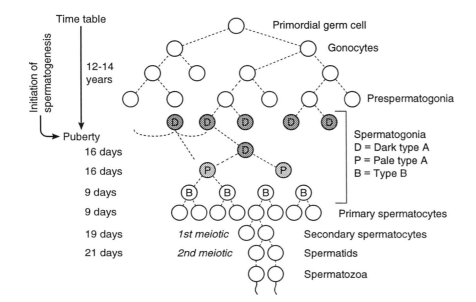

FIG. 15-10. The process of spermatogenesis is initiated at the time of puberty and involves cell division and differentiation. From one original spermatogonium, 64 spermatids can be produced in approximately 74 days. An additional 10–21 days is required for sperm transport.

Spermatogenesis begins with the formation of spermatogonia, classified as long, pale or dark type A and type B cells depending on the morphologic characteristics of the nucleus (Figs. 15-10 and 15-11). These spermatogonia are smaller than either prespermatogonia or gonocytes and are arranged along the basal lamina of the seminiferous tubules. By the time of puberty, the number of spermatogonia per testis is approximately 6×10^8. Each spermatogonium (type A dark) undergoing differentiation gives rise to two additional dark type A spermatogonia, each of which differentiates into two pale type A spermatogonia. Each pale type A spermatogonia divides to form two type B spermatogonia, which are located either at the tubular periphery or adjacent to the type A cells. Each type B spermatogonium then yields two primary spermatocytes. Thus, each spermatogonium undergoing differentiation gives rise to 16 primary spermatocytes. Each day, approximately, 1.5–3 million spermatogonia begin this differentiation process.

Differentiation of the spermatogonia occurs in the seminiferous tubules in an organized fashion. Because certain cellular types are always associated with each other, it is likely that contiguous groups of spermatogonia undertake spermatogenesis simultaneously. In the human seminiferous tubules, six typical cellular associations or stages have been identified (Fig. 15-12). Since these six stages or associations are repeated throughout the seminiferous tubule, the succession of the six stages in any one area of the tubular epithelium constitutes *one cycle of the seminiferous epithelium*. Four "passages" through the cycle of the seminiferous epithelium are needed to transform a spermatogonium A into spermatids (S_2) (see Fig. 15-12).

The primary spermatocytes that result from the final spermatogonial division undergo a long first meiotic division (approximately 19 days) in the same fashion as the oocytes (see Figs. 15-10 and 15-11). Leptotene, zygotene, pachytene, and diplotene stages of the first meiotic prophase are distinguished by the chromatin arrangement and changes in cell size. During this time, spermatocytes enlarge, synthesis of RNA and DNA becomes intense, unique membrane proteins appear, and the Golgi complex expands as the nucleus goes through metaphase, anaphase,

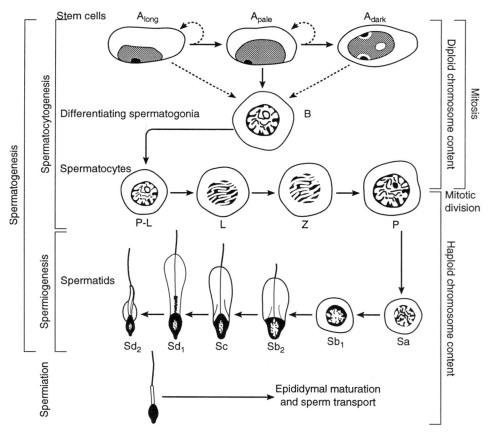

FIG. 15-11. The process of spermatogenesis can be subdivided into spermatocytogenesis and spermiogenesis. Spermatozoon release into the lumen of the seminiferous tubule is called spermiation. During these processes, as the cells pass through pachytene (P), leptotene (L), and zygotene (Z), the number of chromosomes is reduced to the haploid state and the nuclear and cytoplasmic portions of the spermatids are reorganized as indicated by changes in their morphology.

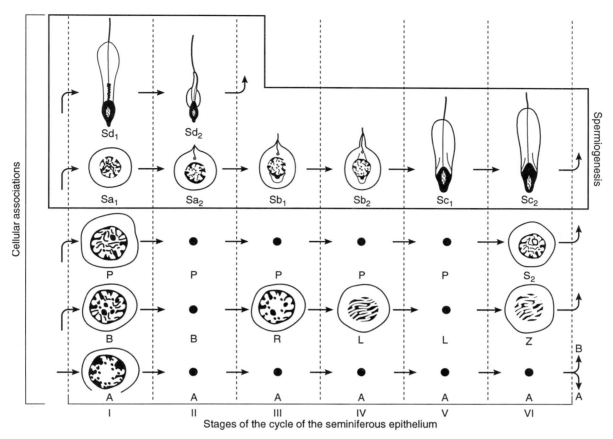

FIG. 15-12. Differentiation of the spermatogonia occurs within the seminiferous tubules in an organized manner. In the human, six cellular associations (stages) are repeated in any one area of the tubule. The succession of these six stages constitutes one cycle of the seminiferous epithelium. Transformation of cell types Sa1 to Sd2 is referred to as spermiogenesis. Leptotene (L), zygotene (Z), and pachytene (P) are subdivisions of prophase.

and telophase of the first maturation division to yield two secondary spermatocytes. The secondary spermatocytes have a short life span of several hours and, without duplicating their DNA, they enter the second meiotic division. This second maturation division results in the formation of two haploid spermatids. Because each of the haploid spermatids contains only 23 chromosomes, two of them will contain 22 autosomes and an X chromosome and the other two 22 autosomes and a Y chromosome.

Ultimately, the spermatids undergo a series of metamorphic changes resulting in highly differentiated spermatozoon. This process whereby the spermatid is transformed into a spermatozoa is known as *spermiogenesis* (Figs. 15-11 to 15-13). Frequently, the first stage of formation of spermatozoa in which the spermatogonia develop into spermatocytes and then into spermatids is referred to as spermatocytogenesis. Thus, spermatogenesis, the process of formation of spermatozoa, can include spermatocytogenesis and spermiogenesis.

During spermiogenesis, the spermatid (characterized by a small spherical nucleus) is transformed into the elon-

gated shape of the spermatozoon. Using hematoxylin and eosin stains, approximately eight steps are described in human spermiogenesis. These steps are classified according to the stage of the seminiferous epithelium and the cell type (see Fig. 15-12). Thus, spermiogenesis begins with the transformation of stage I [type Sa_1 cells (round spermatids)], progresses to stage II (type Sa_2), and is completed at stage II [type Sd_2 cells (spermatids with tails and little cytoplasm)]. During stage I, the *Golgi*, visible adjacent to the nucleus in the type Sa_1 spermatid, begins to elaborate small granules referred to as *proacrosomic granules* (see Fig. 15-13). These coalesce to form a spherical acrosomic granule associated with the nuclear membrane. The *head cap* expands around the acrosomic granule. As spermiogenesis continues, the nucleus becomes eccentric, the chromatin condenses, the cell elongates, and the *axial filament* forms. Following reduction of the cytoplasm around the axial filament, the mitochondria become associated with the proximal portion of the tail. The excess cytoplasm separates from the cell and becomes the residual body (cytoplasmic droplet) seen

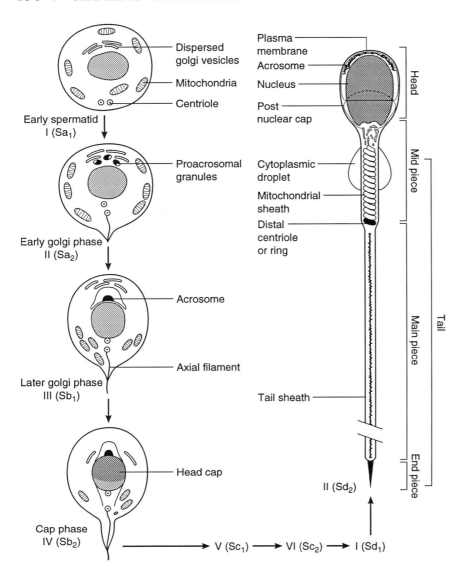

Early spermatid
I (Sa₁)

Dispersed
golgi vesicles

Mitochondria

Centriole

Early golgi phase
II (Sa₂)

Proacrosomal
granules

Later golgi phase
III (Sb₁)

Acrosome

Axial filament

Cap phase
IV (Sb₂)

Head cap

→ V (Sc₁) → VI (Sc₂) → I (Sd₁)

Plasma
membrane

Acrosome

Nucleus

Post
nuclear cap

Head

Cytoplasmic
droplet

Mitochondrial
sheath

Distal
centriole
or ring

Mid piece

Tail sheath

Main piece

Tail

End piece

II (Sd₂)

FIG. 15-13. Spermiogenesis, the transformation of the spermatid (Sa1) into a spermatozoon (Sd2), involves nuclear and cytoplasmic changes and rearrangement of numerous organelles to form the elongated, compacted nuclear shape of the spermatozoon.

along the flagellum in what is now termed a mature spermatid (see Fig. 15-13). Disturbances of spermiogenesis result in altered nuclear shape and lead to abnormal sperm forms.

The process whereby a mature spermatid frees itself from its association with the Sertoli cells and enters the lumen of the seminiferous tubule as a spermatozoon is referred to as *spermiation*. Under ideal conditions, each spermatogonium undergoing differentiation can yield 64 spermatozoa. However, nearly half of the potential sperm are lost during meiosis in a similar fashion to oocytes lost to atresia. Irrespective of sperm loss, approximately 2×10^8 sperm are produced each day from the time of sexual maturity until advanced age. When the spermatozoa leave the testes they are immature. During their journey through the epididymis they develop the capacity for sustained motility. The structural state of the nuclear chromatic and tail organelles become modified and they loose the rem-

nant of spermatid cytoplasm known as the cytoplasmic droplet. These final maturational changes are critical factors influencing their ability to fertilize an oocyte.

Hormonal Control of Spermatogenesis

Hormonal factors necessary for *initiation* of spermatogenesis are different from those needed for its *maintenance* or reinitiation. Since spermatogenesis does not occur in a hypophysectomized individual, initiation of spermatogenesis requires both LH and FSH. FSH binds to the Sertoli cells in the seminiferous tubule resulting in stimulation of adenylate cyclase, increased intracellular cyclic AMP, activation of protein kinases, and increased phosphorylation of a variety of proteins (such as activin and inhibin). FSH may also influence the sensitivity of the testis to LH by regulation of LH receptor numbers of the Leydig cells. LH enhances testosterone synthesis in the Leydig cells. The androgens that are produced bind to high-affinity cytoplasmic and nuclear receptors in the spermatogenic tubule to cause the expression of specific genes necessary for the process of sperm differentiation. The gonadotropins also stimulate the seminiferous tubule to produce such substances as transferrin and androgen-binding protein. It has been proposed that testosterone is necessary for meiosis in the male and that FSH is involved in the completion of spermatid development. Thus, spermatogenesis is initiated by FSH and LH and is maintained by LH alone.

SUGGESTED READING

Oogenesis and Embryogenesis

Adashi EY. The ovarian life cycle. In: Yen SSC, Jaffe RB, eds. *Reproductive Endocrinology: Physiology, Pathophysiology, and Clinical Management,* 3rd ed. Philadelphia: WB Saunders, 1991;181.

Baker TG, Scrimgeous JB. Development of the gonads in anencephalic human fetuses. In: Coutts JRT, ed. *Functional Morphology of the Human Ovary.* Baltimore: University Park Press, 1981;13.

Byrd W, Wolf DP. Oogenesis, fertilization and early development. In: Wolf DP, Quigley MM, eds. *Human In Vitro Fertilization and Embryo Transfer.* New York: Plenum Press, 1984;213.

Erickson GF. An analysis of follicle development and ovum maturation. In: Speroff L, ed. *Seminars in Reproductive Endocrinology,* vol. 4. New York: Thieme, 1986;233.

Gondos B. Oogenesis and spermatogenesis. In: Meisami E, Timiras PS, eds. *Handbook of Human Growth and Developmental Biology, vol 2, Endocrines, Sexual Development, Growth, Nutrition, and Metabolism.* Boca Raton: CRC Press, 1989;137.

Paulson RJ. Oocytes, from development to fertilization. In: Mishell DR, Davajan V, Lobo RA, eds. *Infertility, Contraception and Reproductive Endocrinology,* 3rd ed. Boston: Blackwell Scientific, 1991;140.

Plachot M, Mandelbaum J. Oocyte maturation, fertilization and embryonic growth in vitro. *Br Med Bull* 1990;46:675.

Seibel MM, ed. Oocyte maturation and follicle development. In: *Infertility: A Comprehensive Text.* Norwalk, CT: Appleton and Lange, 1990;37.

Speroff L, Glass RH, Kase NG, eds. The ovary: embryology and development. In: *Clinical Gynecologic Endocrinology and Infertility,* 5th ed. Baltimore: Williams and Wilkins, 1994;93.

Tsafriri A, Bar-Ami S, Lindner HR. Control of the development of meiotic competence and of oocyte maturation in mammals. In: Beier HM, Lindner HR, eds. *Fertilization of the Human Egg In Vitro.* Berlin: Springer-Verlag, 1983;3.

Spermatogenesis

Aitken RJ. Evaluation of human sperm function. *Br Med Bull* 1990;46:654.

DeKretser DM. Morphology and physiology of the testis. In: Becker KL, Bilezikian JP, Bremner WJ, Hung W, Kahn CR, Loriaux DL, Rebar RW, Robertson GL, Wartofsky L, eds. *Principles and Practice of Endocrinology and Metabolism.* Philadelphia: JB Lippincott, 1990;928.

Stevens RW. Basic spermatozoon anatomy and physiology for the clinician. In: Acosta AA, Swanson RJ, Ackerman SB, Kruger TF, van Zyl JA, Menkveld R, eds. *Human Spermatozoa in Assisted Reproduction.* Baltimore: Williams and Wilkins, 1990;1.

Clinical Reproductive Medicine,
Edited by Bryan D. Cowan and David B. Seifer
Lippincott-Raven Publishers, Philadelphia © 1997

CHAPTER 16

Implantation Biology

Bryan D. Cowan

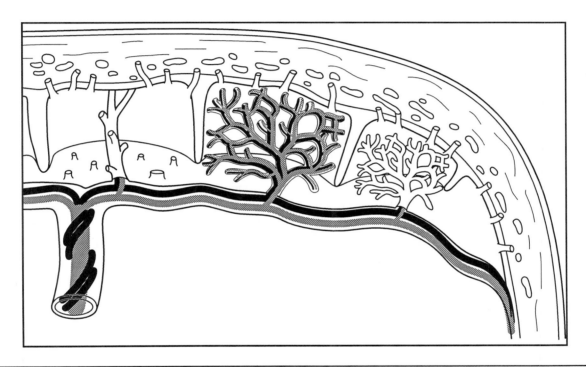

Implantation
Comparative Placental Development
The Human Villous Structure
Trophoblast Regulation of Maternal
    Immunotolerance of Pregnancy

Adhesion Molecules and Implantation
Summary
Suggested Reading

B. D. Cowan: Division of Reproductive Endocrinology, Department of Obstetrics and Gynecology, University of Mississippi Medical Center, Jackson, MS 39216-4505

The placenta is an organ that is characteristic of mammalian species. Its shape and composition show considerable variation between species but its activities are common to all. The placenta performs biological functions for the fetus such as transfer of respiratory gases and nutrients and elimination of waste products. In adults, these same functions require the lungs, intestines, and kidneys, respectively.

The placenta represents a heterotrophic allograft, containing both maternal and paternal antigens. In the uterus, the placenta forms a barrier between the maternal and fetal circulations. This "junction" serves not only for nutrient and gas exchange but as a mediator against maternal immunologic rejection. While much of the exchange physiology of the placenta has been understood during the last 20 years, we are only beginning to appreciate the complexities of maternal immunologic recognition and acceptance of the allograft.

IMPLANTATION

After ovulation, the ovum is captured in the distal portion of the fallopian tube. Here fertilization occurs and the developing zygote travels down the fallopian tube to enter the uterus approximately 4 days after ovulation. Embryonic cleavage occurs during the first 4 days of development. In this process, the embryonic cells divide to produce daughter cells of half the original size. Since no new cell growth occurs during these first 4 days, the embryo remains the size of the original fertilized oocyte (approximately 150 μm).

After entering the uterus, the embryo develops different growth strategies. First it differentiates into two distinct cell types. One cell type is the inner cell mass (destined to become the embryo) and the second is the trophoblast (destined to become the placenta). Cell growth now occurs after each cell division. As a result, the embryo begins to enlarge.

Implantation is the process of embryonic attachment to the uterine wall. Implantation occurs about day 7 to 8 after ovulation in humans. The embryo probably targets its attachment to special sites on the epithelial surface of the uterine cavity. It was once believed that the human embryo "fell" into the glandular crypts of the endometrium, but this is not the case. Instead, the embryo targets hypoepithelial vessels on the surface of the endometrium. It is purported that these hypoepithelial vessels transform the surface of the endometrium to a receptive environment and that this environment attracts the embryo (see section on cell adhesion molecules, below).

Not every species implants after the embryo enters the uterus. Several species demonstrate *delayed* implantation. Two forms of delayed implantation have been observed: *facultative* and *obligate*. Facultative delayed implantation occurs in some species (rat, red kangaroo) only during stress (such as lactation, starvation, or injury). If stress is not present, implantation occurs unimpeded. Obligate delayed implantation occurs (Alaskan fur seal, mink, bear) during each cycle. In either case, the embryo is represented by a free-floating compacted morula/nonexpanding blastocyst that displays minimal metabolic activity. Removing stress in facultative delay reinitiates embryogenesis and implantation, but most of the initiators of implantation after obligate delay are unknown. Curiously, the light cycle controls the duration of the delay in mink. Delayed implantation is not known to occur in primates or humans.

After identifying the implantation site, the embryo attaches. There are at least three distinct mechanisms by which the mammalian trophoblast can invade the endometrium. The trophoblast may penetrate between the uterine epithelial cells (intrusive penetration), directly replace the epithelial cells (displacement penetration), or fuse directly with endometrial cells (fusion penetration) (Table 16-1). Intrusive penetration is observed in the ferret, guinea pig, and possibly the rhesus monkey. Displacement penetration is observed in mouse and rat placentation. Fusion penetration has only been observed in rabbits. The mode of invasion in humans has not yet been identified but is probably related to *intrusive* penetration as observed in the rhesus monkey.

The morphologic sequence of events associated with human implantation is outlined in Fig. 16-1. Although the embryo initially attaches to the uterine epithelium, the ultimate target for implantation is the decidua. The trophoblast cells attach to the epithelium, then penetrate to the decidua. The initial cytotrophoblast cells that lead the invasion process fuse to form a syncytium (syncytiotrophoblast). Penetration then continues for about 4 days, until the embryo is completely buried within the endometrium. It is important to remember that the uterine stroma does not simply make space for the invading embryo. This tissue undergoes changes in response to the embryo that include cell growth and differentiation.

COMPARATIVE PLACENTAL DEVELOPMENT

The nature and interaction between the trophoblast and the maternal tissues (implantation site) show considerable variation between species. For example, in humans the bulk of the fetal syncytiotrophoblast comes into direct contact with maternal blood. In sheep, fetal blood comes into contact with maternal epithelium instead. The most

TABLE 16-1. *Mechanisms of trophoblast attachment to the endometrium*

Type	Examples
Intrusive penetration	Ferret, guinea pig, primate
Fusion penetration	Rabbits
Displacement penetration	Mouse, rat

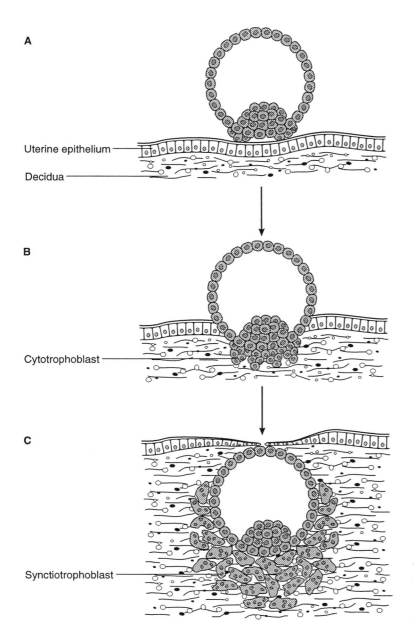

A

Uterine epithelium

Decidua

B

Cytotrophoblast

C

Synctiotrophoblast

FIG. 16-1. Human implantation. The embryo attaches to the surface epithelium at the embryonic pole **(A)**, penetrates the epithelium by intrusion led by cytotrophoblast **(B)**, and establishes a trophoblast bed in the decidua with fused syncytiotrophoblast **(C)**.

useful scheme to categorize these different anatomies was introduced by Grosser. He described three fundamental types of placentae (Table 16-2). The chorial plate is considered to be the fetal unit, and descriptors of the attachment interface describe the placenta. The chorionic plate is composed of three tissue types: capillary endothelium, mesodermal connective tissue, and trophoblast epithelium. The *epitheliochorial* placenta preserves maternal epithelia and endothelia. When only maternal endothelium is preserved, the placenta is classified as *endotheliochorial*. When maternal blood comes into contact with trophoblast, the placenta is termed *hemochorial*. The hemochorial class is subdivided by the number of layers of trophoblast between the maternal blood and fetal en-

dothelium. When only one such layer is encountered (as in humans), then the placenta is classified as *hemomonochorial* (Fig. 16-2).

THE HUMAN VILLOUS STRUCTURE

The hemomonochorial placenta establishes both the exchange mechanism between the mother and fetus, and the protection zone against lethal maternal immunologic recognition. The human fetal circulation is separated from the maternal circulation by only three fetal cell layers: capillary endothelium, connective tissue, and trophoblast epithelium. The vessels in the placenta penetrate as a tree-like structure into a sinusoid within the maternal

TABLE 16-2. *Grossner classification of placentae*

Type	Examples	Maternal structure	Fetal structure
Epitheliochorial	Sow, Mare	Epithelium, Endoethelium	Chorionic plate
Endotheliochorial	Carnivores	Endothelium	Chorionic plate
Hemochorial	Human	None	Chorionic plate
-mono-		None	1 trophoblast layer
-di-		None	2 trophoblast layers
-tri-		None	3 trophoblast layers
Hemoendothelial	Rat, guinea pig, rabbit	None	Vessel endothelium

decidua. Here the finger-like structures are bathed in a pool of maternal blood where gas exchange occurs (Fig. 16-3). The cells in the villous structure perform both anatomic and physiologic functions. The villous anchoring plate attaches the fetal tissues to the maternal decidua and creates the villous compartment. At the same time, the trophoblast cells that line the villous spaces are specialized and probably secrete important regulatory substances, particularly in early pregnancy (Table 16-3). Perhaps the most notable regulatory factor is human chorionic gonadotropin (hCG), the luteotrophic factor of pregnancy in humans. Immunoregulatory factors are also present in trophoblast. These factors probably provide immunologic protection within the villous by guarding against foreign antigen invasion and may modulate maternal cell-mediated immunity.

TROPHOBLAST REGULATION OF MATERNAL IMMUNOTOLERANCE OF PREGNANCY

The trophoblast contributes to pregnancy immunotolerance by limiting expression of major histocompatibility (MHC) antigens (*trophoblast invisibility*). The human trophoblast does not express classical MHC antigens. Classical (HLA-A, B, C) class I MHC genes encode highly polymorphic, cell surface glycoproteins that are associated with β_2-microglobin. Nonclassical class I genes (HLA-E, F, and G) are relatively nonpolymorphic and encode smaller glycoproteins. Of the three "nonclassical" class I genes, HLA-G is currently the most interesting in relation to pregnancy immunotolerance. HLA-G is expressed in first-trimester extravillous cytotrophoblasts, term chorioamnion, and first-trimester villous mesenchyme cells. Villous trophoblast exhibits more variable expression, with higher levels of HLA-G in the villous cytotrophoblast than syncytiotrophoblast. The role of HLA-G in the immunology of pregnancy is undefined, but several lines of evidence suggest that HLA-G may restrict antigen presentation and thereby reduce maternal cell-mediated responses to the fetus.

Immunotolerance of human pregnancy may also depend on *trophoblast resistance* to maternal effector cells. Human trophoblasts are resistant to killing by either antibody, cytotoxic T cells, natural killer (NK) cells, macro-

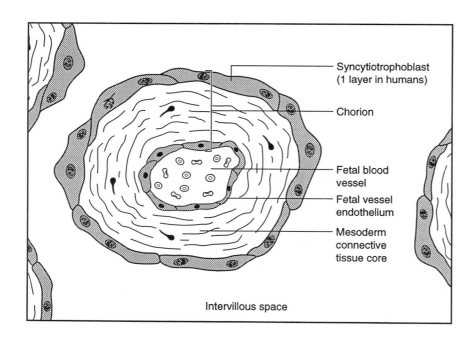

FIG. 16-2. Human hemomonochorial villous structure, transverse view.

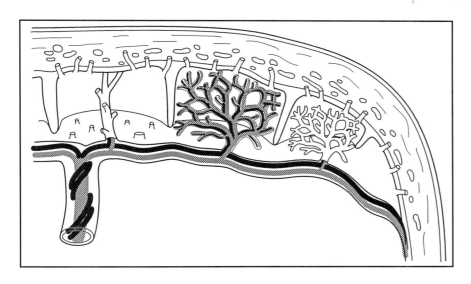

FIG. 16-3. Essential features of the villous structure. Each cotyledon is separated by a septum of decidual tissue. Maternal blood is provided from the decidual arteries and emptied by the veins. The trophoblast is anchored to the decidua by a trophoblast column, the villous plate.

phages, and the decidua-associated large granular lymphocyte (LGL) with NK-like killing activity. This resistance of trophoblast to LGL/NK killing has been attributed to a lack of NK target structures on the trophoblast surface.

A third proposal concerning pregnancy immunotolerance states that maternal rejection responses are regulated (*self-defense*) by trophoblast-derived factors acting at the maternal–fetal interface. The trophoblast may ensure its own immunologic survival by the release of local immunomodulatory factors. The factor(s) mediating this response remain largely uncharacterized. However, interferons (IFNs) and specialized cytokines (IL-10) have demonstrated important biological functions in the placenta. In all species studied, IFN activity can be detected

in tissues of the maternal–fetal interface. Human pregnancy is characterized by enhanced class I IFN expression (IFN-α and β) and decreased IFN-γ (class II) production. IFN-α has been localized to villous syncytiotrophoblast and extravillous trophoblast. Class I IFNs suppress immune effector cell proliferation and function, and may play an important role in the regulation of cell surface antigen expression by human trophoblast. A potent immunoregulatory cytokine, IL-10, may also be expressed by fetal trophoblast. IL-10 was originally described in mice as a factor produced by class II T-helper cells (T$_H$2) that suppressed proinflammatory cytokines [IL-2, IFN-γ, and tumor necrosis factor (TNF)-α] production by class I T-helper cells (T$_H$1). Through this regulation of the cytokine network, IL-10 may bias the maternal immune response toward antibody production and away from cell-mediated immunity at the maternal–fetal interface.

The human decidua is a rich source of growth factors that affect the balance between the mother and fetus (Table 16-3). Decidual growth factors currently known to influence trophoblast function include colony stimulating factors, epidermal growth factors, transforming growth factor-β (TGF-β), and IL-1. The colony-stimulating factors (CSF-1, GM-CSF, and IL-3) are widely purported as beneficial to trophoblast development and function. Both CSF-1 and GM-CSF increase trophoblast growth, and GM-CSF increases IFN-γ synthesis by the sheep trophoblast. The epidermal growth factors include TGF-α and epidermal growth factor (EGF). These growth factors increase hCG secretion by choriocarcinoma cell lines and normal trophoblasts. TGF-β is a multifunctional cytokine that can stimulate or inhibit cellular function depending on the target cell type. TGF-β expression in the human uterus is correlated with reproductive status, with low expression during the proliferative phase, an increase during the secretory phase, and a subsequent greater increase

TABLE 16-3. *Some important placental regulatory factors*

	Hormonal	Immunologic	Growth
Trophoblast:			
hCG	x		
hpL	x		
Estradiol	x		
Estriol	x		
Progesterone	x		
IFN-α		x	
IL-10		x	
HLA-G		x	
Decidua:			
CSF-1			x
GM-CSF			x
IL-3			x
TGF-α			x
EGF			x
TGF-β		x	x
IL-1		x	x

during early pregnancy. TGF-β inhibits proliferation of first-trimester human trophoblast while stimulating formation of multinucleated syncytiotrophoblast. Another decidua-derived cytokine proposed as a mediator of trophoblast development and function is IL-1. IL-1 mRNA and protein have been detected in the human placenta, endometrium, and decidua. IL-1 is produced by preimplantation embryos and blockage of the receptor inhibits blastocyst attachment.

ADHESION MOLECULES AND IMPLANTATION

The roles of adhesion molecules in implantation are just being investigated. Several classes of adhesion molecules are known (integrins, selectins), but integrins are better studied in reproduction.

The integrins are a large family of cell adhesion *receptors* that are involved in cell-to-cell and cell-to-matrix reactions. Currently, at least 21 different integrin molecules are known and expressed in an astonishing variety of cells throughout the body. The integrins function to anchor cells to a specific location and transmit information to the cell. Integrins are thus involved with diverse cellular processes such as immunologic homing, metastatic spread, healing, and embryologic development.

The integrin molecules are heterodimers, composed of an α and β subunit. Thus, an intact integrin will be described as the combination of the α and β subunit, such as $\alpha_1\beta_1$. The interaction of integrins with their respective ligands requires the presence of both α and β subunits. Ligand specificity is determined by the αβ heterodimer and is unlike the binding in traditional specific ligand–receptor conditions. Most integrins interact with more than one matrix, and many matrix molecules interact with more than one integrin receptor. Important matrix ligands include fibronectin and laminin. No fewer than seven different integrins bind to fibronectin

TABLE 16-4. *Integrins and possible functions during reproduction*

Integrin		Site	Effect
β_1	α_4	Endometrium	Cyclic expression
β_3	α_5	Endometrium	Cyclic expression
β_3	—	Endometrium	Infertility?
β_1	—	Embryo	Inner cell mass involution
β_1	α_1	Trophoblast	Limits invasion
β_1	β_5	Trophoblast	Accelerates invasion

and six bind to laminin (Fig. 16-4). This redundancy may provide important advantages for cell–cell and cell–matrix binding.

The contributing cells of implantation (maternal endometrium and fetal trophoblast) express integrins. Our understanding of the role for integrins during implantation is just now unfolding, but some preliminary and exciting observations are noteworthy. Three important biological behaviors of integrins in reproduction have been identified (integrin *expression*, *polarity*, and *switching*).

During the ovarian menstrual cycle, certain endometrial integrins are expressed constitutively whereas others are phasic and hormonally regulated. The expression of two cycle-dependent endometrial integrins ($\alpha_4\beta_1$, $\alpha_5\beta_3$) is framed during the implantation window in humans. A defect in the *endometrial* expression of one of these integrins (β_3) has been postulated to cause infertility. Additionally, a defect in *embryonic* expression of β_1 causes involution of the inner cell mass but preserves the trophoblast (Table 16-4). In addition to *expression* of the integrin, *polarity* of the integrin distribution over the cell may be an important regulator during implantation. Human uterine epithelium displays distinct polarization

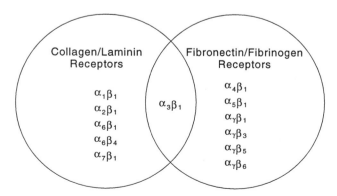

FIG. 16-4. Extracellular matrix binding of the integrin family. No fewer than six integrins bind collagen and seven bind fibronectin. Only $\alpha_3\beta_1$ has overlapping binding.

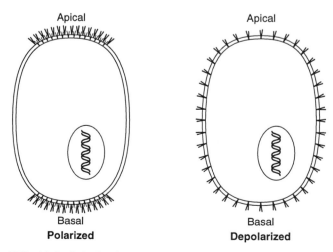

FIG. 16-5. Polarized and nonpolarized configuration of distributed integrins. The nonpolarized configuration appears to promote endometrial-trophoblast associations.

regarding the distribution of integrins. Loss of apical-basal polarity (Fig. 16-5) appears to promote trophoblast–endometrial association whereas a polarized configuration inhibits association. The trophoblast also demonstrates *switching* of integrin expression. The invading first trimester trophoblast expresses $\alpha_5\beta_1$ but integrin expression switches in later pregnancy to $\alpha_1\beta_1$. It is believed that this switching regulates the invasiveness of the trophoblast.

SUMMARY

The human placenta is structurally composed of a hemomonochorion. This structure forms after cell-to-cell and cell-to-matrix adhesion of the trophoblast to the endometrium. Integrins probably play a vital role in establishing this interface. Immunomodulatory factors derived from both the trophoblast and decidua maintain this privileged allograft.

SUGGESTED READING

Arey LB. *Developmental Anatomy.* 7th ed. Philadelphia: WB Saunders, 1974.

Bavister BD. *Preimplantation Embryo Development.* New York: Springer-Verlag, 1993.

Cheresh DA, Mecham RP. *Integrins.* San Diego: Academic Press, 1994.

Damsky CH, Librach C, Lim KH, Fitzgerald ML, McMaster MT, Janatpour M, Zhou Y, Logan SK, Fisher SJ. Integrin switching regulates normal trophoblast invasion. *Development* 1994;120:3657–3666.

Glasser SR, Mulholland J, Psychoyos A. *Endocrinology of Embryo–Endometrium Interactions.* New York: Plenum Press, 1994.

Ilesanmi AO, Hawkins DA, Lessey BA. Immunohistochemical markers of uterine receptivity in the human endometrium. *Microsc Res Tech* 1993; 15:208–222.

Lessey BA, Castelbaum AJ, Buck CA, Lei Y, Yowell CW, Sun J. Further characterization of endometrial integrins during the menstrual cycle and in pregnancy. *Fertil Steril* 1994;62:497–506.

Stephens LE, Sutherland AE, Klimanskaya IV, Andrieux A, Meneses J, Pedersen RA, Damsky CH. Deletion of β_1 integrins in mice results in inner cell mass failure and peri-implantation lethality. *Genes Dev* 1995;9: 1883–1885.

Tabibzadeh S. Regulatory roles of IFN-γ in human endometrium. *Ann NY Acad Sci* 1994;734:1–6.

Thie M, Arrach-Ruprecht B, Sauer H, Fuchs P, Albers A, Denker HW. Cell adhesion to the apical pole of epithelium: a function of cell polarity. *Eur J Cell Biol* 1995;66:180–191.

Clinical Reproductive Medicine,
Edited by Bryan D. Cowan and David B. Seifer
Lippincott-Raven Publishers, Philadelphia © 1997

CHAPTER 17

Infertility Evaluation

Bryan D. Cowan

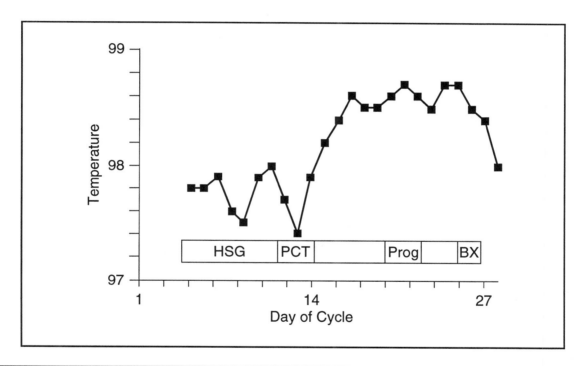

Infertility Testing
  Male Factor Evaluation
  Ovulation Factors
  Tuboperitoneal Evaluation
  Uterine Factors
Timing of Studies
Strategy of Evaluation
Measures of Fertility Treatment Success

Treatment Options
  Male Factor Treatments
  Tubal Disease
  Ovulation Defects
  Unexplained Infertility
Impact of Age of Reproduction
Summary
Suggested Reading

B. D. Cowan: Division of Reproductive Endocrinology, Department of Obstetrics and Gynecology, University of Mississippi Medical Center, Jackson, MS 39216-4505

Approximately 2.5 million married couples are affected by subfertility during their reproductive lives. The reasons for this high prevalence of subfecundity are complex but include time-dependent acquired diseases (sexually transmitted diseases and endometriosis), age-dependent decreasing fecundity, and population demographics (eg, the "baby boomers"). The fertility rate in the United States has been nearly constant for several years at 2.1 live births per reproductive age female. This rate matches the ideal fertility rate to maintain a population profile consistent with "zero population growth." As such, there is great emphasis in our society on having only the number of children desired at the time in our reproductive lives that is most convenient. Thus, many couples seek fertility services to overcome acquired diseases, enhance the natural decreasing fertility associated with age, and accommodate lifestyle agendas.

INFERTILITY TESTING

Infertility is established when a couple has unencumbered coital exposure for 12 months without conception. In general, three major potential etiologic factors are assessed to uncover the causes of infertility. Although reported infertility populations vary, it is convenient to consider that about 20% of couples will have male factor dysfunction; that ovulation defects affect 30%; and female anatomic abnormalities are present in 40% (Table 17-1). Thus, it is appropriate to assess male factors, ovulation factors, and tuboperitoneal factors in every couple with infertility.

Male Factor Evaluation

The history of the male should include the usual medical information, as well as information concerning history of previously fathered pregnancies, trauma, testicular mumps, environmental exposure, and heat exposure. If a physical examination can be performed, the genitalia should be inspected to assess developmental stage and testicular size. Palpation for scrotal masses, varicocele, and inguinal hernia should be performed.

The single most important laboratory test is the semen analysis. The semen analysis should report important information including volume, total ejaculated sperm, percent motility of sperm, and percent normal forms (Table

TABLE 17-1. *Etiologic factors in infertility*

Defect	Percentage
Male factors	20
Tubal factors	40
Ovulation defect	30
Unexplained	10

TABLE 17-2. *Semen analysis norms*

Volume	2–6 ml
Sperm per ejaculate	60–200 million
Motile sperm	≥50%
Grade of motility (0–4)	≥3+
Oval morphology	≥50%

17-2). The cycle of sperm production lasts approximately 70–80 days. This is important to consider when evaluating male factors because acute illnesses may have adverse consequences on an isolated semen analysis. Abnormalities of a semen analysis should be confirmed by repeat testing on two or three additional occasions. Repeat testing should be accomplished in a new "sperm cycle." Although commonly used, the hamster zona-free oocyte penetration test, cervical mucous penetration test, postcoital test, and others provide limited information beyond the semen analysis. Because some of these tests are difficult to perform, interpretation is highly variable, and their ability to predict fertility is inconclusive, we recommend that these tests be used only in special circumstances when they can enhance the information obtained from a quality-controlled semen analysis.

Ovulation Factors

Ovulation defects occur in two forms. Anovulation is the easiest form to recognize. Ovulatory dysfunction (luteal phase defect, low-serum progesterone) is more difficult to establish and is subject to continued controversy.

Women with 28- to 32-day cycles are probably (99.8%) ovulatory. This essential information is deemed reliable because only 2–3 of 1000 women with this history will be discovered to be anovulatory. Thus, the careful establishment of a menstrual history is fundamental to determining ovulatory status. However, this important history is subjective information, and objective information is usually requested to confirm ovulation. Objective measures of ovulation include basal body temperature chart monitoring, serum progesterone measurements in the luteal phase, and endometrial biopsy of secretory endometrium.

Basal body temperature monitoring will commonly reveal a temperature elevation of 0.2–0.6°F after ovulation. This temperature rise is associated with the release of luteal phase progesterone and the resetting of the hypothalamic thermoregulator. The temperature remains elevated throughout the luteal phase, and the typical "biphasic" profile is demonstrated repeatedly. Unfortunately, ovulatory defects are difficult to establish with this monitoring. Neither the luteal length nor the magnitude of temperature rise correlates with other measures of luteal dysfunction (progesterone, endometrial biopsy). Thus, basal body temperature monitoring is a good tool to establish ovulation but is limited by its inability to assess luteal dysfunction.

Serum progesterone measurements >5 ng/ml confirm ovulation. Most clinicians use serum progesterone to both confirm ovulation and establish the adequacy of ovulation. Controversy surrounds the threshold value of serum progesterone that establishes an ovulatory defect. In general, a serum progesterone obtained 6–8 days prior to the onset of menses that is >5 ng/ml but <10 ng/ml is interpreted as ovulatory but associated with luteal dysfunction. Similarly, a serum progesterone >20 ng/ml drawn at the same mid-luteal time is associated with adequate luteal function. It is important to remember that it is the timing of the progesterone measurement (6–8 days prior to the onset of menses) that is critical to its interpretation for ovulatory adequacy. Unfortunately, there is no consensus on what serum progesterone between 10 and 20 ng/ml reflects concerning luteal dysfunction or adequacy. However, these values indicate that ovulation has occurred.

Endometrial biopsy is also used to establish ovulation and the adequacy of luteal function. It is typically performed 2–3 days prior to the onset of menses. Luteal phase defect is established if the maturation of the endometrium lags the chronologic duration of the cycle by more than 2 days. The original description of luteal phase defect based on endometrial maturation required two biopsies for confirmation. However, this practice is inconvenient, and most patients object to the extra cost and discomfort. Unfortunately, low progesterone does not correlate with endometrial immaturity.

Adjuncts to ovulatory assessment include urinary measurements of midcycle luteinizing hormone (LH) surge and follicular sonography. Although these tests are helpful for planning strategies such as insemination, hormonal manipulation, or fertility testing, they are used only to predict ovulation and suffer from lack of measuring the event of interest (ovulation).

Tuboperitoneal Evaluation

Evaluation for tuboperitoneal disease should include a history that includes information regarding previous exposure to sexually transmitted diseases, abdominal or pelvic surgery, and previous method of contraception. Two important tests are used to establish normalcy of tuboperitoneal status.

The hysterosalpingogram (HSG) is a contrast study that provides information about both the internal uterine contour and tubal patency. It is an office-based procedure and associated with minimal discomfort. Historically, the test was of great value in determining the type of subsequent surgical treatment or evaluation for tuboperitoneal disease. If a normal HSG was observed, then diagnostic laparoscopy was performed. If an abnormal study was observed (eg, hydrosalpinx), then laparotomy was recommended. Today most tubal disorders are treated with laparoscopy. Therefore, there is little need for the HSG to

be used in the decision algorithm for surgery. Its advantage now is to disclose unsuspected proximal disease (occlusion or salpingitis isthmica nodosa) and to alert the operating surgeon to the extent of distal disease that could be encountered during endoscopic evaluation and treatment.

Both aqueous and oil-based contrast medium are available. Although HSG is generally not considered a therapeutic tool, some evidence suggests that fertility is enhanced if oil-based reagent is used. Unfortunately, the oil-based reagent occasionally produces a syndrome associated with multiple disseminated lipid droplets. Patients complain of joint pain, respiratory compromise, intense fatigue, and neurologic changes. Chest X ray is usually diagnostic (contrast in the lungs) and treatment is supportive. Fatalities have occasionally been reported.

In general, patients at high risk for sexually transmitted disease should receive antibiotic prophylaxis (doxycycline 100 mg BID × 5 days) after HSG. If hydrosalpinx is detected, antibiotic therapy should be initiated because these women are at high risk for postprocedure infection. Women without these two risk factors probably do not benefit from antibiotic therapy. Active infection with gonorrhea or chlamydia is a contraindication for the procedure.

Laparoscopy currently represents the standard of diagnostic modalities for tuboperitoneal status. With this instrument, adhesions, hydrosalpinx, endometriosis, and ovarian pathology can be assessed and treated (see Chapter 21).

Uterine Factors

Mullerian anomalies infrequently cause infertility, but some notable examples include transmural fibroids, submucosal fibroids, intrauterine polyps, and uterine septum (a cause of repetitive pregnancy loss). Physical exam and hysterogram will usually disclose many of these abnormalities. Two additional adjuncts to the evaluation of Mullerian defects include sonography and hysteroscopy. Hysteroscopy can be used to cannulate the fallopian tube and correct some cases of proximal tubal occlusion, or for direct resection of intrauterine lesions. Sonography or sonohysterography can detect the location of intrauterine or mural anatomic defects. Magnetic resonance imaging (MRI) visualization, although expensive, can detect aberrant Mullerian structures with high accuracy as well.

TIMING OF STUDIES

An efficient and cost-effective fertility investigation can be performed within two cycles. Figure 17-1 shows the timing of tests based on the ovarian menstrual cycle. Semen analysis can be performed at any time. HSG and laparoscopy/hysteroscopy should be performed after the

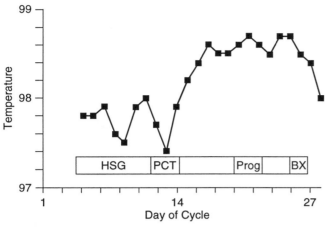

FIG. 17-1. Timing of fertility tests in an ovarian menstrual cycle. The strategy is to avoid invasive procedures when an unrecognized pregnancy could occur (eg, after ovulation). Prog, progesterone; BX, biopsy; PCT, postcoital test; HSG, hysterosalpingogram.

TABLE 17-3. *Infertility testing*

Basic tests	Adjunctive tests
Male: Semen analysis	Postcoital test, antisperm antibodies, sperm penetration tests
Female: Ovulation history, progesterone, BBT, endometrial biopsy	Follicular ultrasound, prolactin, thyroid panel, follicle-stimulating hormone

BBT, basal body temperature

menstrual cycle but before ovulation. This is to reduce contamination of the pelvis with menstrual blood and to eliminate the possibility of testing during early conception. Serum progesterone is typically obtained 6–8 days prior to the onset of menses, and endometrial biopsy is performed 2–3 days prior to the onset of menses.

At our institution, we recommend a "basic profile" that consists of a semen analysis to evaluate male gametes and basal body temperature chart or serum progesterone to assess ovulation. We perform HSG or sonohysterography if the likelihood of advancing to laparoscopy is low (eg, candidates for insemination or advanced follicular stimulation with a negative history for pelvic conditions). Laparoscopy is used to diagnose and treat tuboperitoneal disease in women that possess "long-term ovarian reproductive reserve." This concept cannot be quantitated presently, but in general we recommend that women >39 years of age forego laparoscopy. This is because these women may not be able to benefit from therapeutic surgery prior to a substantial reduction in their remaining fertility (see below).

Although other tests exist (Table 17-3), it is important to remember that these tests are used to explain "unexplained infertility." Little evidence suggests that "findings" in these tests will be advantageous. The basic fertility investigation outlined in Table 17-3 will usually lead to the cause of infertility in 85–90% of couples.

STRATEGY OF EVALUATION

The strategy of evaluation is based on the level of clinical care required for proper treatment of a couple's fer-

tility disorders. For our discussions, it seems convenient to consider three levels of care (basic, complex level I, complex level II).

In the first level of care (basic) the strategy is based on the successful treatment of the anovulatory patient and referral of patients with complex disorders to higher levels. As seen in Fig. 17-2, women >35 years of age should be referred to higher level evaluation and treatment facilities. Therefore, only women <35 years of age are candidates for the basic evaluation. At this level of evaluation, a semen analysis is performed on the male and an assessment of ovulation performed on the female. If an ovulation defect exists, clomiphene therapy is initiated for 4–6 months. Thyroid and prolactin screening is performed to

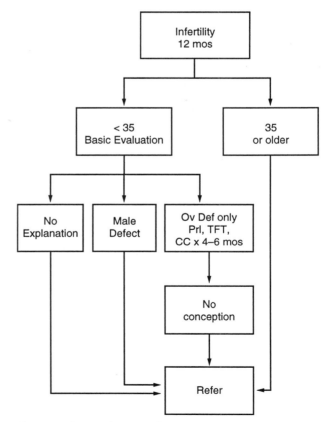

FIG. 17-2. Basic algorithm for the management of infertility. CC, clomiphene; TFT, thyroid function tests; Prl, prolactin; Ov Def, ovulation defect.

TABLE 17-4. *Complex level 1*

Condition	Treatments
Male	AID, AIH
	Urology consult
	Adoption counseling
Ovulation	Clomiphene
	Glucocorticoids
	HMG
	hCG
	Sonograms
	Estradiol
Tubal	Laparoscopy
	Adhesiolysis
	Salpingostomy
	Tubal anastomosis
	Tubal cannulation
	Uterotubal implantation
	Cystectomy
	ART counseling
Uterine	Hysteroscopy
	Septum division
	Myomectomy
	Unification procedures

AID, artificial insemination—donor; AIH, artifical insemination—husband; hMG, human menopausal gonadotropin; hCG, human chorionic gonadotropin; ART, assisted reproductive technology.

exclude correctable endocrine dysfunction. If male factor abnormalities are detected, these couples should be referred to higher order facilities. Additionally, if no disorder is found, referral is appropriate.

In complex level 1 (Table 17-4), the strategy is to treat diagnosis-related conditions (male factor, tuboperitoneal disease, and complex anovulation) with specific diagnosis-related procedures. This involves a comprehensive evaluation of tubal and Mullerian abnormalities, and the ability to treat couples with insemination, advanced follicular stimulation, and advanced endosurgical management. It makes little sense to perform expensive and time-consuming diagnostic procedures such as laparoscopy if the operating surgeon does not possess the skills to properly treat the conditions detected.

Complex level 2 represents the application of diagnosis-independent treatments (gamete technologies) to correct infertility (see Chapter 22). Here the wide array of assisted reproductive technologies (Table 17-5) are ap-

TABLE 17-5. *Complex level 2*

Endogenous ART
  In vitro fertilization
  GIFT
  PROST
  TET
  ICSI
Cooperative ART
  Oocyte donation
  Surrogate

GIFT, gamete intrafallopian transfer; PROST, pronuclear ovum stage transfer; TET, tubal embryo transfer; ICSI, intracytoplasmic sperm injection; ART, assisted reproductive technology.

plied. In general, patients are offered these treatments when they have failed conservative therapies at the basic and complex level 1, or enter treatment when the woman is older (see Chapter 22).

MEASURES OF FERTILITY TREATMENT SUCCESS

Fertility treatment success is time-dependent and related to the number of female ovulatory cycles. As such, two parameters have been established to discuss fertility success. *Fecundity* is the measure of pregnancy rate per single ovulatory cycle. *Cumulative probability* of pregnancy represents the expectation of conception within a population. That expectation is time-dependent and, for example, may occur within 6 months or 6 years. As such, analytic tools have been developed that assess the per cycle fecundity, maximum cumulative probability of pregnancy, and duration of time required to achieve the therapeutic effect.

Essentially, two models are used today to estimate fecundity and cumulative probability. The more traditional model is life table analysis. While this model is useful in analyzing time-dependent data, it has an inherent weakness when used to analyze fertility data. In traditional life table analysis, the event of interest is life or death, and eventually the entire population is affected. However, in the pregnancy model, it is rare to see a population have a 100% pregnancy success rate. Because of this weakness, logistic models have been developed. These logistic models fit the data better, and allow easy calculations of cycle fecundity and cumulative probability (Fig. 17-3).

Table 17-6 compares the fecundity and cumulative probability of conception for various treatment options that correct fertility disorders. These relative comparisons serve as the bases for both the initiation of treatment and the rational discontinuation of further efforts.

TREATMENT OPTIONS

Treatment options can be classified as diagnosis-related or empiric. Diagnosis-related treatments are provided for couples affected by disordered male factors, tubal factors, or ovulation defects. Empiric therapy is provided to couples with unexplained infertility.

Male Factor Treatments

The cornerstone of male factor treatment is insemination. Two types of insemination are provided based on the severity of the defect. Homologous washed intrauterine insemination (AIH) uses sperm gathered from the husband. The sperm is submitted to a laboratory process to eliminate seminal fluid (wash), and often the enhanced

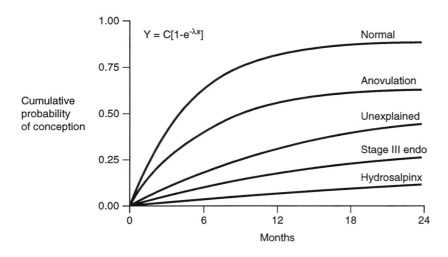

FIG. 17-3. Typical logistic graphical analysis of five types of fertility treatment outcome. The equation for logistic analysis is Y = C[1 − e$^{-\lambda x}$] where ^{x} represents the interval in time (usually a month) and Y is the cumulative probability. The variables of interest are λ (the monthly fecundity rate) and C (the maximum expected cumulative probability of pregnancy). Using this model, important estimates of fertility outcome after treatment can be obtained.

motile fraction is purified from immotile sperm (swim-up). The washed and enriched specimen is then placed in the uterus just before or at the time of ovulation. In general, AIH has a per-cycle fecundity that ranges from 3% to 9% and a cumulative probability that approaches 30% to 35% over approximately 8–12 months.

Donor insemination (AID) relies on contributed gametes from an alternate male. Current recommendations for AID state that this sperm should be obtained from individuals who have no history of genetic diseases and are negative for sexually transmitted diseases (eg, HIV, hepatitis, gonorrhea, and syphilis). The sperm is obtained, frozen, and quarantined for 6 months. The donors are then rescreened for transmittable diseases, and if negative after the quarantine, the sperm is released.

The sperm is stored frozen in liquid nitrogen vapors and thawed prior to insemination. One insemination per ovulatory cycle is as effective as two inseminations, but intrauterine inseminations are better than intracervical inseminations. Inseminations should be performed just before or at ovulation. The expected fecundity for AID is approximately 12–18% per month, and cumulative pregnancy success rates approach 70% after six to eight treatment cycles.

In isolated cases, the new ART technologies have demonstrated efficacy for men with restrictive oligospermia (see Chapter 22). Lastly, retrograde ejaculation and electrostimulatory ejaculation, as well as testicular aspiration/biopsy, have granted acquisition of sperm for use in ART programs.

Tubal Disease

Tubal disease that impairs fertility is caused by pelvic adhesions or endometriosis. Although the diseases are different, the surgical approach for each is the same. The strategy is to optimize the pelvic anatomy to the greatest extent possible using meticulous surgical technique (see Chapter 21).

The extent of pelvic adhesions determines the prognosis for affected patients. Women who require only adhesiolysis have a pregnancy success rate of nearly 50% with a per-cycle fecundity ranging from 6% to 8%. On the other hand, women who require neosalpingostomy for hydrosalpinx have a per-cycle fecundity of <3% and an overall expected maximum probability of pregnancy ≤25%. Another curious feature of those patients who undergo neosalpingostomy is that the time from operation to the time the pregnancies start occurring is delayed. The maximum pregnancy success rate after surgery requires approximately 2 and even 3 years of continued observation. As such, maturing women may not be candidates for reparative tubal surgery.

Endometriosis is classified into stages based on the extent of disease present. Pregnancy success rates in women with stage I disease appear to be independent of the therapy provided. The fecundity rate in patients with stage I disease is approximately 8% each month, with a maximum probability of pregnancy at 60%. In contrast,

TABLE 17-6. *Comparison of fertility treatment success*

Condition	Treatment	Fecundity (λ)	Maximum Probability (c)
Normal	Observation	0.20	0.90
Anovulation	Clomiphene	0.16	0.65
Hydrosalpinx	Neosalpingostomy	0.04	0.20
Stage III–IV endometriosis	Surgery	0.06	0.35
Unexplained infertility	Observation	0.06	0.60
Male factor	AIH	0.03	0.30
Male factor	AID	0.12	0.70

AIH, artificial insemination—husband; AID, artifical insemination—donor.

women with stage III and IV disease benefit from surgery. The monthly fecundity is approximately 5% with a cumulative probability of 35% in 30 months. Stage II disease is intermediate. Once again, maturing women may not be able to take advantage of the time frame required to see a benefit from surgery.

Tubal anastomosis is commonly performed after previous sterilization but may be performed for patients with obstructive proximal tubal disease (salpingitis isthmica nodosa). In general, pregnancy rates approach 70% after one year and occur with a per-cycle fecundity of 12–18% per month.

Ovulation Defects

The detailed description of the management of patients with ovulation defects is described in Chapter 24. However, for our considerations, we will describe the expected outcome of clomiphene and human menopausal gonadotropin (hMG) therapy.

Clomiphene citrate is used to correct ovulatory disturbances. On this therapy, approximately 85% of patients will ovulate and approximately 65% will achieve a pregnancy in 4–6 months. The per-cycle fecundity is approximately 12%.

hMG therapy (Metrodin, Pergonal, Humegon) has been used to treat estrogenized/androgenized chronic anovulation (PCOD) that is resistant to clomiphene therapy and women afflicted with hypogonadotropic hypogonadism. Curiously, the latter group (hypogonadotropic hypogonadism) has an excellent response to hMG therapy. Approximately 90% of these patients will achieve a pregnancy in approximately 6 months of therapy with a per-cycle fecundity of 35%. This represents the highest fertility treatment option available to clinicians. Fortunately, patients with hypogonadotropic hypogonadism are seen rarely, but their response to therapy is very favorable. In contrast, patients with chronic anovulation who fail to ovulate on clomiphene citrate fair much worse. The expected maximum probability of pregnancy is approximately 35–40%, and per-cycle fecundities range from 6% to 8%.

Unexplained Infertility

The strategy of unexplained infertility is based on the desire to shorten the duration to maximum probability of pregnancy and to increase the per-cycle fecundity. In general, these diagnosis-independent strategies involve multiple follicular stimulation (see Chapter 24), insemination, and gamete technologies (see Chapter 22). If not treated, couples with unexplained infertility have a 60% probability of pregnancy within 5 years and a per-cycle fecundity of approximately 5–7%. Follicular stimulation with insemination shortens the interval of time and increases per cycle fecundity. Similarly, gamete technologies accomplish the same goals.

IMPACT OF AGE OF REPRODUCTION

Female aging (maturity) is associated with two detrimental reproductive events. As the prophase I oocyte ages, it appears to acquire increasing risk for nondysjunction events that lead to trisomy 21 (Table 17-7). Additionally, reproductive efficiency, as estimated by population fertility rates, is also dramatically influenced by age. Little evidence regarding natural fertility rates is available from concurrent societies because developed societies choose to limit reproduction (contraception) and developing societies are nutritionally depleted and have poor records. For these reasons, historical records of unencumbered societies that did not limit reproduction have served as the demographic basis for unencumbered fertility rates. Two such societies have been studied: the Mormons of the 1800s and the European aristocracy of the 17th and 18th centuries. Figure 17-4 shows the age-related decline in fertility rates in Mormon women. The rate declines slowly from 25 to 35 years of age, but then declines dramatically thereafter. The reasons for this declining reproductive efficiency are not known but probably include an increase in spontaneous abortion, altered

TABLE 17-7. *Age-specific risk for cytogenetic disorders*

Maternal age	Risk of Down's syndrome
20	1/1923
21	1/1695
22	1/1538
23	1/1408
24	1/1299
25	1/1205
26	1/1124
27	1/1053
28	1/990
29	1/935
30	1/885
31	1/826
32	1/725
33	1/592
34	1/465
35	1/365
36	1/287
37	1/225
38	1/177
39	1/139
40	1/109
41	1/85
42	1/67
43	1/53
44	1/41
45	1/32
46	1/25
47	1/20
48	1/16
49	1/12

Data are from Hook and Chambers (1977) and Hook (1981). Because the sample size for some intervals is relatively small, 95% confidence limits are sometimes relatively large. Despite this, these figures indicate genetic counseling.

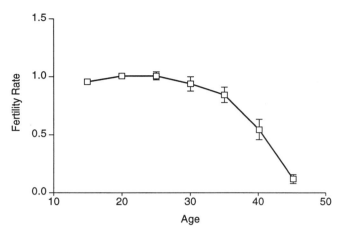

FIG. 17-4. Age-specific fertility.

hypothalamic-pituitary-ovarian dynamics, oocyte depletion, oocyte aging, and uterine aging.

SUMMARY

Infertility affects a large proportion of reproductive-aged couples. An efficient basic evaluation will diagnose the cause of infertility in 85–90% of couples. Ovarian age is a fundamental factor in evaluating treatment strategies and determining prognosis. Information concerning success of fertility treatment should be a part of the strategies to treat infertile couples.

SUGGESTED READING

Ovulation

Dawood MY. Corpus luteal insufficiency. *Curr Opin Obstet Gynecol* 1994; 6:121–127.
Olive DL. The prevalence and epidemiology of luteal-phase deficiency in normal and infertile women. *Clin Obstet Gynecol* 1991;34:157–166.
Palermo R, Albano C, Agrifoglio V, Giambanco L, Napoli P. Anovulatory infertility. *Acta Europea Fertilitatis* 1994;256:93–106.

Male

Aitken RJ, Baker HW, Irvine DS. On the nature of semen quality and infertility. *Hum Reprod* 1995;10:249.
Baker DJ, Paterson MA. Marketed sperm: use and regulation in the United States. *Fertil Steril* 1995;63:947–952.
Baker HW. Male infertility. *Endocrinol Metabol Clin North Am* 1994;23: 783–793.
Bhasin S, deKretser DM, Baker HW. Clinical review 64: Pathophysiology and natural history of male infertility. *J Clin Endocrinol Metab* 1994;79: 1525–1529.
Howards SS. Treatment of male infertility. *N Engl J Med* 1995;332: 312–317.
Irvine DS, Aitken RJ. Seminal fluid analysis and sperm function testing. *Endocrinol Metab Clin North Am* 1994;23:725–748.
Jenkins CS, Williams SR, Schmidt GE. Salpingitis isthmica nodosa: a review of the literature, discussion of clinical significance, and consideration of patient management. *Fertil Steril* 1993;60:599–607.

Markham SM, Waterhouse TB. Structural anomalies of the reproductive tract. *Curr Opin Obstet Gynecol* 1992;4:867–873.
Marshburn PB, Kutteh WH. The role of antisperm antibodies in infertility. *Fertil Steril* 1994;61:799–811.
Schlesinger MH, Wilets IF, Nagler HM. Treatment outcome after varicocelectomy. A critical analysis. *Urol Clin North Am* 1994;21:517–529.
Wolff H. The biologic significance of white blood cells in semen. *Fertil Steril* 1995;63:1143–1157.
Yavetz H, Yogev L, Hauser R, Lessing JB, Paz G, Homonnai ZT. Retrograde ejaculation. *Hum Reprod* 1994;9:381–386.

Tubal

Acosta AA. Process of fertilization in the human and its abnormalities: diagnostic and therapeutic possibilities. *Obstet Gynecol Surv* 1994;49: 567–576.
Cates W Jr, Wasserheit JN. Genital chlamydia infections: Epidemiology and reproductive sequelae. *Am J Obstet Gynecol* 1991;164:1771–1781.
Feichtinger W. Results and complications of IVF therapy. *Curr Opin Obstet Gynecol* 1994;6:190–197.
Gomel BV, Wang I. Laparoscopic surgery for infertility therapy. *Curr Opin Obstet Gynecol* 1994;6:141–148.
Haney AF. Endometriosis–associated infertility. *Baillieres Clin Obstet Gynaecol* 1993;7:791–812.
Healy DL, Trounson AO, Andersen AN. Female infertility: Causes and treatment. *Lancet* 1994;343:1539–1544.
Honore LH. Pathology of female infertility. *Curr Opin Obstet Gynecol* 1994;6:364–371.
Soper DE. Pelvic inflammatory disease. *Infect Dis Clin North Am* 1994;8: 821–840.
Westrom LV. Sexually transmitted diseases and infertility. *Sex Transm Dis* 1994;21:S32–37.
Yoder IC, Hall DA. Hysterosalpingography in the 1990s. *Am J Roentgenol* 1991;157:675–683.

Unexplained

Confino E, Radwanska E. Tubal factors in infertility. *Curr Opin Obstet Gynecol* 1992;4:197–202.
Krysiewicz S. Infertility in women: Diagnostic evaluation with hysterosalpingography and other imaging techniques. *Am J Roentgenol* 1992; 159:253–261.
LaSala GB, Cittadini E. Unexplained infertility. *Acta Europaea Fertilitatis* 1994;25:7–17.
Markham S. Cervico-utero-tubal factors in infertility. *Curr Opin Obstet Gynecol* 1991;3:191–196.
Marrero MA, Ory SJ. Unexplained infertility. *Curr Opin Obstet Gynecol* 1991;3:205–210.
Negro-Vilar A. Stress and other environmental factors affecting fertility in men and women: overview. *Environ Health Persp* 1993;101:59–64.
Toner JP, Glood JR. Fertility after the age of 40. *Obstet Gynecol Clin North Am* 1993;20:261–272.

Outcome

Chandra A, Gray RH. Epidemiology of infertility. *Curr Opin Obstet Gynecol* 1991;3:169–175.
Cordero JF. The epidemiology of disasters and adverse reproductive outcomes: lessons learned. *Environ Health Persp* 1993;101:131–136.
Hull MG. Effectiveness of infertility treatments: Choice and comparative analysis. *Int J Gynaecol Obstet* 1994;47:99–108.
Jaffe SB, Jewelewicz R. The basic infertility investigation. *Fertil Steril* 1991;56:599–613.
Mineau G, Trussell J. A specification of marital fertility by patents' age, age at marriage, and marital duration. *Demography* 1982;19:335–350.
Rojansky N, Brzezinski A, Schenker JG. Seasonality in human reproduction: an update. *Hum Reprod* 1992;7:735–745.
Speroff L. The effect of aging on fertility. *Curr Opin Obstet Gynecol* 1994; 6:115–120.
Vandekerckhove P, O'Donovan PA, Lilford RJ, Harada TW. Infertility treatment: from cookery to science. The epidemiology of randomised controlled trials. *Br J Obstet Gynaecol* 1993;100:1005–1036.

Clinical Reproductive Medicine,
Edited by Bryan D. Cowan and David B. Seifer
Lippincott-Raven Publishers, Philadelphia © 1997

CHAPTER 18

Endometriosis

Steve London

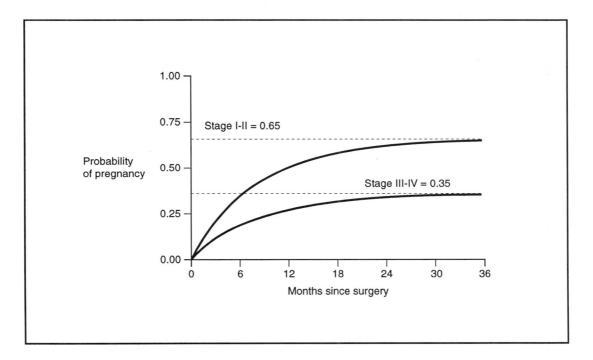

Epidemiology and Diagnosis
Pathogenesis
Pathology
Endometriosis and Pain

Endometriosis and Fertility
Extrapelvic Endometriosis
Summary
Suggested Reading

S. London: Department of Obstetrics and Gynecology, Louisiana State University Medical Center, Shreveport, LA 71130-3932

Endometriosis is the presence of endometrial glands and stroma at ectopic sites. Dr. Sampson brought endometriosis to clinical attention in the 1920s. Since that time, approximately 5000 articles have been written about this subject. Despite our large body of literature, the etiology, pathogenesis of symptoms, and best method of treatment remain controversial. The purpose of this chapter is to review specific clinical controversies and suggest management plans based on our current understanding of the disease.

EPIDEMIOLOGY AND DIAGNOSIS

The exact prevalence of endometriosis in the general population is unknown. It has been estimated that 10% of women aged 15–50 have endometriosis. The prevalence of endometriosis may be higher than 10% depending on the patient group studied. In patients with infertility, approximately 40% will be found to have endometriosis. In women with pelvic pain, approximately 20% will have endometriosis. Adolescents complaining of secondary dysmenorrhea/pelvic pain may have an incidence as high as 50% (Table 18-1). Reproductive-aged women who are evaluated for pelvic mass will be found to have endometriosis approximately 7% of the time.

First-degree relatives of women with endometriosis have a 3- to 10-fold increased risk of having endometriosis when compared to the general population. If a first-degree relative is involved, the patient tends to develop more advanced stage disease. Another group of women at greater risk for endometriosis are those with obstruction to menstrual outflow such as a noncommunicating rudimentary horn or a transverse vaginal septum.

Unfortunately, there is no specific patient profile obtainable by history, physical exam, or laboratory that allows the physician to determine who will develop endometriosis. The precise clinical diagnosis is difficult because there is no reliable test short of laparoscopy that establishes the diagnosis. Women who have endometriosis frequently have antiendometrial antibodies. However, the heterogenic nature of these antibodies and variability in production quantity makes measuring these antibodies unreliable for clinical diagnosis. Recently, CA-125 has been noted to be elevated in women with endometriosis. The higher the titer, usually the more extensive the disease. Unfortunately, many women with mild and moderate disease have normal CA-125 levels. The endometrial secretory protein PP-14 has also been shown to be elevated in women with endometriosis. However, PP-14's utility as a screening test remains unproved.

Even diagnosis by direct visualization is less than perfect. Endometriosis has both a typical (classic) and an atypical (non-classical) appearance. The classic lesion is described as that of a "powder burn" that is dark blue and raised. However, it is now recognized that atypical appearances such as clear vesicles, white or yellow spots (nodules), circular folds of peritoneum (pockets), and visually normal peritoneum can contain endometriosis. Therefore, surgical diagnosis of endometriosis is dependent on a surgeon's experience for identifying the disease and his or her index of suspicion at the time of procedure.

PATHOGENESIS

The etiology of endometriosis is unknown. Several theories have been offered over the years to explain its occurrence, but none adequately explains all situations. Three useful theories (Table 18-2)—reflux menstruation (Sampson's theory), hematogenous/lymphatic transport, and celomic metaplasia (Meyer's theory)—have been commonly cited to explain endometriosis. Retrograde or reflux menses was attractive because it explained the most common sites of endometriosis. However, this theory could not explain why endometriosis did not develop in all women or how endometriosis in distant sites could occur. To explain these rare situations, some investigators proposed that endometrial tissue was transported by the lymphatics or blood vessels, and then directly implanted. Consistent with this theory, endometrial tissue is often found in the uterine veins and lymphatics. However, this theory does not explain why women without uteri or why women who never menstruate develop endometriosis. Celomic metaplasia, championed by Meyer in the early 1900s, stated that the peritoneum, in response to a noxious stimulus, could undergo metaplasia into endometrial tissue. This was attractive because it explained both local and distant disease. However, the noxious metaplasia-inducing agent has never been found. If celomic metaplasia is occurring, why do women with infectious processes that irritate the peritoneal cavity not develop endometriosis at a more rapid rate than others? Another problem with the theory of celomic metaplasia is that the thoracic cavity has

TABLE 18-1. *Incidence of endometriosis in certain patient groups*

Patient group	Incidence (%)
Overall	10
Infertility	40
Pelvic pain	20
Pelvic mass	7
Adolescents with secondary dysmenorrhea	50

TABLE 18-2. *Etiology of endometriosis*

Old	New
Celomic metaplasia	Transport
Reflux menstruation (Sampson's theory)	
Hematogenous/lymphatic	

the same epithelium as the peritoneal cavity, yet thoracic endometriosis is rare. Furthermore, if celomic metaplasia were to occur, then a background endometriosis rate should exist in men. Therefore, these three theories have been combined into one that encompasses features of each and is unified under the name "transport theory." The transport theory states that in genetically susceptible individuals, transportation of menstrual blood to remote sites (peritoneum, pleura, vagina, nasal mucosa) by any mechanism can incite the development of endometrial glands and stroma in ectopic locations.

PATHOLOGY

Endometriosis is the presence of endometrial glands and stroma outside the uterus. It is variable in gross appearance and is most frequently found on the peritoneum and ovaries. The gross appearance of endometriosis undergoes a natural progression. The earliest lesion is usually red, petechial, and on the peritoneal surface. With further growth, detritus accumulates within the lesion giving a cystic dark brown/blue–black appearance. This creates an inflammatory response and the peritoneal surface becomes thickened and scarred, giving the classic powder burn implants. At this stage, adhesions may develop, and if the implants are on the ovary, "endometriomas/chocolate cysts" may also form. The implants may erode into the underlying tissues but appear to be minimal on the surface of the peritoneum. This erosion may extend into the supporting tissue, particularly the rectovaginal septum.

Microscopically, the lesions appear to be endometrial glands and stroma. Even though they look similar, the two tissues are functionally different. The characteristic changes of estrogen and progesterone receptors throughout the menstrual cycle are absent in ectopic locations compared to the normal endometrium. Endometriotic implants contain estrogen receptors but the expression of progesterone receptors is variable, thus explaining why the response of implants to progesterone therapy is highly variable.

ENDOMETRIOSIS AND PAIN

Endometriosis-associated clinical symptomatology is so variable that it essentially must be considered in the differential diagnosis of every complaint of reproductive age women (Table 18-3). Still, the primary symptom of women with endometriosis is pain. The pain produced by endometriosis is difficult to categorize. The literature reports dysmenorrhea, lower abdominal pain, rectal pain, low-back pain, dyspareunia, and dysuria due to endometriosis.

The exact type of pain may depend on the implant's location and the impact on the patient's life may depend on her tolerance to pain. Several theories have been pro-

TABLE 18-3. *Symptoms of endometriosis*

Pain
Infertility
Pelvic mass
Abnormal bleeding
Ovarian cyst
Premenstrual spotting

posed to explain how endometriosis may cause pain. Peritoneal irritation from leaking endometriomas or menstrual detritus, prostaglandin or interleukin production by the implant, or scarring and retraction that occurs with endometriotic implants have all been offered as explanations. Additionally, endometriosis may involve the bowel or bladder and give rise to pain from these viscera.

Women with "chronic pelvic pain" will have endometriosis at least 20% of the time. Despite this increased prevalence, there is uncertainty as to whether the endometriosis itself causes the pain. This possibility must be considered as some patients will not respond to any form of therapy including hysterectomy. Finally, the amount of pain experienced by a patient does not correlate well with the extent of disease.

How best to counsel for pain is difficult. There are very few studies in the literature where the measured outcome is pain relief. Observation with simple analgesic therapy may be best for patients with mild discomfort. Many physicians when treating a young patient remote from childbearing recommend aggressive medical therapy to "preserve her childbearing capacity" and "prevent disease progression." The appropriateness of this is controversial as there is little evidence to predict if the endometriosis will interfere with fertility. Additionally, although endometriosis progresses in many women, it does not progress universally.

The physician has many choices when considering medical therapy of endometriosis (Table 18-4). The rationale behind medical therapy for endometriosis is to stimulate a condition that causes endometrial atrophy and/or regression. Such naturally occurring conditions are pregnancy and menopause. Additionally, androgen will cause endometrial atrophy.

The physician has three groups of drugs: (1) those that mimic pregnancy; (2) those that mimic menopause; and

TABLE 18-4. *Medical therapy for endometriosis*

Medication	Average relative cost
Oral contraceptives	1.0
Oral medroxyprogesterone acetate 40 mg/day	0.84
Depo-Provera 150 mg every 12 weeks	1.48
Danocrine 800 mg/day	7.4
GnRH agonists	14

GnRH, gonadotropin-releasing hormone.

(3) those that possess androgen. In general, it is best to start with the least expensive and the least toxic therapy possible. If the patient is young and suffering from significant dysmenorrhea, oral contraceptives are the drug of choice. Oral contraceptives will commonly alleviate the pain. If the patient fails to respond to oral contraceptives, then progestin-only therapy should be considered. Although this is not the "pseudopregnancy" regimen used many years ago, it still provides a level of progestin that will induce endometrial atrophy. Medroxyprogesterone acetate 20–40 mg daily is given continuously (ie, no hormone-free intervals). If the patient tolerates this, then Depo-Provera 150 mg every 3 months can be substituted. Progestins will relieve pelvic pain in approximately half of patients. Bloating, depression, weight gain, and breakthrough bleeding are frequent side effects. Progestins should be tried as the first agent in long-term pain management due to their low cost and lack of serious side effects.

Androgens such as testosterone and Danocrine can alleviate pain in up to 90% of patients. Methyltestosterone used in doses of 5–10 mg/day may control the pain of endometriosis within 2 weeks. Unfortunately, androgen side effects of the patient limits its long-term application. Therefore, testosterone is not used today. Danocrine acts directly on the implant as an androgen and indirectly as a gonadotropin suppressor. Danocrine also inhibits steroidogenic enzymes in the ovary, thereby decreasing estrogen stimulation of the lesion. Danocrine is usually used for 6–9 months and is usually started at 800 mg/day to achieve amenorrhea. The 800-mg dose should be given as 200 mg four times daily. Pain relief usually is accomplished within 2–3 weeks. When relief occurs, the dose can be decreased to 600 mg daily for 3–4 weeks, then to 400 mg daily unless there is a return of symptomatology. Using the least effective dose to control the pain is designed to minimize the androgen side effect. Many women experience acne, oily skin, deepening of the voice, weight gain, and edema that leads to patient dissatisfaction and noncompliance. When the dose goes below 800 mg daily, other contraceptive measures must be used. Danocrine is superior to pseudopregnancy oral contraceptives in terms of pain relief. The recurrence of pain following medical treatment with Danocrine is approximately 33% at 5 years, comparable with conservative surgery.

Pseudomenopause is best accomplished with gonadotropin-releasing hormone (GnRH) agonists. GnRH agonists are available in preparations that will last for a month. After a brief period of pituitary stimulation, the agonist blocks luteinizing hormone (LH) and follicle-stimulating hormone (FSH) production and induces a state of hypogonadism due to lack of gonadotropin stimulation of the ovaries. As estrogen levels fall, endometrial stimulation diminishes and pain relief occurs. Approximately 90% of patients placed on GnRH agonist will receive clinically significant pain relief. The side effects of

the drug are those of severe hypoestrogenism such as hot flashes, vaginal dryness, insomnia, and irritability. A small but clinically detectable loss of bone mass occurs if treatment continues for more than 6 months. Concern about this problem and other long-term effects of hypoestrogenism limits the duration of GnRH agonist therapy to 6 months. Add-back therapies using small amounts of estrogen and/or progestin to prevent bone loss and restore lipid profiles may reduce bone demineralization and allow GnRH agonist therapy to be extended.

Several therapies have been tried in Europe that are not available in the United States. Gestrinone is an antiestrogen, antiprogesterone steroid with effects similar to those of Danocrine, but with fewer androgen side effects. Additionally, gestrinone has the advantage of only requiring twice-weekly oral administration. Cyproterone acetate is a 17-hydroxyprogesterone derivative that has progestinal activity. Cyproterone when combined with estrogen causes pain relief in patients with endometriosis. RU-486, a synthetic steroid with antiprogesterone/antiglucocorticoid activities, can antagonize endometrial effects of exogenous estrogen. Whether or not this drug will be useful clinically needs further study.

Surgical therapy is grouped into two categories: conservative and definitive. Conservative surgery refers to resection and/or ablation of the endometrial implants leaving childbearing capacity intact. Definitive therapy refers to hysterectomy, bilateral salpingo-oophorectomy. Conservative surgery for pain has a recurrence rate of 13% by 3 years and 40% by 5 years. Recently, laser ablation of endometrial implants at the time of laparoscopy has become popular to control pain. While this may be appropriate for women desiring to conceive, pain recurs in 30–70% of women after 1 year.

Hysterectomy remains a viable choice for women with recalcitrant pain and have no further desire for childbearing. Interestingly, neither age, stage of diagnosis, nor conception following surgery predicts who will have a recurrence and who will not. If a decision has been made to proceed with hysterectomy, the ovaries are usually removed at the same time. There has been some concern that removal of ovaries in young women may make them at greater risk for the complications of hormone replacement. However, to date, there does not appear to be any adverse effect associated with hormone replacement in these women. If the ovaries are left behind, approximately 25% of women will require further surgery for recurrence of endometriosis or related symptoms.

ENDOMETRIOSIS AND FERTILITY

When endometriosis interferes with ovum pick-up or causes tubal occlusion, the etiology of infertility is clear (ie, mechanical). However, how endometriosis affects human fertility in minimal and mild disease without anatomic distortion is speculative (ie, chemical). It appears that the endometrial implants secrete products into the tubal/peritoneal environment that are toxic to reproduction. These products may have direct toxic effects on sperm, sperm motility, sperm–egg interaction, tubal transport, and may lead to an increase in early embryo wastage. The most likely candidates of toxic factors are prostaglandins and stimulation of macrophage secretory products. Therefore, it is highly probable that even minimal endometriosis adversely affects human reproduction.

In general, the treatment of choice for endometriosis for patients who desire fertility is surgery. Medical management has not been shown to enhance fertility beyond the expected pregnancy rate of observation alone. Additionally, medications cannot relieve the anatomic distortion caused by more extensive lesions. At the present time, laparoscopic treatment is the preferred surgical approach for endometriosis. However, value of destroying *minimal* lesions at the time of laparoscopy is undecided. Most surgeons feel that because the patient already had an anesthetic for diagnosis, safe surgical ablation of disease is appropriate to eradicate disease and prevent possible progression of the endometriosis. Patients who have laser vaporization of endometriosis may become pregnant more quickly than those who do not have these lesions removed. There is no evidence to suggest that treating the patient medically preoperatively or postoperatively will enhance her overall pregnancy rate. Pregnancy rate after surgery in women with minimal to mild disease is 60% (Fig. 18-1) and occurs over a 5-year interval. Curiously, this response is nearly identical to unexplained couples (see Fig. 18-1).

In women with severe disease or adhesions, surgical resection is the treatment of choice. This surgery attempts to remove all endometriotic tissue and restore pelvic anatomy to its best possible condition. Pregnancy rates are approximately 35% after 2 years (see Fig. 18-1). In

the past, presacral neurectomy with anterior uterine suspension was included in the surgical approach. The routine inclusion of these procedures in asymptomatic patients is controversial.

EXTRAPELVIC ENDOMETRIOSIS

Extrapelvic endometriosis occurs at a considerably lower frequency than pelvic endometriosis. Extrapelvic endometriosis may be grouped into four areas of occurrence in decreasing order of occurrence. These are: (1) intestinal tract endometriosis with sigmoid, descending colon, and rectum; (2) urinary tract endometriosis, usually involving the bladder and ureter; (3) thoracic cage and pulmonary endometriosis; and (4) endometriosis of other sites such as the Bartholin gland, scar, or obturator fossa. The true prevalence of endometriosis is probably underestimated as intestinal endometriosis may go undiagnosed for long periods of time. In women with severe pelvic endometriosis, as many as 50% have been reported to have some degree of bowel involvement. In all locations, acute relief of symptoms can usually be achieved by hormonal manipulation. If the lesion is isolated and identifiable, surgery is the best long-term therapy.

SUMMARY

Endometriosis affects 10% of all women, although its prevalence can be up to 50% in women with pain and infertility. The only way to diagnose endometriosis conclusively is by visualization or biopsy. Pain from endometriosis is best treated with medical therapy. Endometriosis may become more extensive over time. However, not all patients experience progression and the time course of progression is not predictable. Although the cause of endometriosis-associated infertility is un-

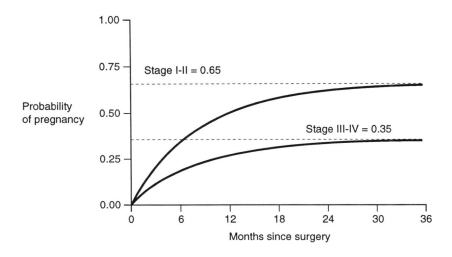

FIG. 18-1. Cumulative pregnancy rates of women with endometriosis treated by surgery. Women with minimal to mild disease achieve a 60% pregnancy rate within 5 years. Women with moderate to severe disease achieve a 35% pregnancy rate in 24 months.

clear, conception can be accomplished after surgery. The extent of disease is a predictor of pregnancy success.

SUGGESTED READING

Adamson GD, Pasta DJ. Surgical treatment of endometriosis-associated infertility: meta analysis compared with survival analysis. *Am J Obstet Gynecol* 1994;171:1488–1505.

Bergquist A, Ferno M. Estrogen and progesterone receptors in endometriotic tissue and endometrium: comparison according to localization and recurrence. *Fertil Steril* 1993;60:63–68.

Canadian Consensus on Endometriosis. *Journal SOGC* (Special Supplement). April 1993:3–35.

Olive D, ed. Endometriosis. *Infertil Reprod Med Clin North Am* 1992;3.

Sutton CJG. A critical evaluation of the management of pelvic pain. In: Brosens I, Downey J, eds. *Current Status of Endometriosis Research and Management.* New York: Parthenon, 1993;425–436.

Waller KG, Shaw RW. Endometriosis, pelvic pain, and psychological functioning. *Fertil Steril* 1995;63:796–800.

Clinical Reproductive Medicine,
Edited by Bryan D. Cowan and David B. Seifer
Lippincott-Raven Publishers, Philadelphia © 1997

CHAPTER 19

Mullerian Anomalies

Harriette L. Hampton

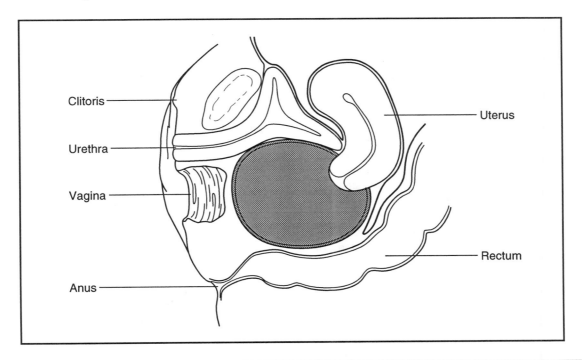

Embryology of the Mullerian System
Classification of Mullerian Anomalies
Important Clinical Presentations
  Obstructive Anomalies
  Imperforate Hymen
  Transverse Vaginal Septum
  Longitudinal Vaginal Septum

  Vaginal Atresia
  Mullerian Agenesis
  Anomalies of the Uterine Cervix
  Incomplete Mullerian Fusion
Obstetric Consequences of Uterovaginal Anomalies
Conclusions
Suggested Reading

H. L. Hampton: Department of Obstetrics and Gynecology, University of Mississippi Medical Center, Jackson MS 39216-4505

Congenital anomalies of the uterus, cervix, and vagina (Mullerian ductal system) occur in 2–3% of women. The majority of these malformations are subtle, but dramatic alterations in reproductive anatomy can obstruct menstrual outflow, produce cyclic or acyclic menstrual disorders, or make coitus difficult. Major Mullerian anomalies usually present during the adolescent years. Although some congenital malformations of the Mullerian system are obvious, the diagnosis of most defects requires a high index of suspicion. Prompt recognition, treatment, and counseling assures the preservation of reproductive function when feasible and allows patients to develop a positive attitude regarding their own sexuality. Delayed diagnosis can result in permanent sterility and inappropriate psychological adaptation. Here we will discuss the basic embryologic development of the Mullerian system and current diagnostic and treatment modalities for important congenital Mullerian anomalies.

EMBRYOLOGY OF THE MULLERIAN SYSTEM

Three important embryologic sites contribute to the development of the normal female genital system. The ovarian oocytes are derived from yolk sac derivatives (Chapter 4), the lower genital tract evolves from urogenital tissue, and the fallopian tubes, uterus, and upper vagina are derived from the Mullerian ductal system.

The fallopian tubes, uterus, cervix, and upper portion of the vagina originate from a pair of Mullerian ducts that develop on the lateral portion of the embryonic abdomen and subsequently fuse in the midline. The cephalad portions of the Mullerian ducts remain separate and form the fallopian tubes. The caudad portions, however, fuse into a Y-shaped uterovaginal primordium consisting of a uterine and vaginal segment (Fig. 19-1). A rudimentary uterus is recognizable at 9 weeks gestation. The vaginal segment of the fused uterovaginal primordium makes contact with the endoderm of the urogenital sinus. This contact leads to the formation of the sinovaginal bulbs, which subsequently fuse to form the vaginal plate. Degeneration of the cells of the vaginal plate forms the vaginal canal leaving squamous epithelium as its lining. Vaginal canalization begins at 11 weeks gestation and is completed at 20 weeks gestation. The hymen initially serves to separate the vaginal from the urogenital sinus. During late fetal development, the hymen canalizes, leaving behind the characteristic hymenal ring at the introitus. Aberrant migration, fusion, or canalization of the Mullerian ducts in the early developmental period produces Mullerian anomalies.

The Mullerian ducts (paramesonephric) develop as invaginations on the lateral surface of the Wolffian (mesonephric) ducts (Fig. 19-2). In the presence of androgen stimulation, the mesonephric ducts develop into the male reproductive ductal system. In the absence of androgen stimulation, Wolffian ducts regress in the female. Because of the close relationship between the Mullerian and Wolffian ducts, cystic Wolffian duct remnants (eg, epoophoron, paroophoron, duct of Gartner) may normally be found in the broad ligaments. The genital tract has a shared embryologic origin with the renal system, which accounts for the high percentage of renal abnormalities found in association with Mullerian anomalies.

External genital differentiation begins at approximately 4 weeks of fetal development. The genital tubercle, lateral labioscrotal, and urogenital folds are the first external structures to form (see Fig. 19-1). In the absence of androgenic stimulation, the genitalia develop as female. By the sixth week of gestation, the urorectal septum fuses with the cloacal membrane and divides the cloaca into ventral and dorsal portions. The anus develops from the dorsal portion and the ventral portion becomes urogenital folds. In females, the urogenital folds form the labia minora, the labioscrotal folds form the labia majora, and the genital tubercle becomes the clitoris. These structures are responsive to androgens and form the scrotum and penis during normal male development.

CLASSIFICATION OF MULLERIAN ANOMALIES

A basic classification scheme divides Mullerian anomalies into three groups: agenesis, vertical fusion defects, and lateral fusion defects. In 1983, Buttram classified Mullerian anomalies into six subgroups: (1) agenesis (vagina, cervix, uterine fundus, fallopian tube, and any combination thereof); (2) unicornuate uterus (connected, nonconnected, without a cavity, without a horn); (3) uterus didelphys; (4) bicornuate uterus (complete, partial, arcuate); (5) septate uterus (complete, partial); and (6) those resulting from the use of diethylstilbestrol (T-shaped). The American Society for Reproductive Medicine (formerly the American Fertility Society) has adopted a similar classification system (Fig. 19-3). Despite the attraction of classification systems that emphasize embryologic genesis, the clinician is tasked with evaluating clinical presentations. We have therefore organized this chapter by clinical presentations of Mullerian anomalies.

IMPORTANT CLINICAL PRESENTATIONS

Obstructive Anomalies

Most women with Mullerian duct and urogenital sinus anomalies undergo normal secondary sexual development because gonadal function is unaffected by these conditions. The usual presentation in women with obstructive anomalies (Table 19-1), therefore, is absent or abnormal menses with otherwise normal growth and secondary sexual characteristics (breasts, external genitalia). Obstructive symptoms such as pelvic mass (hematocolpos, hematometra) or pelvic pain (endometriosis) often

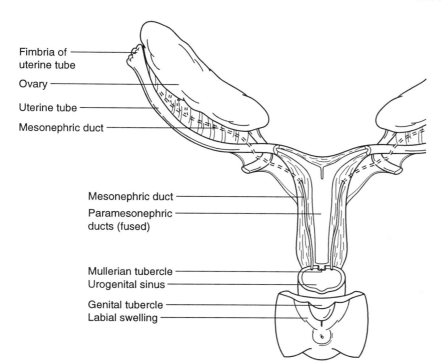

Fimbria of
uterine tube

Ovary

Uterine tube

Mesonephric duct

Mesonephric duct

Paramesonephric
ducts (fused)

Mullerian tubercle
Urogenital sinus

Genital tubercle
Labial swelling

FIG. 19-1. A reconstruction of the anterior aspect of the genital ducts in a 48-mm female human fetus.

result when the diagnosis of obstructive lesions is delayed. Because of the embryologic association of the Mullerian duct with the developing renal system, uterine anomalies are frequently associated with renal anomalies. As such, a urologic examination is an obligatory part of the evaluation of patients with a Mullerian anomaly. A few examples of Mendelian inheritance of Mullerian anomalies exist, and some are associated with recognized somatic syndromes (Table 19-2). However, most forms of Mullerian duct and urogenital sinus abnormalities are inherited in a polygenic-multifactorial fashion.

Imperforate Hymen

Imperforate hymen is not an infrequent clinical entity, reported in 1 of 5000 live female births. The diagnosis of an imperforate hymen should be made before adolescence as a part of routine neonatal and infant examinations. However, when detected after menarche, the classic presentation is primary amenorrhea and pelvic pain. In these cases, a diagnostic delay of 12 months is not unusual. The thickness of the membrane is quite variable but with Valsalva a characteristic bulge is observed at the

TABLE 19-1. *Obstructive Mullerian anomalies*

Imperforate hymen
Transverse vaginal septum
Longitudinal vaginal septum
Vaginal agenesis

introitus. When the diagnosis is suspected prior to menstruation, a mucocolpos can be detected with abdominal or transperineal sonography.

Surgical therapy for imperforate hymen involves a cruciate incision into the hymenal membrane extending to the 10, 2, and 6 o'clock positions. In dense hymens, a triangular section of the membrane may be excised. Hemostasis is secured with needle-tip electrocautery and fine suture as needed. Prophylactic antibiotic therapy is not required. In rare instances, a bulging mucocolpos is appreciated in the immediate newborn period. Local anesthesia for hymenotomy and drainage should be performed when this neonatal condition is detected. When imperforate hymen is detected during childhood, surgical therapy should be deferred until the hymenal boundaries can be accurately appreciated. This usually occurs at Tanner IV development when mucocolpos develops and orients the hymen and the vagina.

Transverse Vaginal Septum

Transverse vaginal septum, unlike imperforate hymen, is uncommon. It is estimated to occur in 1 in 75,000 live female births. Transverse vaginal septae are most often located at the junction of the upper and middle third of the vagina but can be encountered at any level along the vaginal canal (Fig. 19-4). There is marked variation in the clinical presentation varying from a small annular ring to a completely obstructed membrane of variable depth.

Clinical symptoms depend both on the width and location of the anomaly. A narrow annular septum has no

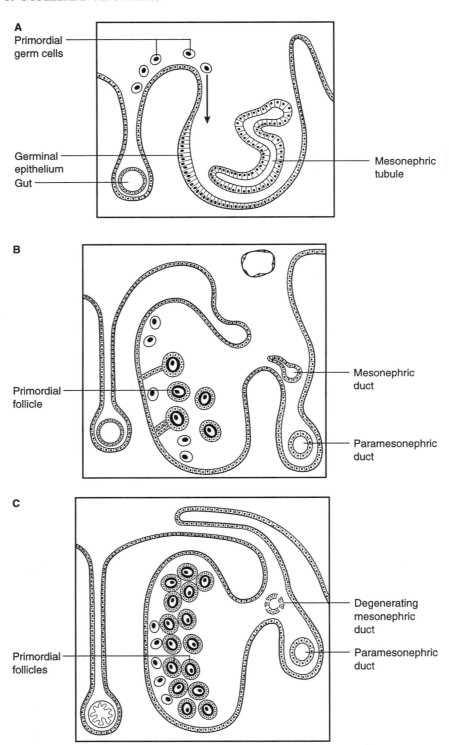

FIG. 19-2. Schematic representation of the early embryologic development of the mesonephric (Wolffian) and paramesonephric (Mullerian) ducts. In the female, the absence of gonadal androgen causes the mesonephric duct to develop. Additionally, the absence of gonadal Mullerian inhibiting substance causes the Mullerian system to persist.

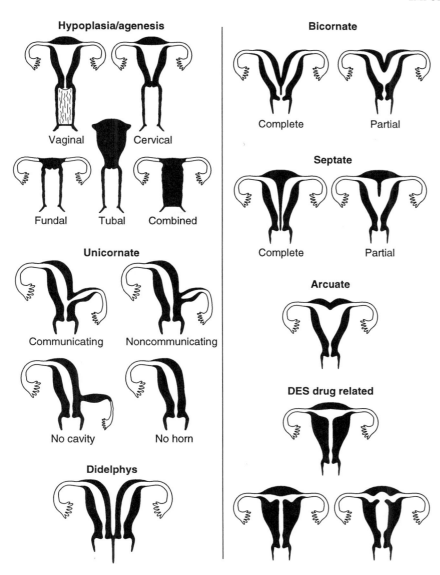

Hypoplasia/agenesis

Vaginal   Cervical

Fundal   Tubal   Combined

Unicornate

Communicating   Noncommunicating

No cavity   No horn

Didelphys

Bicornate

Complete   Partial

Septate

Complete   Partial

Arcuate

DES drug related

FIG. 19-3. Classification of uterine anomalies according to the American Society for Reproductive Medicine (formerly the American Fertility Society).

clinical significance and usually does not require treatment. Conversely, primary amenorrhea and pain in cases of complete obstruction require prompt surgical therapy. When a small fistula connects the upper and lower vagina, symptoms range from dysmenorrhea and irregular spotting to pelvic inflammatory disease secondary to ascending infection. A perforate septum low in the vaginal canal is a frequent cause of dyspareunia.

Surgical repair of a transverse septum is quite challenging. Correction of this defect requires removal of the septum and anastomosis of the upper and lower vagina. It is important to preserve mucosa to successfully anasto-

TABLE 19-2. *Heritable disorders associated with Mullerian anomalies*

Mode of inheritance	Disorder	Associated Mullerian defect
Autosomal dominant	Camptobrachydactyly	Longitudinal vaginal septa
	Hand–food–genital	Incomplete Mullerian fusion
Autosomal recessive	Kaufman–McCusick	Transverse vaginal septa
	Johnson–Blizzard	Longitudinal vaginal septa
	Renal–genital–middle ear anomalies	Vaginal atresia
	Fraser syndrome	Incomplete Mullerian fusion
Polygenic multifactorial	Mayer–Rokitansky–Kuster–Hauser syndrome	Mullerian aplasia
X-linked		

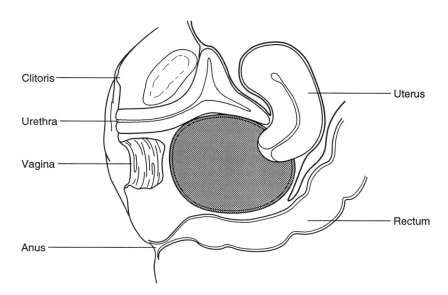

FIG. 19-4. Sagittal view of hematocolpos associated with complete transverse vaginal septum.

mose wide defects. It is necessary to completely release the constrictive band commonly found at the septal site. Circumferential small incisions with a scalpel held at a 45° angle to the mucosa help to release the stricture. In the event that the septum is wide and the mucosa cannot be joined without tension, a split-thickness skin graft can be fashioned to bridge the defect. In repair of a thick high vaginal septum, an abdominal incision may be necessary to orient the cervix.

Transvaginal sonography during the preoperative evaluation of a transverse septum can outline the depth of the septum and help estimate the need for skin grafting when a hematocolpos (menstrual blood in the vagina) is present. A vaginal sonogram is helpful in assessing proximal mucosal depth and width of the obstruction in women with a microperforate transverse septum. Instillation of saline or Sinograffin® through the perforation will define the upper space on sonogram or with plain films.

In order to prevent a stricture in the postoperative period, a small mold or tampon can be inserted vaginally. Daily cleansing and mold change are required until healing is confirmed. When vaginal grafting is required the duration of dilation is for 4 months, as with a McIndoe vaginoplasty.

Longitudinal Vaginal Septum

In addition to a transverse orientation, vaginal septae also occur in the longitudinal axis, in either a coronal or a sagittal plane (Fig. 19-5). Longitudinal septa most often

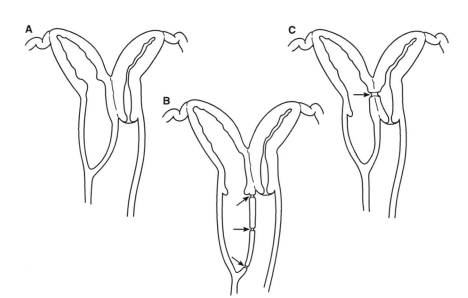

FIG. 19-5. Three examples of uterus didelphys with imperforate longitudinal vaginal septum. In **A**, a complete obstruction to outflow of the right system exists. In **B**, microperforations in the imperforate vaginal septum allow menstrual egress. In **C**, a communication between the left and right uterine horns allows menstrual egress.

occur in association with abnormalities of uterine fusion but may sometimes develop as an isolated malformation. As with transverse septae, most longitudinal septae have a sporadic occurrence but both autosomal dominant and recessive inheritance patterns have been reported. Longitudinal septae usually are asymptomatic but may cause prolongation or arrest of the second stage of labor by mechanical obstruction. Excision of the membrane is indicated with complaint of dyspareunia or when childbearing is anticipated. Imperforate or obstructed longitudinal septum is associated with ipsilateral renal agenesis and is now recognized as a syndrome.

Vaginal Atresia

The clinical presentation of vaginal atresia, in which the inferior portion of the vagina is replaced by fibrous tissue, should be distinguished from Mullerian aplasia. Vaginal atresia results from the failure of the urogenital sinus to contribute to the inferior vagina, but the Mullerian structures (including cervix) are intact. The classic presentation is primary amenorrhea and a midline pelvic mass and cyclic pain (Fig. 19-6). Sonography will confirm hematocolpos, hematometra, and the vaginal obstruction. Prompt vaginoplasty (described below) is the treatment of choice.

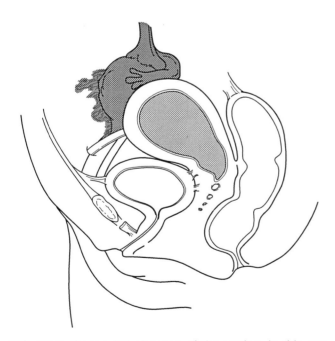

FIG. 19-6. Congenital absence of the vagina. In this syndrome, the vagina is replaced by fibroconnective tissue. The cervix, uterus, and fallopian tubes are present. This represents the variant of congenital absence of the vagina associated with a uterus. This syndrome is differentiated from congenital cervical agenesis by the presence of cervical stroma.

Mullerian Agenesis

Mullerian agenesis, often called Rokitansky–Kuster–Hauser syndrome, is defined as congenital absence or hypoplasia of the uterine corpus, uterine cervix, and proximal portion of the vagina. The incidence ranges from 1/4000 to 1/10,000 live female births. Ovaries are normal and fallopian tubes are usually present bilaterally. Complete vaginal agenesis occurs in 75% of patients with this syndrome. Approximately 25% of patients have a short vaginal pouch. With repeated attempts at intercourse, additional vaginal depth may be developed. Unfortunately, some women develop urethral dilatation as a result of attempted intercourse.

The classic presentation of Rokitansky–Kuster–Hauser syndrome is primary amenorrhea with normal breast and pubic hair development. Physical examination usually confirms Mullerian agenesis. Rectal examination demonstrates a characteristic midline band in the region where the uterus would normally be palpated. Pelvic sonography confirms uterine agenesis or hypoplasia and usually identifies bilateral ovarian structures. Uterine remnants should be excised when pelvic pain is part of the syndrome, even though functional endometrium is rare. In the majority of cases, however, laparoscopic diagnosis is not necessary.

Treatment of Mullerian agenesis can be either medical or surgical. A nonoperative method of vaginal construction involves the use of dilators mounted on a specially designed bicycle seat. Progressive dilator sizes can create a functional vagina in a period of as little as 8 weeks, but usually 4–6 months is required to produce a satisfactory result. In patients with a vaginal depth of 3–4 cm, dilator therapy is the treatment of choice.

The gold standard for surgical correction of Mullerian and vaginal agenesis is McIndoe vaginoplasty, a procedure in which a split-thickness skin graft (obtained from the buttock) is placed into the newly dissected vaginal canal. At our institution, vaginoplasty is usually performed during the summer vacation months. The average age is 16 years with a range of 11–20 years. Preoperative counseling includes a slide review of the procedure and an opportunity to meet other patients who have undergone the procedure. Patients should be made aware that graft failure and fistula formation are recognized complications of the procedure. Sexual relations are satisfactory in most patients who undergo McIndoe vaginoplasty.

It is interesting that regardless of technique, the neovagina develops many features of the normal vagina. The new vaginal epithelium evolves a hormonally responsive stratified squamous epithelium with glycogen production. Cornification occurs normally throughout the menstrual cycle. Papanicolaou surveillance is required in these patients because squamous carcinoma of the neovagina can occur. Isolated cases of vaginal prolapse have been observed in patients undergoing vaginal construction by both nonoperative and McIndoe procedures.

There is a select group of patients requiring vaginoplasty secondary to androgenic stimulation in utero, whether from congenital adrenal hyperplasia, male pseudohermaphroditism, or true hermaphroditism. Clinically, these patients have a flat perineum with microphallus or clitoromegaly and no vagina. The surgical dissection in these cases is more difficult than in cases of vaginal agenesis. While functional results with McIndoe vaginoplasty are satisfactory, the cosmetic result does not approach that of Rokitansky patients.

New techniques for vaginal construction without grafting utilize tissue expanders in the labia minora. The tissue expanders preoperatively enlarge labial skin to the appropriate diameter to line a newly canalized vagina. In addition, a laparoscopic procedure, referred to as modified Vecchetti, utilizes a suprapubic anchor for a vaginal pessary. The pessary expands the vaginal dimple to a 10-cm vagina over a 2-week period in an outpatient setting. Finally, full-thickness free pedicle grafts from the scapula and the rectus abdominis are used to line a dissected vaginal canal. Though technically difficult, these procedures benefit the patient by not requiring postoperative dilatation.

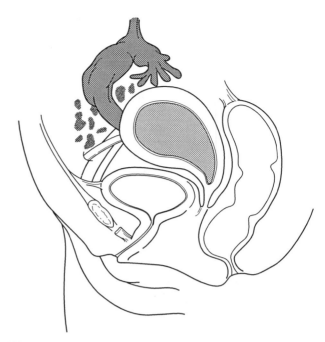

FIG. 19-7. Cervical agenesis. Here only the uterus and fallopian tube remain. The cervix is absent, and the uterus is connected to the vaginal fibroconnective tissue without interpositional cervical stroma.

Anomalies of the Uterine Cervix

Failure of Mullerian fusion and canalization is responsible for isolated cases of cervical agenesis or hypoplasia in combination with a normal uterine corpus. Clinical symptoms include primary amenorrhea, pelvic mass, and pain. Transvaginal sonography and/or magnetic resonance imaging (MRI) of the pelvis are invaluable in delineating the presence of cervical stroma (Fig. 19-7). Reports of significant morbidity and even mortality after surgical repair in the 40 recorded cases in the English literature make management decisions difficult. It is our opinion that only patients with partial atresia (i.e., the presence of some cervical stroma) are candidates for conservative management. Cervical split-thickness grafts in combination with a cervical stent may optimize outcome after conservative correction of this defect. Hysterectomy remains the treatment of choice for congenital absence of the cervix.

Incomplete Mullerian Fusion

The abnormalities of uterovaginal fusion that are diagnosed during adolescent years are most commonly obstruction. Uterine didelphys with unilateral imperforate vagina and ipsilateral renal agenesis is the most common fusion defect presenting at this time (see Fig. 19-5). The classic adolescent presentation is progressive dysmenor-

rhea with a paravaginal mass. Patients with an anatomic communication at the level of the cervix or incomplete vaginal obstruction may report a persistent foul-smelling discharge that worsens after their menstrual cycle. Once the diagnosis has been confirmed, the vaginal septum can be excised.

The second most common obstructive fusion defect is a unicornuate uterus with a contralateral blind horn, either rudimentary or of normal size. Once confirmed (by sonography and/or MRI), surgical correction involves either a unification metroplasty (rare), or hemihysterectomy, depending on the size of the obstructed horn.

The more common fusion defects, including uterus unicornis, uterus arcuatus, uterus subseptus, uterus septus, uterus bicornis unicollis, uterus bicornis bicollis, and uterus didelphys (see Fig. 19-3) are infrequently diagnosed during adolescent years because they are nonobstructive in nature. These conditions are usually associated with obstetric consequences (embryonic loss, preterm labor, or malpresentation) but are not usually associated with pain or abnormal bleeding.

OBSTETRIC CONSEQUENCES OF UTEROVAGINAL ANOMALIES

Uterovaginal anomalies may affect fertility and obstetric outcome (Table 19-3). Patients with Mullerian agenesis and complete cervical atresia requiring hysterectomy

TABLE 19-3. *Obstetric consequences of Mullerian anomalies*

Anomaly	Sterility	Impaired fertility	Obstetric complications
Mullerian aplasia	Yes	N/A	N/A
Complete cervical atresia	Yes	N/A	N/A
Imperforate hymen	No	No	No
Transverse vaginal septum	No	Yes	No
Partial cervical atresia	No	Yes	No
Vaginal atresia	No	Yes	No
Didelphys	No	No	Yes
Rudimentary horn	No	No	Yes
Uterine septum	No	No	Yes

are functionally sterile. Assisted reproduction and surrogate parenting have been successful in this select patient population. Secondary to the high pelvic location of ovaries, laparoscopic rather than transvaginal egg retrieval was required. In contrast, patients with imperforate hymen treated with hymenotomy do not have impaired fertility or obstetric sequelae.

Subfertility is documented in cases of transverse vaginal septum, partial cervical atresia, and vaginal atresia. Pregnancy rates of only 50% are reported after correction of a transverse vaginal septum. The etiology of this subfertility may relate to endometriosis from delayed diagnosis and retrograde menstrual flow. Once pregnancy reaches term in patients with a perforate transverse septum, the obstetric risk is limited to soft tissue dystocia from vaginal constriction or, more commonly, vaginal lacerations. The reproductive outcome of patients with corrected vaginal atresia has not been reported, but we may infer rates similar to transverse vaginal septae. Successful pregnancy after canalization procedures in patients with cervical agenesis has resulted in only 3 pregnancies in 40 reported cases. Impaired fertility may result from sequelae of postoperative ascending infection, endometriosis, or cervical dysfunction.

In contrast to vaginal and cervical anomalies, the obstetric sequelae of uterine anomalies may be catastrophic. Patients with an asymmetric uterus and a rudimentary horn generally have unimpaired fertility. The obstetric outcome depends on whether the pregnancy is in the normal hemiuterus or in the rudimentary horn. If the pregnancy is located in the normal uterine horn, the only obstetric risk is fetal malpresentation. If the pregnancy occurs in the rudimentary horn, a high rate of uterine rupture (89%) has been observed.

Patients with uterine didelphys or unilateral horn do not have reduced fertility. The reproductive consequences related to these two anomalies are preterm labor or malpresentation. The Strausman-type unification metroplasty is only rarely performed for persistent poor obstetric outcome.

In contrast, women with a uterine septum can suffer from repeated early pregnancy loss as well as preterm labor and malpresentation. A decade ago, the technique of transcervical hysteroscopic septum (resection) was introduced (Fig. 19-8). This technique has been associated with excellent reproductive outcome (>70% delivered) and low surgical morbidity, replacing transabdominal resection metroplasty.

CONCLUSIONS

The recognition of an adolescent with an obstructive Mullerian anomaly is an infrequent occurrence for most practitioners. A high index of suspicion for Mullerian defects in young women with primary amenorrhea, abnormal bleeding, pelvic pain, dysmenorrhea, or dyspareunia is prudent. The surgical repair of Mullerian anomalies requires expertise for optimal outcome. Reproductive conservation is the paramount surgical objective. The emotional impact of impaired reproductive anatomy must be appreciated. Treating physicians should provide appropri-

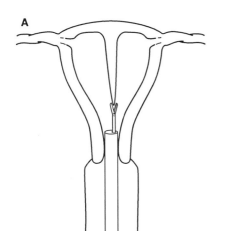 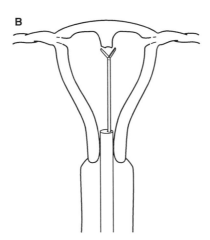

FIG. 19-8. Transcervical hysteroscopic division of a uterine septum. Division of the septum begins with sharp incisions at the most inferior portion **(A)** and is complete when the septum has been divided at the level of the fundus **(B)**.

ate counseling and psychological support for these very anxious patients and their parents.

SUGGESTED READING

Anonymous. The American Fertility Society classifications of adnexal adhesions, distal tubal occlusion, tubal occlusion secondary to tubal ligation, tubal pregnancies, mullerian anomalies and intrauterine adhesions. *Fertil Steril* 1988;49:944–955.

Ansbacher R. Uterine anomalies and future pregnancies. *Clin Perinatol* 1983;10:295–304.

Batzer FR, Corson SL, Gocial B, Daly DC, Go K, English ME. Genetic offspring in patients with vaginal agenesis: Specific medical and legal issues. *Am J Obstet Gynecol* 1992;167:1288–1292.

Bergh PA, Breen JL, Gregori CA. Congenital absence of the vagina: the Mayer–Rokitansky–Küster–Hauser syndrome. *Adol Pediatr Gynecol* 1989;2:73–85.

Buss JG, Lee RA. McIndoe procedure for vaginal agenesis: Results and complications. *Mayo Clin Proc* 1989;64:758–761.

Golan A, Langer R, Bukovsky I, Caspi E. Congenital anomalies of the mullerian system. *Fertil Steril* 1989;51:747–755.

Hampton HL. Role of the gynecologic surgeon in the management of urological anomalies in adolescents. *Curr Opin Obstet Gynecol* 1990;2:812–818.

Johnson N. The free-flap vaginoplasty: a new surgical procedure for the treatment of vaginal agenesis. *Br J Obstet Gynaecol* 1991;98:184–188.

Keckstein J. Laparoscopic creation of a neovagina: Modified Vecchietti method. *Endosc Surg* 1995;3:93–95.

Lilford RJ. Use of tissue expansion techniques to create skin flaps for vaginoplasty. Case report. *Br J Obstet Gynaecol* 1988;95:402–407.

Lin CC, Chen AC, Chen TY. Double uterus with an obstructed hemivagina and ipsilateral renal agenesis: report of 5 cases and a review of the literature. *J Formosan Med Assoc* 1991;90:195–201.

Scanlan KA, Pozniak MA, Fagerholm M, Shapiro S. Value of transperineal sonography in the assessment of vaginal atresia. *AJR* 1990;154:545–548.

Sherer DM, Beyth Y. Ultrasonographic diagnosis and assisted surgical management of hematotrachelos and hematometra due to uterine cervical atresia with associated vaginal agenesis. *J Ultrasound Med* 1989;8:321–323.

Tolhurst DE, van der Helm TW. The treatment of vaginal atresia. *Surg Gynecol Obstet* 1991;172:407–414.

Wagner BJ, Woodward PJ. Magnetic resonance evaluation of congenital uterine anomalies. *Semin Ultrasound Comput Tomogr Magnet Reson Imag* 1994;15:4–17.

Clinical Reproductive Medicine,
Edited by Bryan D. Cowan and David B. Seifer
Lippincott-Raven Publishers, Philadelphia © 1997

CHAPTER 20

Ectopic Pregnancy

Bryan D. Cowan

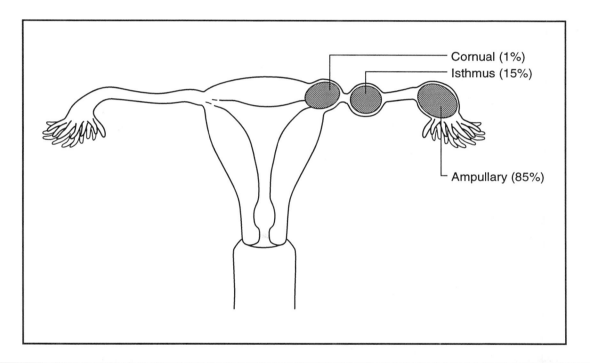

Epidemiology
Histopathology
Diagnosis
Surgical Treatment
   Operations for Distal Tubal Pregnancy
   Operations for Proximal Tubal Pregnancy

Complications
Subsequent Reproduction
Nonsurgical Treatment
Summary
Suggested Reading

B. D. Cowan: Division of Reproductive Endocrinology, Department of Obstetrics and Gynecology, University of Mississippi Medical Center, Jackson, MS 39216-4505

EPIDEMIOLOGY

Ectopic pregnancy is a significant cause of maternal mortality, adversely affects future reproduction, and contributes significantly to the economic burden of health care for women. The National Hospital Discharge Survey obtains comprehensive data regarding ectopic pregnancies that is compiled by the Centers for Disease Control (Table 20-1). From 1970 to 1987, the incidence of ectopic pregnancy in the United States generally increased every year. More than 70,000 ectopic pregnancies occur annually, and the incidence is nearly 20 per 1000 live births.

The reasons for the increase of ectopic pregnancies are not clearly understood but can be attributed in part to better reporting, improved diagnostic tools for the detection of this condition, and acquired risks for this disease in the reproductive population of women (Table 20-2). The most significant risk factor is scarring of the tubes and ovaries from infection. The incidence of pelvic infection has increased during recent years. *Chlamydia* and *Neisseria* gonorrhea represent the most important and frequently occurring genital tract pathogens. Reparative pelvic surgery, previous sterilization, gamete technology (gamete/zygote intrafallopian or intrauterine placement), congenital tubal anomalies, diethylstilbestrol (DES) exposure in utero, and transperitoneal migration of the ovum also contribute to the pool of ectopic pregnancies. However, these factors are much less important than prior infection or surgery. Finally, as a national trend, many women are deferring childbirth until late in their reproductive lives. The risk for ectopic gestation is greater in older women, and this sociologic shift has occurred with sufficient magnitude to become an important contributor to the incidence of ectopic pregnancy.

Complications from ectopic pregnancy remain a leading cause of maternal death in the United States today. Fortunately, the death rate has decreased in the years from 1970 to 1987. The case-fatality rate for these years was 3.4 deaths/10,000 ectopic pregnancies. In 1984, 39 women died as a result from ectopic pregnancy; 33 died in 1985, 36 died in 1986, and 30 died in 1987. A study of 86 deaths among 102,100 cases of ectopic pregnancy that occurred in the United States during 1979–1980 revealed that 77% of those women sought medical care, 100% complained of pain, and the cause of death was acute hemorrhage in 85% of cases. Errors in diagnosis occurred in 49% of the cases. Commonly, gastrointestinal disorders, intrauterine pregnancy, or pelvic inflammatory disease confused the diagnosis. More than half of these deaths might have been prevented if patients or providers acted more expeditiously.

TABLE 20-2. *Risk factors for ectopic pregnancy*

Prior pelvic infection
Adhesions
Pelvic/abdominal surgery
Endometriosis
Failed sterilization
Prior or concomitant IUD use
Gamete technology
External migration of the ovum
Congenital tubal anomalies (including exposure to diethylstilbestrol)
Advanced maternal age

HISTOPATHOLOGY

Approximately 90% of ectopic pregnancies occur in the oviduct, and most of these are ampullary implantations (Fig. 20-1). Regardless of the implantation site, the invading trophoblast usually mimics the same biological responses as trophoblast invading the decidua of the endometrium. The trophoblast destroys the epithelium and invades the muscularis. Most of the invading trophoblast proliferates below the mucosa of the lumen within the muscularis. Penetration of the muscularis to the peritoneum is rare because trophoblast growth is usually restricted by the muscularis. Focal bleeding into the implantation site is a common sequela of oviductal nidation and is believed to be responsible for distension, intermittent pelvic pain, and ultimate rupture.

The ampullary muscularis is considerably thinner than the corresponding site of the isthmus and interstitium. The depth of the "submucosal" area that can be invaded is therefore considerably less in ampullary ectopic gestations compared to isthmic sites. As such, ampullary ges-

TABLE 20-1. *Numbers and rates of ectopic pregnancies by year, United States, 1970–1987*

| Year | Number | Rates | | |
		Reported pregnancies	Live births	Females aged 15–44
1970	17,900	4.5	4.8	4.2
1971	19,300	4.8	5.4	4.4
1972	24,500	6.3	7.5	5.5
1973	25,600	6.8	8.2	5.6
1974	26,400	6.7	8.4	5.7
1975	30,500	7.6	9.8	6.5
1976	34,600	8.3	11.0	7.2
1977	40,700	9.2	12.3	8.3
1978	42,400	9.4	12.8	8.5
1979	49,900	10.4	14.3	9.9
1980	52,200	10.5	14.5	9.9
1981	68,000	13.6	18.7	12.7
1982	61,800	12.3	17.0	11.5
1983	69,600	14.0	19.2	12.6
1984	75,400	14.9	20.6	13.6
1985	78,400	15.2	20.9	14.0
1986	73,700	14.3	19.7	12.8
1987	88,000	16.8	23.1	15.3
Total	878,800	16.8	14.0	9.7

[1]Rounded to nearest 100.
[2]Rate per 1000 reported pregnancies.
[3]Rate per 1000 live births.
[4]Rate per 10,000 females.

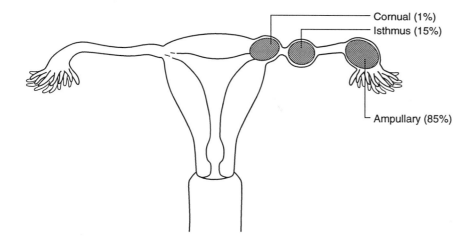

FIG. 20-1. Common tubal pregnancy implantation sites. Approximately 65% of tubal pregnancies attach to the distal half of the tube (ampullary) and 35% attach to the proximal portion (isthmus).

tations are more amenable to conservative removal of the ectopic pregnancy without tubal resection. Those pregnancies arising in the isthmus or interstitium are more difficult to remove without resecting the tube. Additionally, isthmic and interstitial implantations commonly injure the narrow lumen, and extraction of these gestations without resection of the tube leads to a high incidence of repeat ectopics.

DIAGNOSIS

Patients with ectopic pregnancy are encountered in two different clinical settings. Women with symptoms of ectopic pregnancy are usually seen in the emergency room. Symptoms of tubal pregnancy are abdominal pain (95%), vaginal bleeding (60%), or a palpable adnexal mass (35%). These findings, however, are often present in women with other diagnoses. Pain occurs from peritoneal stretching of the distended tube or blood in the peritoneal cavity from tubal rupture or regurgitation. Vaginal bleeding occurs as a result of insufficient hormonal support of the decidualized endometrium. In the past patients with tubal rupture accounted for 85% of all cases of ectopic pregnancy. This was especially true when diagnosis was based on the classic triad of pelvic pain, abnormal vaginal bleeding, and an adnexal mass. Unfortunately, this triad occurs in only one third of patients with ectopic pregnancy. Asymptomatic patients present earlier in the course of their disease through their obstetrician or during an infertility investigation. The latter group provides the greatest opportunity for early diagnosis and conservative intervention.

Improvements in diagnostic measures for early detection of ectopic pregnancy have greatly influenced the morbidity and mortality of affected patients. Human chorionic gonadotropin (hCG) measurements and high-resolution pelvic sonography have been employed to de-

tect ectopic pregnancies early. Additionally, serum progesterone measurements have shown a promising capability for predicting early gestational complications. With these detection methods, a substantial proportion of ectopic pregnancies are now diagnosed prior to the onset of symptoms or tubal rupture.

The hCG concentration can be highly predictive of gestational abnormalities. During the first 40 days of pregnancy, the serum hCG concentration doubles approximately every 2 days. The amount of hCG produced varies with the gestational age. The hCG doubling is more rapid in early gestation (1.4–1.5 days to double) than in the pregnancy approaching 7–8 weeks (3.3–3.5 days to double). After approximately 7–8 weeks of gestation, the hCG titer peaks and then declines. As a consequence, hCG doubling is generally not helpful after 7–8 weeks gestation. A single quantitative serum hCG determination has limited value in predicting gestational normalcy. The quantitation of hCG can be established in either of two ways: Second International Standard (Standard IS) or the International Reference Preparation (IRP). It is important to know which hCG reference is used when correlating hCG levels with clinical interpretation and other diagnostic modalities. For estimates of conversion, IRP values are approximately twice as high as the Second IS. Approximately 85% of patients with a normal hCG doubling will have a normal intrauterine pregnancy and ultimately deliver. Approximately 75% of patients with abnormally slow hCG doubling will have an intrauterine abortion or ectopic pregnancy. Human chorionic gonadotropin determinations cannot discriminate between an ectopic pregnancy and an intrauterine abortion. The formula to calculate hCG doubling time is shown in Fig. 20-2. The calculation of hCG doubling times is clumsy for clinical applications. For patient management purposes, it is more convenient to estimate hCG increments over time. The *minimum* expected increment is of greater interest than the *average* increment. The minimum expected increases in normal

$$DT \text{ days} = \frac{\log_{10}(2) \ (Day_2 - Day_1)}{\log_{10}(hCG_2 \, / \, hCG_1)}$$

FIG. 20-2. Calculation of human chorionic gonadotropin (hCG) doubling times. Day 1 is the initial sample of hCG (hCG_1) and day 2 is the second sample (hCG_2).

TABLE 20-3. *Minimal increments of hCG over time*

Sampling interval (days)	Minimum expected increase in hCG (%)
2	65
3	100

hCG, human chorionic gonadotropin.

pregnancies at 2- and 3-day sampling intervals are approximately 65% and 100%, respectively (Table 20-3).

Ultrasonography allows the clinician to visualize the site of the gestation. A *positive* sonographic diagnosis can be made by identifying an extrauterine fetus. A *presumptive* diagnosis of ectopic pregnancy can be made by failure to visualize an intrauterine gestation when the hCG titer is above the "discriminatory hCG zone." The discriminatory hCG zone is defined as the range of hCG concentrations above which a normal intrauterine gestation will be visualized. If an intrauterine gestational sac is not seen when the hCG concentration exceeds the discriminatory level, ectopic pregnancy occurs in 85% of cases. Transvaginal sonography has higher resolution than transabdominal sonography, lowers the discriminatory hCG zone, and allows earlier identification of abnormal gestations. As a result, gestational sacs can be visualized (Fig. 20-3) when the hCG level reaches approximately 1500 mIU/ml (IRP) or 1000 mIU/ml (Second IS). Because there is variability among hCG assays and the resolution of different imaging systems, each laboratory and clinical service must establish its own discriminatory zones for both transabdominal and transvaginal sonography.

As an additional diagnostic test, *progesterone monitoring* in abnormal pregnancies has been investigated. Progesterone production is decreased in ectopic pregnancies compared to intrauterine gestations of the same gestational age. Unfortunately, there is no agreement as to the "discriminatory value of progesterone," which defines an abnormal gestation. Furthermore, a progesterone determination cannot distinguish between an abnormal intrauterine gestation (missed abortion) and ectopic pregnancy. Data at our institution indicate that the best discriminatory progesterone is 10 ng/ml (Fig. 20-4). If the progesterone concentration is <10 ng/ml, most of these pregnancies will be abnormal. Thus, progesterone monitoring during early gestation can identify pregnancies at risk without the need for multiple testing.

Figure 20-5 outlines a systematic evaluation of early pregnancy. This diagnostic algorithm utilizes the contemporary tools of serial hCG monitoring and vaginal sonography. In the absence of pain, evaluation of the patient in an ambulatory environment is appropriate. Hospitalization is necessary if pain is a presenting complaint. The role of serum progesterone measurements is not completely established as this predictor of ectopic pregnancy has not been included in the algorithm.

SURGICAL TREATMENT

Prior to the development of safe anesthesia for surgical treatment, expectant management of ectopic pregnancies resulted in a mortality rate of nearly 70%. Salpingectomy

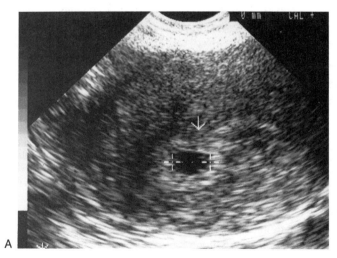
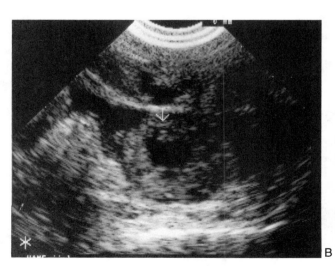

FIG. 20-3. Transvaginal sonography. The view in **A** shows an 8-mm intrauterine gestational sac with an hCG titer of 1,420 mIU/ml. The view in **B** shows a tubal pregnancy with an hCG titer of 1840 mIU/ml.

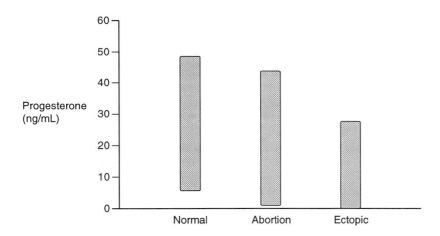

FIG. 20-4. Serum progesterone in normal, abortive, and ectopic pregnancies. Relative operating characteristic curve analysis (data not shown) indicates that 10 ng/ml is the best discriminatory progesterone concentration. Although there is considerable overlap, most pregnancies are abnormal.

for surgical treatment was first described in 1884, and the remarkable effectiveness in reducing maternal mortality from ectopic pregnancy made extirpative surgery standard treatment. In 1953, the first case of conservative surgical treatment for ectopic pregnancy was reported in the English literature. Since then many methods for the conservative advances in endoscopic instrumentation and techniques have allowed successful surgical treatment via endoscopy. This surgical approach has reduced operative morbidity and hospital costs, and allowed the patient to return to normal activities in a shorter time than the postoperative recovery from a laparotomy.

Conservative or nonconservative tubal surgery for treatment of the ectopic must be individualized for each patient and surgeon. For conservative management, the patient should desire future fertility, be hemodynamically stable, and have an unruptured and surgically accessible gestation. Appropriate equipment and instruments must be available (Chapter 21), and the surgeon as well as the operating room team must be properly trained. If the fallopian tube is ruptured or the patient is hemodynamically unstable, more urgent and nonconservative surgical treatment is usually required to manage the patient expeditiously. The selection of the operation is guided by the location of the ectopic pregnancy, the capabilities of the surgeon, and the availability of operating room resources.

Operations for Distal Tubal Pregnancy

Salpingostomy is commonly performed to treat unruptured ampullary gestations. In this technique, a linear incision is performed in the antimesenteric portion of the fallopian tube, and the ectopic gestation is expressed through this incision (Fig. 20-6A). To minimize bleeding and thereby optimize the success of this procedure, cauterization of the serosal vessels at both sides of the anticipated incision is often performed. Additionally, a dilute solution of vasopressin (20 U/ml mixed with 10–20 ml normal saline) can be injected into the mesosalpinx below the ectopic pregnancy. After the incision has been performed, small bleeding vessels can be ligated or cauterized.

To perform salpingostomy through the laparoscope, a three-puncture technique is usually required (Chapter 21). Two suprapubic punctures are used for operative instruments that stabilize and manipulate the ectopic gestation. An atraumatic grasping forceps should be used to elevate and stabilize the pregnancy. A 2- to 4-cm incision is created and the ectopic gestation teased from the decidual bed. Excessive grasping at the bed of the ectopic gestation can damage the tube and increase bleeding. Salpingotomy is performed in the same fashion as salpingostomy, but in this technique the edges of the incision are approximated with fine interrupted suture. Despite the aesthetic appeal of reapproximating the serosal edges, there is no evidence that salpingotomy is superior to salpingostomy, and the additional surgery at the site of the ectopic pregnancy may increase adhesions to the fallopian tube. Fimbrial expression of the ectopic pregnancy has been reported as treatment for distal ampullary ectopic pregnancies to avoid opening the oviduct. However, this approach may be associated with a higher incidence of persistent trophoblast tissue. As such, it should be reserved for those patients with fimbrial pregnancies that are already in the process of spontaneous abortion.

Tubal rupture and overt hemorrhage commonly require salpingectomy (complete or partial) to provide rapid treatment and prevent serious morbidity and mortality. The removal of the involved ovary is not recommended, as was once the common practice, unless the ovary is involved with the ectopic pregnancy or other ovarian pathology exists.

Operations for Proximal Tubal Pregnancy

Segmental resection has been the preferred operation for tubal pregnancies located in the isthmus of the fallopian

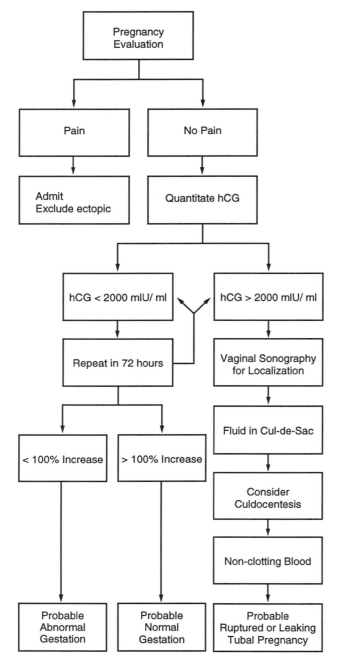

FIG. 20-5. Evaluation of early pregnancy. This algorithm uses serial hCG monitoring and vaginal sonography to aid in establishing a diagnosis. An important aspect of this algorithm is the exclusion of patients who have pain. See text for details.

tube (Fig. 20-6B). The tubal lumen is narrow and the site of the ectopic pregnancy is difficult to identify. The muscularis is commonly invaded by the ectopic gestation at this site, and the subsequent inflammatory response after salpingostomy leads to an increased rate of proximal tubal obstruction. Additionally, the incidence of repeat ectopic pregnancy in patients with isthmic ectopic pregnancies

treated with linear salpingotomy is nearly 50%. Therefore, removal of the tubal segment containing the gestation is advised when the ectopic is found in this location. The smallest portion of fallopian tube necessary to include the gestation is resected. Although tubal anastomosis has been performed at the time of resection, most authors prefer to perform a second operation after edema and inflammation from the ectopic pregnancy have resolved.

The surgical treatment of cornual (interstitial) ectopic pregnancy is associated with hemorrhage that may require hysterectomy. The cornual gestation is better protected in the interstitium than in the remainder of the tube, and as a result these pregnancies are usually more advanced than other tubal pregnancies when diagnosed. Cornual resection and repair can be performed in only about 50% of such cases. Hysterectomy is required for the remainder. In general, hysterectomy is recommended for multiparous women over 35 years old, and conservative treatment for nulliparous or young women. The surgical technique requires a V-shaped wedge of uterine tissue to be removed.

COMPLICATIONS

Conservative treatment for ectopic pregnancy, whether by salpingotomy or fimbrial expression, has the potential to preserve fertility and reduce operative morbidity. The major problems associated with conservative surgery are hemorrhage at the implantation site and subsequent persistent trophoblast with compression of the site or injection of the mesosalpinx with dilute vasopressin. Occasionally, small bleeding vessels can be identified within the implantation bed and cauterized or ligated. If these therapies fail, salpingectomy or resection of the involved segment is performed.

Women who undergo surgical removal of the ectopic pregnancy without the removal of the affected tube are at risk for "persistent ectopic pregnancy," or "persistent ectopic trophoblast." Although the etiology of this condition is not clear, it is generally believed that the trophoblast continues to grow in the tube from which it was incompletely removed at the time of surgical extraction or that trophoblast implants develop at sites in the pelvis where the ectopic pregnancy touched during surgical excision. This complication is estimated to occur in 5–15% of conservative operations. To confirm that surgical treatment for ectopic pregnancy was successful, patients who have salpingostomy or ampullary expression of an ectopic should be monitored with hCG titers. In general, if the trophoblast tissue is completely resected, hCG titers disappear in approximately 12–24 days. If left untreated, the clinical course of women with persistent ectopic trophoblast is unclear. However, the cases reported in the literature are often associated with pain, adnexal mass, tubal rupture, hypotension, and hemoperitoneum. There-

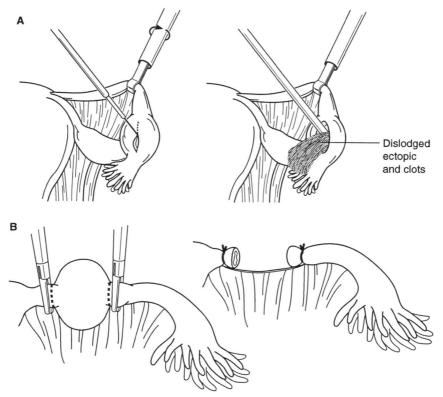

Dislodged ectopic and clots

FIG. 20-6. Surgical options for the management of distal tubal pregnancy. **A:** Linear salpingostomy—a small incision is placed directly over the distal ectopic pregnancy, and bleeding points are cauterized. The ectopic pregnancy is extruded from the tube, and the edges of the incision are not approximated. **B:** Partial salpingectomy—removal of the ectopic and the affected portion of the tube. The tube immediately adjacent to the ectopic pregnancy is cauterized or sutured bilaterally to establish hemostasis. The tube is divided and the mesosalpinx directly beneath the ectopic is cauterized or sutured. The tubal gestation is then resected. An alternative method is to apply a loop suture that incorporates the ectopic pregnancy.

fore, treatment for persistent trophoblast should be initiated if hCG titers persist or rise. Treatment of persistent trophoblast has been limited to surgery or medical therapy (see below).

SUBSEQUENT REPRODUCTION

Subsequent reproduction after surgery for ectopic pregnancy is independent of the technique of management. DeCherney compared intrauterine and ectopic pregnancy rates in women treated with salpingostomy to those treated with salpingectomy. There was not a significant difference between the groups. Approximately 40% in both groups had a subsequent intrauterine gestation, and 12% in each group had a recurrent ectopic pregnancy. This information is different from that reported for conservative surgery a decade ago where the incidence of ectopic pregnancy was greater in women who had conservative management of their fallopian tube rather than salpingectomy. At that time, conservative surgical treat-

ment of tubal pregnancies was only performed on patients with abnormal or absent contralateral tubes. This operation was considered "a rescue" surgical procedure to save reproductive function because a salpingectomy would sterilize the patient. In recent years, the indications for conservative surgery have been expanded to include women with normal contralateral anatomy, and recent data reflect these trends. Postoperative infertility after conservative surgery is associated with previous sterility, coexistent periadnexal adhesions or tubal disease, rupture of the ectopic pregnancy, and older age.

NONSURGICAL TREATMENT

Tubal pregnancies may resolve spontaneously without the need for medical or surgical intervention. This has been particularly well documented in recent clinical series where patients with an ectopic had resolution of their disease without the need for surgical management. Case reports of tubal rupture during rapidly declining hCG titers or of low hCG titers associated with chronic ectopic pregnancies emphasize the need for caution in the non-surgical management of these patients.

Recently, there has been an interest in medical therapy for treatment of unruptured tubal pregnancy. This treatment avoids surgical intervention, potentially preserves reproductive potential, and reduces the cost of medical care. Methotrexate, a folinic acid antagonist, was the first drug used to treat tubal pregnancies nonsurgically. To date, the outcome of over 200 patients treated with methotrexate have been reported in the literature. The cure rate with this therapy is over 90%, and little toxicity occurs.

In general, candidates for methotrexate therapy should have an unruptured ectopic pregnancy, an hCG titer <15,000, a desire for future reproduction, or severe medical diseases that would be compromised by surgery (Table 20-4). In addition to the primary treatment of ectopic pregnancy with methotrexate, this agent has been advocated as the treatment of choice for persistent trophoblast after conservative tubal surgery for ectopic pregnancy.

Several routes of methotrexate treatment have been used (intramuscular, oral, direct injection). The most common is intramuscular injection. Most physicians are familiar with this route of administration, the technique is not associated with vesication complications, and the drug is readily available. The dose of methotrexate used to treat ectopic pregnancies has been determined empirically, principally modeled after the experience with treatment of gestational trophoblastic disease. The most common regimen used in this country has been a single dose of 50 mg/M^2. However, additional experience with this protocol suggests that the cure rate may not be as optimistic as previously reported. Alternative commonly used dosages include 1 mg/kg on alternate days for 2–3 injections (eg, days 1, 3, and 5).

In addition to methotrexate, local injection of prostaglandin at the time of laparoscopy has been used successfully to treat unruptured ectopic pregnancies. Prostaglandin was injected under laparoscopic guidance if the tube was visualized, the transverse diameter of the oviduct over the conceptus was <2.5 cm, the serosa over the site of the pregnancy was intact, and there was no fresh bleeding from the tubal ostium. Over 90% of treated women were cured.

TABLE 20-4. *Selection criteria for methotrexate treatment of unruptured tubal pregnancy*

An ectopic <3 cm
Desires for future fertility
hCG <15,000 mIU/ml (IRP)
No pain suggesting potential rupture
No active bleeding

hCG, human chorionic gonadotropin; IRP, International Reference Preparation.

SUMMARY

The incidence of ectopic pregnancy has increased between 1970 and 1992. Approximately 100,000 tubal pregnancies and 30 deaths occur annually. Historically, most ectopic gestations were diagnosed late in their course, often only after rupture occurred. Human chorionic gonadotropin assays and transvaginal sonography have improved our ability to detect ectopic pregnancies before symptoms or rupture occur. Early detection and a desire to preserve reproductive potential in women affected with tubal pregnancies has led to the development of conservative surgery and medical treatment for this condition. Nearly 45% of women with an ectopic pregnancy treated conservatively carry a subsequent pregnancy to term.

SUGGESTED READING

Anonymous. Ectopic pregnancy: United States, 1990–1992. *MMWR* 1995; 44:46–48.

Breen JL. A 21-year survey of 645 ectopic pregnancies. *Am J Obstet Gynecol 1979;*106:1004.

Cowan BD. Evaluation and treatment of ectopic pregnancy. *J Clin Pract Sexual* 1991;7:8.

Goldner TE, Lawson HW, Xia Z, Atrash HK. Surveillance for ectopic pregnancy: United States, 1970–1989. *MMWR* 1993;42:73–85.

Grimes DA. The morbidity and mortality of pregnancy: still risky business. *Am J Obstet Gynecol* 1994;170:1489–1494.

Leach RE, Ory SJ. Modern management of ectopic pregnancy. *J Reprod Med* 1989;34:324.

Parmley TH. The histopathology of tubal pregnancy. *Clin Obstet Gynecol* 1987;30:119.

Soper DE. Pelvic inflammatory disease. *Infect Dis Clin North Am* 1994;8: 821–840.

Westrom LV. Sexually transmitted diseases and infertility. *Sex Transm Dis* 1994;21:S32–37.

Diagnosis

Barnhart K, Mennuti MT, Benjamin I, Jacobson S, Goodman D, Coutifaris C. Prompt diagnosis of ectopic pregnancy in an emergency department setting. *Obstet Gynecol* 1994;84:1010–1015.

Brown DL, Doubilet PM. Transvaginal sonography for diagnosing ectopic pregnancy: positivity criteria and performance characteristics. *J Ultrasound Med* 1994;13:259–266.

Buster JE, Carson SA. Ectopic pregnancy: new advances in diagnosis and treatment. *Curr Opin Obstet Gynecol* 1995;7:169–176.

Cacciatore B, Stenman UL, Ylostalo P. Early screening for ectopic pregnancy in high-risk symptom-free women. *Lancet* 1994;343:517–518.

Cowan BD. Ectopic pregnancy. *Curr Opin Obstet Gynecol* 1993;5: 328–332.

Isaacs JD, Whitworth NS, Cowan BD. Relative operating characteristic analysis in reproductive medicine: comparison of progesterone and human chorionic gonadotropin doubling time as predictors of early gestational normalcy. *Fertil Steril* 1994;62:452–455.

Kadar N, Bohrer M, Kemmann E, Shelden R. The discriminatory human chorionic gonadotropin zone for endovaginal sonography: a prospective, randomized study. *Fertil steril* 1994;61:1016–1020.

Kutluay L, Vicdan K, Turan C, Barioglu S, Oguz S, Godmen O. Tubal histopathology in ectopic pregnancies. *Eur J Obstet Gynecol Reprod Biol* 1994;57:91–94.

Lopez HB, Micheelsen U, Berendtsen H, Kock K. Ectopic pregnancy and its associated endometrial changes. *Gynecol Obstet Invest* 1994;38: 104–106.

McKennett M, Fullerton JT. Vaginal bleeding in pregnancy. *Am Fam Physician* 1995;51:639–646.

Ooi DS, Perkins SL, Claman P, Muggah HF. Serum human chorionic gonadotropin levels in early pregnancy. *Clin Chim Acta* 1989;181:281.

Pittaway DE, Reish RL, Wentz AC. Doubling times of human chorionic gonadotropin increase in early viable intrauterine pregnancies. *Am J Obstet Gynecol* 1985;152:299.

Ransom MX, Garcia AJ, Bohrer M, Corsan GH, Kemmann E. Serum progesterone as a predictor of methotrexate success in the treatment of ectopic pregnancy. *Obstet Gynecol* 1994;83:1033–1037.

Storring PL, Gaine-Des RE, Bangham DR. International reference preparation of human chorionic gonadotropin for immunoassay: potency estimates in various bioassays and protein binding assay systems and international reference preparation of the alpha and beta subunits of human chorionic gonadotropin for immunoassay. *J Endocrinol* 1980;84:295.

Surgery

DeCherney A, Boyers A. Isthmic ectopic pregnancy: segmental resection as the treatment of choice. *Fertil Steril* 1985;44:307.

Donnez J, Nisolle M. Endoscopic management of ectopic pregnancy. *Baillieres Clin Obstet Gynaecol* 1994;8:707–722.

Kamrava MM, Taymor ML, Berger MJ, Thompson IE, Seibel MM. Disappearance of human chorionic gonadotropin following removal of ectopic pregnancy. *Obstet Gynecol* 1983;62:486.

Pouly J, Mahnes H, Mage G, et al. Conservative laparoscopic treatment of 321 ectopic pregnancies. *Fertil Steril* 1986;46:1093.

Stangel JJ, Gomel V. Techniques in conservative surgery for tubal gestation. *Clin Obstet Gynecol* 1985;23:1221.

Tulandi T. Medical and surgical treatment of ectopic pregnancy. *Curr Opin Obstet Gynecol* 1994;6:149–152.

Vermesh M, Silva PD, Rosen GF, Stein AL, Fossum GT, Sauer MV. Management of unruptured ectopic gestation by linear salpingostomy: a prospective, randomized clinical trial of laparoscopy versus laparotomy. *Obstet Gynecol* 1989;73:400.

Yeko TR, Villa A, Parsons AK, Maroulis GB. Laparoscopic treatment of ectopic pregnancy. Residents' learning experience. *J Reprod Med* 1994;39:854–856.

Medical Management

Fernandez H, Bourget P, Vilele Y, Lelaidier C, Frydman R. Treatment of unruptured tubal pregnancy with methotrexate: pharmacokinetic analysis of local versus intramuscular administration. *Fertil Steril* 1994;62:943–947.

Paulsson G, Kvint S, Labecker BM, Lofstrand T, Lindblom B. Laparoscopic prostaglandin injection in ectopic pregnancy: success rates according to endocrine activity. *Fertil Steril* 1995;63:473–477.

Stovall TG. Medical management of ectopic pregnancy. *Curr Opin Obstet Gynecol* 1994;6:510–515.

Trio D, Strobelt N, Picciolo C, Lapinski RH, Ghidini A. Prognostic factors for successful expectant management of ectopic pregnancy. *Fertil Steril* 1995;63:469–472.

Yeko Tr, Mayer JC, Parsons AK, Maroulis GB. A prospective series of unruptured ectopic pregnancies treated by tubal injection with hypersomolar glucose. *Obstet Gynecol* 1995;85:265–268.

Reproductive Outcome

Gruft L, Bertola E, Luchini L, Azzilonna C, Bigatti G, Parazzini F. Determinants of reproductive prognosis after ectopic pregnancy. *Hum Reprod* 1994;9:1333–1336.

Oelsner G, Goldenberg M, Admon D, Pansky M, Rut-Kaspa I, Rabinovitch O, Carp HJ, Mashiach S. Salpingectomy by operative laparoscopy and subsequent reproductive performance. *Hum Reprod* 1994;9:83–86.

Seifer DB, Silva PD, Grainger DA, Barber SR, Grant WD, Gutmann JN. Reproductive potential after treatment for persistent ectopic pregnancy. *Fertil Steril* 1994;62:194–196.

Complications

Hagstrom HG, Hahlin M, Bennegard-Eden B, Sjoblom P, Thorburn J, Lindblom B. Prediction of persistent ectopic pregnancy after laparoscopic salpingostomy. *Obstet Gynecol* 1994;84:798–802.

Seifer DB, Diamond MP, DeCherney AH. Persistent ectopic pregnancy. *Obstet Gynecol Clin North Am* 1991;18:153–159.

Clinical Reproductive Medicine,
Edited by Bryan D. Cowan and David B. Seifer
Lippincott-Raven Publishers, Philadelphia © 1997

CHAPTER 21

Reproductive Surgery

Michael S. Opsahl and Edwin D. Robins

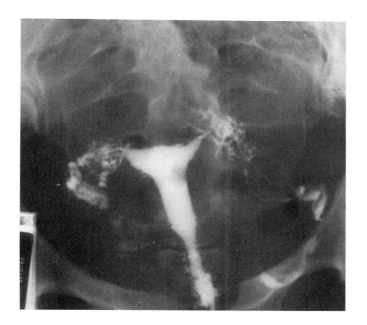

Diagnosis of Pelvic Disease
Principles of Reproductive Surgery
  Endoscopy versus Laparotomy
  Laser versus Conventional Electrosurgery
  Adhesion Prevention
Specific Diseases
  Pelvic Adhesion and Neosalpingostomy

Endometriosis
Leiomyoma
Proximal Tubal Disease
Sterilization Reversal
Uterine Diseases
Ectopic Pregnancy
Suggested Reading

M. S. Opsahl: Uniformed Services University of the Health Sciences, Genetics and IVF Institute, Fairfax, VA 22031

E. D. Robins: Institute of Reproductive Medicine and Sciences, St. Barnabas Hospital, Livingston, NJ 07039

The decision to proceed with surgery for pelvic disease depends largely on the expectation of a live-born child. For advanced and extensive pelvic disease, in vitro fertilization (IVF) provides a greater likelihood of pregnancy than surgery. Furthermore, the time necessary to achieve pregnancy after a reconstructive operation is often delayed for as long as 72 months. Lastly, advanced reproductive age is associated with a decline in fecundity. Thus, maturing women or those with diminished ovarian reserve may not have sufficient opportunity to wait for pregnancy after surgery, but surgery is a viable option of many young couples.

This chapter deals primarily with indications for surgery and expectations for postoperative pregnancy. Several extensive atlases of surgery adequately describe the technical details of individual procedures and such details are beyond our space limitations.

DIAGNOSIS OF PELVIC DISEASE

Appropriate therapy for pelvic disease requires an accurate diagnosis. This includes not only the location and extent of pelvic disease but other associated fertility factors. Approximately 25–35% of couples have multiple diagnoses that affect the therapeutic plan and prognosis for pregnancy. An evaluation can be accomplished in 2–3 months and consists of semen analysis, documentation of ovulation, and assessment of pelvic adhesions and tubal patency. Other fertility testing such as the postcoital examination, endometrial biopsy, and antisperm antibody testing should be considered ancillary tests because they detect subtle and controversial etiologies. Ancillary testing should rarely postpone therapy for significant pelvic disease.

The most meaningful preoperative test for pelvic adhesions and tubal disease is the hysterosalpingogram (HSG). Although the HSG has a reputation for inaccuracy, in our experience certain HSG findings are extremely reliable. We classify HSG results as normal (normal cavity, bilateral tubal fill and spill, and with normal tubal architecture), abnormal (bilateral distal tubal obstruction, with or without tubal dilatation), or suspicious (all others including proximal tubal occlusion, unilateral distal tubal obstruction, or distal tubal spill but with loculation suggesting periadnexal adhesions). The normal HSG has a negative predictive value of 97%, whereas the abnormal HSG has a positive predictive value of 96%. Suspicious films are less reliable for predicting pelvic disease and they have a positive predictive value of only 54%. Nevertheless, suspicious HSGs are often associated with moderate to severe pelvic disease (Table 21-1).

We recommend that patients with an abnormal HSG be counseled for IVF or pelviscopic surgery. Those with suspicious findings require diagnostic laparoscopy. The surgeon should anticipate the need for pelviscopic surgery in

TABLE 21-1. *Correlation of HSG and surgical findings by HSG classification*

HSG	n	Surgical findings	
		Confirmed (%)	Not confirmed (%)
Normal	327	96.6	3.4
Suspicious	336	63.1	36.9
Abnormal	93	95.7	4.3
Totals	756	81.6	18.4

these cases. A normal HSG allows delay of laparoscopy in selected cases to complete a trial of medical therapy when male or ovulatory factors are present (Fig. 21-1).

PRINCIPLES OF REPRODUCTIVE SURGERY

The goal of reproductive surgery is to restore, as nearly as possible, diseased or deformed pelvic structures to their normal anatomic state. Unavoidable consequences of surgery are trauma, bleeding, air drying of serosal surfaces, and tissue reaction that can lead to adhesion formation. To comply with good surgical principals, four areas of well-intended surgical adjuncts have been proposed. Magnification, endoscopy, laser application, and adhesion prevention each offer potential benefits to our patients. However, the body of literature describing these modalities is still evolving, and these techniques presently must be considered developmental. Magnification techniques emphasize delicate tissue handling, fine instruments, magnification, constant irrigation of the pelvic organs, meticulous hemostasis, and less reactive suture material. Magnification has been most valuable in tubal anastomosis procedures. Its value for other disease is less clear because microsurgery does not appear to benefit salpingostomy procedures. The endosalpingeal damage present in cases of severe disease is likely to be the most important factor related to pregnancy failures.

Endoscopy versus Laparotomy

The last decade has seen endoscopic surgery all but replace laparotomy for the surgical treatment of infertility disorders. Endoscopy has several theoretical advantages and disadvantages (Table 21-2). Nevertheless, the most important measure for comparison of endoscopic surgery with standard laparotomy is the pregnancy rate. Endoscopic surgery generally demonstrates comparable but not superior results to laparotomy.

Laser versus Conventional Electrosurgery

Initial enthusiasm for lasers focused on the hope that they were less traumatic, more precise, and associated

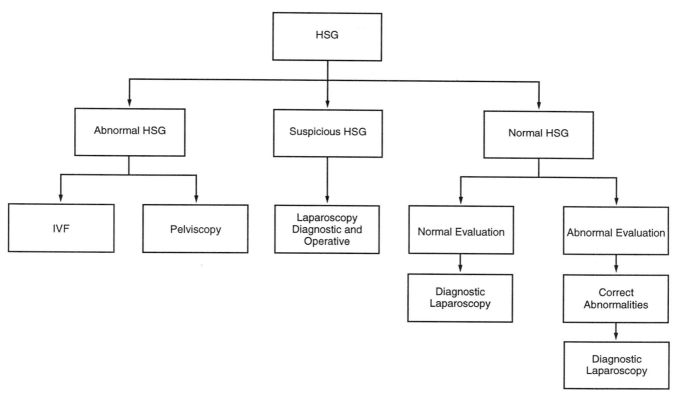

FIG. 21-1. Management algorithm for evaluating infertile couples with hysterosalpingography.

with less postoperative adhesion formation. Recent evidence suggests that lasers should be viewed as merely another surgical tool. In well-designed comparative studies, laser and electrosurgery appear to have similar postoperative results for both periadnexal adhesions and distal tubal obstruction (2-year follow-up).

Adhesion Prevention

Infertility is thought to be secondary to pelvic adhesions in approximately 15–20% of couples. Minimizing adhesion reformation and de novo adhesion formation after reparative surgery is a major concern for the reproductive surgeon. In a multicenter study, the Operative Laparoscopy Study Group noted a reduction in adhesion

scores at second-look laparoscopy but nearly all patients had some adhesion reformation. New adhesion formation occurred infrequently. Thus, with appropriate surgical technique, adhesion scores can be reduced and the incidence of de novo adhesions minimized, but reformation remains the most significant consequence.

Surgical adjuvants used to prevent adhesions may be classified into fibrinolytic agents, anticoagulants, antiinflammatory agents, antibiotics, and barriers. Numerous agents have been evaluated for their ability to reduce postoperative adhesion formation (Table 21-3). Unfortunately, satisfactory results have not been demonstrated in humans with the use of most of these agents. Meticulous surgical technique remains the best method to control postoperative adhesions.

SPECIFIC DISEASES

Pelvic Adhesion and Neosalpingostomy

Pelvic adhesions are associated with infertility and, including endometriosis, account for approximately 25–30% of infertility diagnoses. Pelvic adhesions are generally classified as mild, moderate, and severe. Adhesions are presumed to impair fertility by mechanically preventing normal ovum pick-up and transport. The

TABLE 21-2. *Endoscopic surgery*

Advantages	Disadvantages
Abdomen closed	Additional training
No tissue drying	Surgery difficult
Modest magnification	New instruments
Documentation	Iatrogenic injury
Reduced hospitalization	Reduced tactile sensation
Short recovery time	

TABLE 21-3. *Agents used to prevent adhesions after surgery*

Fibrinolytic	Anticoagulant	Antiinflammatory	Antibiotic	Barrier
Fibrinolysin	Heparin	Corticosteroids	Tetracyclines	Omental graphs
Papain	Citrates	Ibuprofen	Corticosporins	Peritoneal graphs
Streptokinase	Oxalates	Antihistamines		Dextran
Hyaluronidase				Crystalloids
Chymotrypsin				Carboxymethylcellulose
Pepsin				Polytetrafluoroethylene (Gore-Tex)
				Oxidized cellulose fabric (Interceed)

severity of pelvic adhesions does not generally affect the outcome or success of IVF. Two primary factors contribute to the prognosis for pregnancy: the type of adhesion (filmy or dense) and the extent of ovarian involvement (surface area free of adhesions). Reported pregnancy rates are inversely proportional to the severity of adhesions; mild = 50–65%, moderate = 25–45%, and severe = 10–25%.

Distal tubal occlusion is the end result of endosalpingeal inflammation and agglutination. Distal occlusion is associated with moderate-severe pelvic adhesions in 82% of cases. Surgical success rates are often poor (<25–35%) but cumulatively range from 0 to 77% after 5–6 years of observation. The prognostic factors associated with pregnancy include the tubal mucosal pattern on HSG, the extent of adnexal adhesions, and the condition of the tubal mucosa at surgery.

Surgery for pelvic adhesions and distal occlusion can be performed either by laparotomy or laparoscopy with equal success in establishing tubal patency and pregnancy. Pregnancies continue to occur through five to six postoperative years, suggesting progressive regeneration of the endosalpinx.

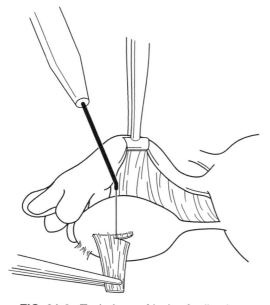

FIG. 21-2. Technique of lysis of adhesions.

The goal of surgery is restoration of normal pelvic organ relationships to enhance ovum capture. Adnexal adhesions are best removed in their entirety rather than merely lysed. Adhesions are lysed by blunt and sharp dissection after placing the adhesion on tension (Fig. 21-2). Aquadissection is an effective method of blunt dissection endoscopically. Dense, vascular adhesions should be coagulated before transection.

Neosalpingostomy for distal tubal obstruction requires an incision into the tubal lumen. This is best accomplished by filling the obstructed tube with fluid and incising the avascular portion of the distal tube with either the laser or microelectrode. The mucosa can then be everted with sutures or by coagulating the external tubal serosa (Fig. 21-3).

Endometriosis

Diagnosis

The etiology and natural course of endometriosis and its impact on fertility remain enigmatic. Surgery plays a crucial role in diagnosis and management. The diagnosis of endometriosis rests on either visualization of disease or biopsy of characteristic lesions at surgery.

The first step in management for the infertile couple is the evaluation of the extent of disease. Several classification systems exist but the Revised American Fertility Society (R/AFS) is arguably the most commonly cited system. All classification schemes assign points to the location and extent of both endometriotic lesions and adhesions. Patients are classified as having minimal, mild, moderate, or severe disease. Surgical assessment should be methodical and thorough, and documentation of disease with videotape or color photographs is encouraged. Some authors recommend preoperative vaginal sonography to screen for occult ovarian endometriomas to supplement the surgical assessment.

Effect of Staging

The effect of endometriosis on infertility is controversial. The pathophysiology is more obvious when endometriosis is associated with anatomic alterations such

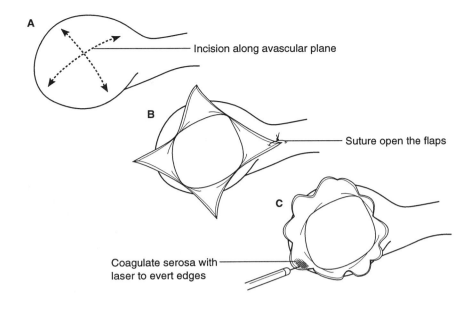

A — Incision along avascular plane

B — Suture open the flaps

C

Coagulate serosa with laser to evert edges

FIG. 21-3. Technique of neosalpingostomy.

as immobility or obstruction of the tubes and ovaries preventing ovum capture. Prospective studies that confirm the association of endometriosis and infertility do not exist.

Surgery

The objective in surgical management of endometriosis for infertility is to reduce gross disease and restore normal anatomic relationships. Diagnostic laparoscopy is necessary to establish the diagnosis and may also provide therapeutic intervention. The limits of laparoscopy are determined by the skill and experience of the surgeon, the available equipment, and the extent of disease. En-

dometriotic implants can be ablated by laser vaporization, electrosurgery, or sharp excision. Aqua- or hydrodissection during laparoscopy to separate the peritoneum from underlying ureters or pelvic vessels can provide added safety before operative excision or ablation (Fig. 21-4). Ovarian endometriomas should be removed or ablated by laser. Endometrioma resection is accomplished by first aspirating the cyst contents and then removing the cyst wall by peeling it free from the ovarian stroma. Laser ablation of the cyst wall, as an alternative or adjunct to excision, is performed after cyst aspiration. Pelvic adhesions are excised as in cases of postinflammatory disease. Judgment should be exercised to avoid dangerous situations that can be treated more effectively or safely by laparotomy.

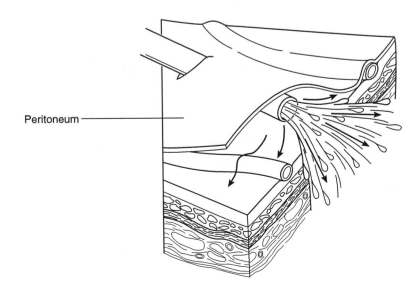

Peritoneum

FIG. 21-4. Technique of aqua- or hydrodissection.

Leiomyoma

Indications for Surgery

Myomectomy is indicated for selected infertile and recurrent spontaneous abortion patients with leiomyomata uteri. The evidence supporting myomectomy for reproductive indications is circumstantial and a prospective randomized study of myomectomy versus expectant management does not exist. Most investigators recommend myomectomy after excluding other causes of infertility or recurrent pregnancy loss. Other criteria for myomectomy include: myoma that is >2–3 cm in diameter; submucous myoma that distorts the uterine cavity; or myoma that obstructs the tubal cornua.

Myomectomy in women with otherwise unexplained infertility accounts for only 1–2% of infertility laparotomies. Subsequent pregnancy rates for this indication range from 16.7% to 70%. Myomectomy for recurrent pregnancy loss is reported to reduce pregnancy wastage. The recurrence of leiomyoma after myomectomy is 15%.

Surgery

Myomectomy is accomplished by shelling out the tumors through a serosal uterine incision. It is important to find the myoma pseudocapsule and use this as the dissecting plane to minimize intraoperative bleeding. Thus the uterine incision extends from the serosal surface until characteristic texture and appearance of the myoma is encountered. The myoma can be grasped for countertraction and delineation of the myoma–myometrium plane during dissection. After removal of the myoma, all dead space should be carefully closed to prevent bleeding and hematoma formation. The serosa should be closed using small calibre absorbable suture. To reduce adhesion formation, the fewest number of uterine incisions should be used, and ideally the incisions should be on the anterior uterine fundus. Although laparoscopic myomectomy has been described, most myomas that are easily removed via laparoscopy are probably of little consequence and transmural myomas that require resection are very difficult to accomplish laparoscopically.

Techniques to prevent bleeding include injecting dilute vasopressin into the surrounding myometrium. We typically dilute 20 units of vasopressin in 20 ml normal saline prior to injection. Occlusive tourniquets on the uterine and ovarian vessels have been advocated in the past, but this technique is clumsy and largely replaced by vasopressin injection. Gonadotropin-releasing hormone agonists (GnRH-a), as a surgical adjuvant, reduce blood loss at myomectomy and facilitate surgical excision. Regrowth of myomas is rapid after discontinuation of medical therapy and myomas return to pretreatment size in <12 months. Postoperative adhesions are perhaps the most important complication.

Hysteroscopic myomectomy for submucous pedunculated myomas involves shaving or resecting the myoma. Hysteroscopic resection of submucous myomas is clearly efficacious.

Proximal Tubal Disease

Salpingitis Isthmica Nodosa

Salpingitis isthmica nodosa (SIN) is a pathologic finding with an unclear etiology and natural history. The most popular etiology is tubal infection. A compelling association exists between infertility, ectopic pregnancy, and SIN. The HSG findings are unmistakable and appear as multiple small diverticular outpouchings in the isthmic portion of the tube (Fig. 21-5). Laparoscopically the tubes appear thickened at the isthmus. Resection of the diseased portion of the tube and microsurgical anastomosis of the remaining tubal segments is indicated in selected cases. Recently, transcervical fluoroscopic tubal recanalization proved successful in some cases of SIN.

Proximal Tubal Occlusion

Proximal tubal occlusion is usually diagnosed by HSG but requires confirmation of occlusion by laparoscopy because of the high incidence of false-positive obstruction. Until recently, surgical treatment was the only treatment option. Correction required either resection of the diseased portion of the tube and microsurgical anastomosis of the remaining tubal segments or macrosurgical tubal implantation. Both techniques require laparotomy,

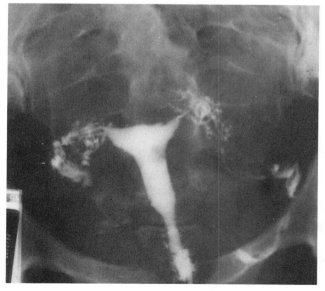

FIG. 21-5. Hysterosalpingogram of typical salpingitis isthmica nodosa.

and tubal implantation mandates caesarean delivery for subsequent pregnancies. Pregnancy rates following tubal implantation range from 30% to 50%; whereas pregnancy rates following microsurgical cornual anastomosis range from 40% to 70%.

Recently, tubal cannulation and balloon tuboplasty have become alternatives to surgery. Successful tubal cannulation by fluoroscopic, hysteroscopic, ultrasound guidance, or falloposcopy have demonstrated the intramural tubal architecture to be relatively linear. Recanalization studies report initial patency rates of 70–90%, 6- to 12-month patency rates of 40–70%, and intrauterine pregnancy rates of 10–40%. Many investigators recommend that tubal cannulation be attempted prior to surgery or IVF in the absence of bipolar tubal disease, ie, distal tubal obstruction coincident with proximal obstruction. Surgery is uniformly unsuccessful for bipolar tubal disease and IVF is the recommended treatment for these women. Cannulation failures imply histologic abnormalities in the tubes and microsurgery or IVF should be considered.

Sterilization Reversal

Sterilization reversal is one of the most successful surgical procedures available to the infertility surgeon. Cumulative pregnancy rates are often 70% but range from 20% to 95%. The prognostic factors influencing the success of the procedure are listed in Table 21-4. Tubal length is the single most important factor because pregnancy rates are directly correlated in all studies. Even previous fimbriectomy is potentially reversible if the tubal remnants are >8 cm and the ampullary width is >1 cm.

Preoperative evaluation should include laparoscopy to assess tubal length only if multiple burn cautery was used for sterilization, the sterilization technique is unknown, or the patient has only one remaining tube. If postpartum Pomeroy, rings, or clips were used, patients have a very small risk of having inoperable tubes (1.5%). Hysterosalpingography is not helpful in determining which patients have operable tubes and thus is not recommended routinely for this group of patients.

Tubal anastomosis for sterilization reversal is one procedure where microsurgery appears to be beneficial. We perform the procedure through a minilaparotomy incision. The pelvic organs are exteriorized and intermittently irrigated with Ringer's lactate solution. Exteriorization serves to elevate the tubes into the operative field and the abdomen provides a platform to stabilize the tissues. The proximal and distal segments are prepared for anastomosis by excising the scar tissue from the distal end of the proximal tubal segment. After confirming tubal patency of the proximal segment, the tubal ends are approximated with a suture in the mesosalpinx. The proximal end of the distal tubal segment is opened with magnification to create a tubal lumen of equal diameter to the lumen on the proximal tubal segment (Fig. 21-6). The anastomosis is performed microscopically in two layers (muscularis-mucosal and serosal) with interrupted 8-0 resorbable suture. Confirmation of tubal patency is performed with chromotubation at the completion of each anastomosis.

Uterine Diseases

Uterine disease associated with reproductive failure includes Mullerian anomalies, intrauterine synechiae, and submucous myomas. Mullerian disorders are discussed in the chapter on recurrent pregnancy loss. Operative hysteroscopy has improved considerably over the last decade with the introduction of a gynecologic resectoscope, improved electrosurgical equipment, and improved video systems that enhance the surgical assistant's view.

Uterine Septum

Repair of a uterine septum is indicated for recurrent pregnancy loss. Little evidence exists to suggest that a septum causes infertility. Nevertheless, given the safety and simplicity of hysteroscopic metroplasty, if a uterine septum is found during a diagnostic endoscopic procedure, metroplasty is a reasonable option.

Hysteroscopic metroplasty is optimally performed in the early follicular phase or after ovarian suppression. Dilute vasopressin injections into the cervix can diminish bleeding and intravasation of distention medium. The septum is incised beginning in the lower uterine segment and extended to the fundus but not into the myometrium. The cavity is most commonly distended with liquid medium such as sorbitol or glycine. Careful monitoring of inflow and outflow volumes are essential to prevent fluid overload. The incision is made with either flexible, semirigid, or rigid scissors, the resectoscope, lasers, or electrocautery. Concurrent laparoscopy is a helpful adjunct to prevent uterine perforation. Postoperatively, most patients receive prophylactic antibiotics. Conjugated estrogens, 2.5–5 mg daily for 30–45 days, followed by progesterone withdrawal are administered to facilitate endometrial overgrowth. Healing of the cavity is complete

TABLE 21-4. *Prognostic factors affecting pregnancy rates with tubal anastomosis*

Tube length at the completion of surgery	
>6 cm	73%
4–6 cm	55%
<4 cm	20%
Use of microsurgery versus macrosurgery	
Macrosurgery	40%
Microsurgery	70%
Method of sterilization	
Noncautery	30–70%
Cautery	40–95%

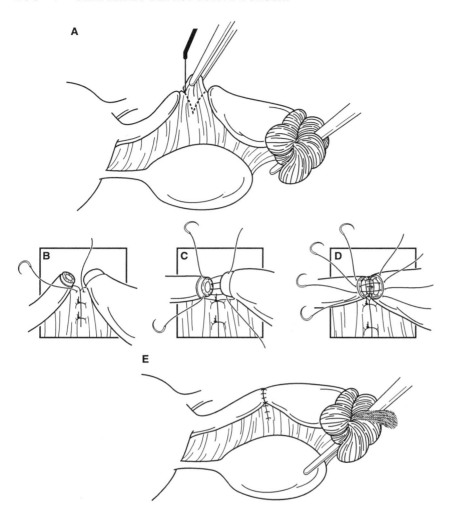

FIG. 21-6. Technique of microscopic tubal anastomosis.

by 2 months postoperatively and further delay in attempting conception is unnecessary.

Complications are uncommon but include bleeding, uterine perforation, incomplete "resection" of the septum, and fluid overload. Most bleeding responds to tamponade. Uterine perforation can limit further surgery but rarely leads to serious complications unless the perforation extends into the uterine vessels. Incomplete resection may require a repeat procedure. Fluid overload occurs from lengthy procedures without accurate intake and output measurement of uterine distention medium.

Intrauterine Synechiae

Intrauterine synechiae are the result of endometrial trauma, typically after pregnancy termination. The adhesions are associated with varying degrees of menstrual disturbances, infertility, or recurrent pregnancy loss. Diagnosis is commonly made with HSG but hysteroscopy may be required to confirm the diagnosis. The synechiae are classified as mild, moderate, or severe. The results of surgery suggest a good postoperative reproductive performance. Hysteroscopy for severe disease is one of the most challenging operations the reproductive surgeon must perform.

Surgical lysis of adhesions is almost always accomplished with scissors rather than with electrosurgery or lasers. Concurrent laparoscopy and attention to fluid status is important. Most surgeons place a pediatric Foley catheter or intrauterine device in the cavity postoperatively to separate the walls during healing and regrowth of the endometrium. Most surgeons also supplement the patient with high-dose conjugated estrogens, 2.5–5 mg daily, for 30–60 days followed by progesterone withdrawal.

Ectopic Pregnancy

Introduction

Ectopic pregnancy is a common complication of reproductive surgery. Risk factors for ectopic pregnancy include previous pelvic infection, tubal surgery, ovulation induction, and assisted reproductive technology (ART). There is no single sign, symptom, or test on which the diagnosis of ectopic pregnancy rests. Avoiding misdiagnosis depends on a high index of suspicion and careful interpretation of the available information in any at-risk woman. A more thorough discussion of the etiology and diagnosis of ectopic pregnancy is included in Chapter 20.

Surgical Therapy

Surgical choices for tubal pregnancy can be classified as radical or conservative. Radical surgery is defined as removal of the entire fallopian tube, whereas conservative surgery includes salpingostomy, salpingotomy, or segmental resection of only the portion containing trophoblast. Both techniques are technically feasible via laparotomy or laparoscopy. The choice of therapy is based on the desires of the patient, her clinical and hemodynamic status at the time of surgery, and the presence of other pelvic pathology.

Indications for a radical procedure include uncontrolled bleeding, an irreparably damaged tube, and a repeat ectopic in the same tube. Visual conformation of a normal-appearing contralateral tube alone should not dictate radical treatment because it may later prove to be obstructed. Salpingectomy by laparoscopy or laparotomy involves resecting from the distal to the proximal end of the tube after ligating or coagulating the vessels in the mesosalpinx (Fig. 21-7). Cornual resection is time consuming, bloody, and of no additional benefit except for true cornual (interstitial) implantations.

Conservative surgery can be accomplished as easily as salpingectomy. Conservative treatment is the only choice for those women with a sole remaining tube who wish to maintain fertility. The main disadvantages of conservative surgery are persistent tubal trophoblast (5%) and repeat ectopic pregnancy in the same tube (15–25%).

A salpingostomy is a linear incision in the antimesenteric surface of the tube. Dilute vasopressin in the mesosalpinx prior to the salpingostomy incision may decrease bleeding. The trophoblast is gently removed with a combination of irrigation and teasing the tissues (Fig. 21-8).

Reoperation/Second-Look Procedures

Unfortunately, reproductive surgery all too often fails to result in a live birth and reoperation is considered. Several questions should be answered before deciding on repeat surgery. First, is the infertility evaluation complete and have all other factors been corrected? Medical record review will answer this question but attention to detail and critical evaluation of previous testing is prudent. Co-

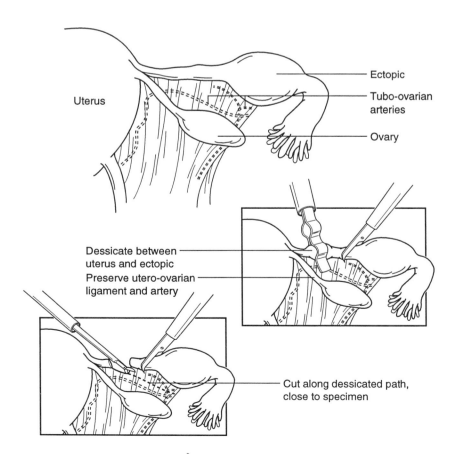

Uterus

Ectopic

Tubo-ovarian arteries

Ovary

Dessicate between uterus and ectopic

Preserve utero-ovarian ligament and artery

Cut along dessicated path, close to specimen

FIG. 21-7. Technique of endoscopic salpingectomy.

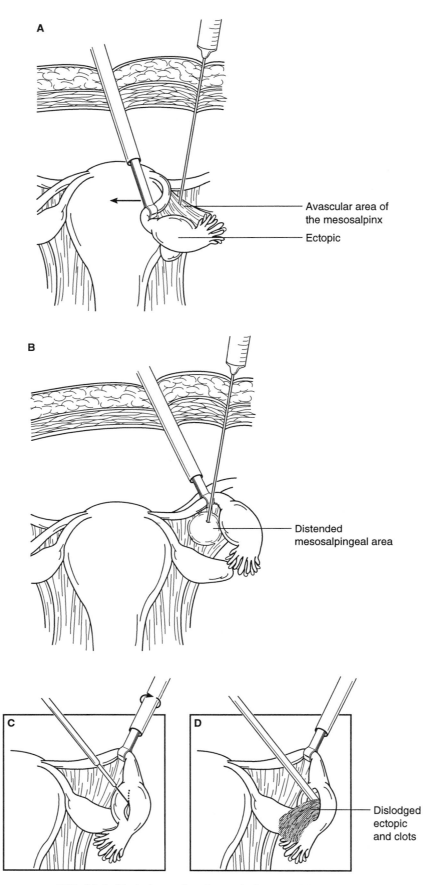

A

Avascular area of
the mesosalpinx

Ectopic

B

Distended
mesosalpingeal area

C

D

Dislodged
ectopic
and clots

FIG. 21-8. Technique of endoscopic linear salpingostomy.

existing infertility factors have a significant effect on fecundity after surgery. Second, would the repeat operation offer a surgical technique that was not previously utilized, such as microsurgery? Review the previous operative report for technical details and determine whether the principles of reproductive surgery were followed and whether a new technology is available for the disease process in question. Third, does the pregnancy success rate for reoperation compare favorably to the success with ART? The live birth rates after reoperation for a variety of diseases range from 0 to 16%. While the cumulative pregnancy rate after surgery is similar to a single IVF cycle, a 3-year postoperative waiting period is necessary.

Second-look laparoscopy is a useful research tool to study pelvic adhesions. Second-look procedures are effective in reducing adhesion scores but not for increasing pregnancy rates.

SUGGESTED READING

General Issues

Heikkinen H, Tekay A, Volpi E, Martikainen H, Jouppila P. Transvaginal salpingosonography for the assessment of tubal patency in infertile women: methodological and clinical experiences. *Fertil Steril* 1995;64:293.

Luciano AA, Maier DB. Electrosurgery and lasers in endoscopic pelvic surgery. *Infert Reprod Med Clin North Am* 1993;4:255.

Operative laparoscopy study group. Postoperative adhesions development after operative laparoscopy: evaluation at early second look procedures. *Fertil Steril* 1991;55:700.

Opsahl MS, Miller B, Klein TA. The predictive value of hysterosalpingography for tubal and peritoneal infertility factors. *Fertil Steril* 1993;60:444.

Tulandi T. Salpingo-ovariolysis: a comparison between laser surgery and electrosurgery. *Fertil Steril* 1986;45:489.

Pelvic Adhesions and Distal Tubal Obstruction

Dlugi AM, Reddy S, Saleh WA, Mersol-Barg MS, Jacobsen G. Pregnancy rates after operative endoscopic treatment of total (neosalpingostomy) or near total (salpingostomy) distal tubal occlusion. *Fertil Steril* 1994;62:913.

Dubuisson JB, Chapron C, Morice P, Aubriot FX, Foulot H, Bouquet de Joliniere J. Laparoscopic salpingostomy: fertility results according to the tubal mucosal appearance. *Hum Reprod* 1994;9:334.

Haney AF, Hesla J, Hurst BS, Kettel LM, Murphy AA, Rock JA, Rowe G, Schlaff WD. Expanded polytetrafluoroethylene (Gore-Tex Surgical Membrane) is superior to oxidized regenerated cellulose (Interceed TC7+) in preventing adhesions. *Fertil Steril* 1995;63:1021.

Mage G, Pouly JL, Joliniere JB, Chabrand S, Riouallon A, Bruhat MA. A preoperative classification to predict the intrauterine and ectopic pregnancy rates after distal tubal microsurgery. *Fertil Steril* 1986;46:807.

Nordic Adhesion Prevention Study Group. The efficacy of Interceed (TC7) for prevention of reformation of postoperative adhesions on ovaries, fallopian tubes, and fimbriae in microsurgical operations for fertility: a multicenter study. *Fertil Steril* 1995;63:709.

Russell JB, DeCherney AH, Laufer N, Polan ML, Naftolin F. Neosalpingostomy: comparison of 24- and 72-month follow-up time shows increased pregnancy rate. *Fertil Steril* 1986;45:296.

Endometriosis

Adamson GD, Pasta DJ. Surgical treatment of endometriosis-associated infertility: meta-analysis compared with survival analysis. *Am J Obstet Gynecol* 1994;171:1488.

Crosignani PG, Vercellini P. Conservative surgery for severe endoemtriosis: should laparotomy be abandoned definitively? *Hum Reprod* 1995;10:2412.

Myomectomy

Goldenberg M, Sivan E, Sharabi Z, Bider D, Rabinovici J, Seidman DS. Outcome of hysteroscopic resection of submucous myomas for infertility. *Fertil Steril* 1995;64:714.

Letterie GS, Coddington CC, Winkel CA, Shawker TH, Loriaux DL, Collins RL. Efficacy of a gonadotropin-releasing hormone agonist in the treatment of uterine leiomyomata: long-term follow-up. *Fertil Steril* 1989;51:951.

Rosenfeld DL. Abdominal myomectomy for otherwise unexplained infertility. *Fertil Steril* 1986;46:328.

Proximal Tubal Obstruction

Patton PE, Williams TJ, Coulam CB. Results of microsurgical reconstruction in patients with combined proximal and distal tubal occlusion: double occlusion. *Fertil Steril* 1987;48:670.

Thurmond AS. Pregnancies after selective salpingography and tubal recanalization. *Radiology* 1994;190:11.

Thurmond AS, Burry KA, Novy MJ. Salpingitis isthmica nodosa: results of transcervical fluoroscopic catheter recanalization. *Fertil Steril* 1995;63:715.

Sterilization Reversal

Dubuisson JB, Chapron C, Nos C, Morice P, Aubriot FX, Garnier P. Sterilization reversal: fertility results. *Hum Reprod* 1995;10:1145.

Groff TR, Edelstein JA, Schenken RS. Hysterosalpingography in the preoperative evaluation of tubal anastomosis candidates. *Fertil Steril* 1990;53:417.

Opsahl MS, Klein TA. The role of laparoscopy in the evaluation of candidates for sterilization reversal. *Fertil Steril* 1987;48:546.

Rouzi AA, McComb PF. A new selection criterion for fimbriectomy reversal. *Fertil Steril* 1995;64:185.

Rouzi AA, Mackinnon M, McComb PF. Predictors of success of reversal of sterilization. *Fertil Steril* 1995;64:29.

Hysteroscopy

Khalifa E, Toner JP, Jones HW Jr. The role abdominal metroplasty in the era of operative hysteroscopy. *Surg Obstet Gynecol* 1993;176:208.

Marabini A, Gubbini G, Stagnozzi R, Stefanetti M, Filoni M, Bovicelli A. Hysteroscopic metroplasty. *Ann NY Acad Sci* 1994;734:488.

March CM, Isreal R, March AD. Hysteroscopic management of intrauterine adhesions. *Am J Obstet Gynecol* 1978;130:653.

Clinical Reproductive Medicine,
Edited by Bryan D. Cowan and David B. Seifer
Lippincott-Raven Publishers, Philadelphia © 1997

CHAPTER 22

Gamete Technologies

Alan S. Penzias

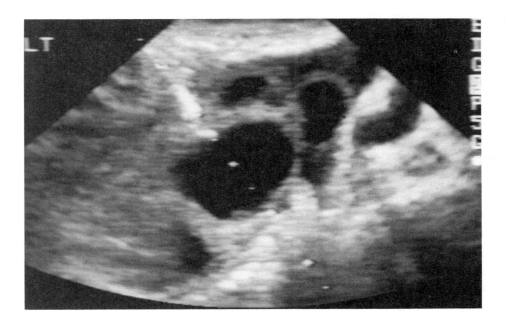

Assisted Reproductive Technology	**Preimplantation Genetic Diagnosis**
The Process of IVF	**Egg Donation**
Assisted Fertilization	**Uterine Surrogacy**
Assisted Embryo Hatching	**Suggested Reading**

A. S. Penzias: Division of Reproductive Endocrinology, Tufts University School of Medicine, Boston, MA 02111

The fastest growing lexicon of acronyms in all of obstetrics and gynecology is found in the area of reproductive endocrinology related to assisted reproduction. GIFT (gamete intrafallopian transfer), ZIFT (zygote intrafallopian transfer), and ICSI (intracytoplasmic sperm injection) are all members of the "club" commonly called assisted reproductive technology (ART). Whereas some authors wax poetic about the art of science, this chapter will explore and describe the science of ART.

Patrick Steptoe and Robert Edwards succeeded in producing the world's first "test tube" baby in 1978. The successful application of in vitro fertilization (IVF) to humans launched a worldwide race to established IVF programs in an attempt to provide state-of-the-art therapy even though the fundamental principles of the process were still being explored. Some practitioners were adept at mastering the process and began producing live births while others faltered. This disparity led to widely discrepant reports of birth rates in the early years of IVF. However, within a relatively short period of time consistent and reproducible results did emerge.

The goal of uniform collection and reporting of treatment outcome largely has been achieved through the Society of Assisted Reproductive Technology (SART) of the American Society of Reproductive Medicine. The annual SART publication of the summary data of its members serves as a reference point for individual programs to judge their own performance and enables public inspection of the achievements and limitations of the specialty.

ASSISTED REPRODUCTIVE TECHNOLOGY

The acronyms of ART can be quite lyrical but don't readily convey the process that they entail (Table 22-1). The centerpiece of ART is IVF. The process of IVF will be discussed in greater depth in a subsequent section; however, in summary, IVF is the mixing of an egg and sperm in a dish "in vitro" followed by incubation in a temperature-controlled, CO_2-enriched environment. If the incubation of sperm and egg is successful, an embryo is generated. Embryogenesis is followed by the transfer of some or all of these freshly generated embryos directly to the patient's uterus through the cervix. Those embryos in excess of the desired quantity for fresh transfer are frozen for the patient's later use. Next to IVF, the procedure that has

gained the most notoriety is gamete intrafallopian transfer. GIFT differs significantly from IVF in that fertilization occurs within the fallopian tubes of the patient and not in a dish in a laboratory incubator. In order to gain access to the fallopian tubes, a laparoscopy is performed. During the laparoscopy, oocytes are retrieved from the ovaries under direct vision by puncture of the ovarian follicles and aspiration of their contents. A suitable number of eggs are then placed into a special catheter. Eggs and sperm are injected into the end of the fallopian tube. Oocytes in excess of the number desired for transfer can be incubated with sperm, just as in IVF, and the resultant embryos frozen for the patient's later use.

The transfer of fertilized ova to the fallopian tubes represents yet another variation of ART. This hybrid of IVF and GIFT has several acronyms that reflect the blend of techniques. Zygote intrafallopian transfer (ZIFT), tubal embryo transfer (TET), and tubal pre-embryo transfer (TPET) are all essentially synonymous but for minor differences. In each of these procedures, eggs are retrieved and mixed in vitro with sperm just as in IVF. Fertilized ova (TPET) or cleaved embryos (ZIFT, TET) are not placed in the uterus, but rather a laparoscopy is performed and the embryos are placed in the fallopian tube. The rationale for employing this variation is to enable the physician to observe fertilization and then transfer only fertilized products to the fallopian tube. In contrast, the fate of eggs transferred to the fallopian tubes in GIFT, vis-à-vis fertilization, is unknown.

Whether or not fertilization occurs is especially important for cases of male factor infertility or unexplained infertility where an assumption regarding the ability of sperm and egg to unite may be questionable. There are, however, several indirect methods for assessing the likelihood of oocyte fertilization in GIFT. When a GIFT procedure yields a large number of oocytes, only a few are delivered with sperm to the fallopian tubes. Those in excess can be incubated with sperm in vitro. If a good percentage of the excess ova fertilize, it may be reasonable to assume that fertilization occurred in vivo within the fallopian tube. If few or none of the excess eggs fertilize in vitro, then one cannot assume that fertilization has occurred in vivo.

The decision to perform GIFT or ZIFT instead of IVF is often based on the reported higher success rates attributed to GIFT and ZIFT than IVF in selected patients. The most recent statistics available indicate that the GIFT procedure resulted in a 28.1% delivery rate per egg retrieval and the ZIFT procedure resulted in a 24.4% delivery rate per egg retrieval compared with 18.6% for IVF (Table 22-2). Several investigators have addressed these differences by performing prospective randomized trials.

In a prospective randomized study of 157 couples with male factor infertility, implantation rates of 12.3% and 10% per replaced embryo were achieved for ZIFT and IVF, respectively. The authors concluded that there was

TABLE 22-1. *ART acronyms*

Acronym	Full term
IVF	In vitro fertilization
GIFT	Gamete intrafallopian transfer
ZIFT	Zygote intrafallopian transfer
TET	Tubal embryo transfer
TPET	Tubal pre-embryo transfer
ICSI	Intracytoplasmic sperm injection

TABLE 22-2. *Comparisons of reported outcomes for all ART procedures in 1993*

	IVF	GIFT	ZIFT	Donor[a]	Cryopreserved ETs[b]
Cycles/procedures[c]	31,900	4,992	1,792	2,766	6,672
Cancellation (%)	14.0	15.8	13.0	14.4	NA[d]
Retrievals	27,443	4,202	1,557	2,368	NA
Transfers	24,410	4,138	1,327	2,446	6,194
Transfers per retrieval (%)	88.9	98.5	85.2	103.3[e]	NA
Pregnancies	6,321	1,472	466	895	984
Pregnancy loss (%)	19	20.6	18,5	20	19.6
Deliveries	5,103	1,182	380	716	791
Deliveries per retrieval (%)	18.6	28.1	24.4	30.2	NA
Singleton (%)	65.9	64.5	61.4	59.9	70.2
EPs	288	61	13	21	11
EP per transfer (%)	1.4	1.5	1.0	0.9	0.2
Birth defects per neonates delivered (%)[f]	2.3	1.2	2.8	1.8	1.8

From Assisted reproductive technology in the United States and Canada: 1993 results generated from the ASRM/SART registry. *Fertil Steril* 1995;64:13–21. Reproduced with the permission of the American Society for Reproductive Medicine.

[a]Donor includes known or anonymous, but not surrogate.

[b]Cryopreserved ET cycles not done in combination with fresh ETs and not with donor egg or embryo.

[c]Includes all cycles, regardless of age or diagnosis.

[d]NA, not available.

[e]Some donors' oocytes used for transfer into more than one recipient.

[f]Birth defect reporting did not account for all neonatal outcomes.

no therapeutic advantage of ZIFT over IVF in male factor infertility. In another prospective randomized trial, 59 couples undergoing oocyte retrieval for nontubal infertility were randomized to ZIFT or IVF. The pregnancy, implantation, and abortion rates did not differ between the groups. In a third prospective, randomized trial, 42 consecutive patients who entered an oocyte donation program were assigned to either uterine embryo transfer or tubal embryo transfer. No differences were observed.

Two additional studies differed in their conclusions regarding the relative success rate of IVF and GIFT or ZIFT. In the first, a total of 150 couples with unexplained infertility, peritoneal endometriosis, or reduced semen quality were assigned to either IVF, ZIFT, or GIFT. The three groups were comparable with regard to age distribution, indications, semen parameters, stimulation regimens, response to stimulation, and number of oocytes retrieved. The pregnancy rate was highest in the two groups in which in vitro fertilization was performed: IVF (45.7%) and ZIFT (37.9%). In comparison, the pregnancy rate for GIFT was 26.2%. In the second study, tubal transfer of cryopreserved embryos proved superior to uterine transfer (58% versus 19%).

Taken together, these studies suggest that the discrepancy in reported pregnancy rates between procedures is likely the result of patient selection bias rather than the inherent superiority of GIFT or ZIFT over IVF.

The success or failure of ART is dependent on a number of factors. However, two elements of the patient profile merit special consideration. The two clinical variables that impact most significantly on ART success are the age of the patient undergoing oocyte retrieval and the presence or absence of male factor infertility. The SART report for 1993 reveals that in patients without male factor infertility, the delivery rate per retrieval was 21.5% for patients under age 40 as compared with 8.6% for women ≥40 years. When male factor infertility was present, the delivery rates per oocyte retrieval were 16.6% and 6.8%, respectively (Table 22-3). The magnitude of the difference in pregnancy rates is made greater when one factors in the cycle cancellation rates. Whereas 12.4% of IVF cycles in women under age 40 without male factor were stopped prior to egg retrieval, the cancellation rate in their counterparts ≥40 years of age was 21.9%. Therefore, recalculating the delivery rate as a function of the number of cycles initiated, the live birth rate per initiated cycle for women under age 40 without male factor is 18.8% compared with 6.7% for women ≥40 years. In the presence of male factor, the live birth rate per initiated cycle for women under age 40 is 14.4% compared with 5.5% for women ≥40 years. Another way to consider these comparative rates is to recognize that once the age of 40 is reached, IVF delivery rates drop by 60–65%.

The great discrepancy in delivery rates above and below age 40 in IVF is no better with the GIFT procedure. In a study of 399 GIFT transfers, one group of investigators reported a 65% drop in the pregnancy rate after the age of 40 had been reached (Table 22-4). Furthermore, the majority of pregnancies and all of the deliveries occurred in women <42 years of age (Table 22-5).

The dramatic decline in pregnancy rates as a function of age has led many investigators to seek out prognostic factors for success in women ≥40 years of age. Although no single determinant is absolutely predictive, an elevated early follicular phase serum concentration of FSH is helpful in identifying particularly poor candidates. In

TABLE 22-3. *Effect of age and diagnosis of male factor on outcome for stimulated IVF cycles in 1993 (%)*

Patient category	No. of retrievals	Cancellations[a] %	Transfers per retrieval %	No. of pregnancies	No. of deliveries[b]	Deliveries per retrieval %
Women <40 years no male factor	17,847	12.4	92.7	4,703	3,833	21.5
Women ≥40 years no male factor	3,120	21.9	87.3	413	268	8.6
Women <40 years male factor	5,198	11.6	80.3	1,076	864	16.6
Women ≥40 years male factor	952	18.8	79.6	113	65	6.8
1993 totals	27,117	13.7	89.3	6,305	5,089	18.8
1992 totals	24,717	14.7	87.7	5,261	4,188	16.9
1991 totals	20,573	14.7	87.7	3,985	3,192	15.5

From Assisted reproductive technology in the United States and Canada: 1993 results generated from the ASRM/SART registry. *Fertil Steril* 1995;64:13–21. Reproduced with the permission of the American Society for Reproductive Medicine.

This table denotes information only on stimulated IVF cycles and excludes unstimulated cycles.

[a]Percentage of stimulated cycles initiated that did not proceed to retrieval.

[b]Deliveries with at least one live-born infant.

summary, when counseling patients who have reached the age of 40 years or beyond, one must be circumspect when quoting success rates.

THE PROCESS OF IVF

The process of IVF ordinarily begins with controlled ovarian hyperstimulation (COH). The goal of COH for ART is to develop several mature eggs in the hope that at least one will result in pregnancy. This aim can be accomplished in a number of ways using medications that are available to the practitioner today, either singly or in combination (Table 22-6).

The medications used for multiple follicular recruitment take advantage of different properties within the follicular developmental cascade and act at different sites including the hypothalamus, pituitary, and ovary. These medications are administered by varied routes including, oral, intravenous, intramuscular, subcutaneous, and by intranasal spray.

The most common stimulation protocols include combinations of gonadotropin-releasing hormone agonist (GnRH-a) and human menopausal gonadotropins (hMGs). GnRH-a is produced by chemically altering

TABLE 22-4. *GIFT treatment pregnancy rates in women under and over age 40*

Group	Age	Pregnancies/transfers
A	≤34	50/170 (29.4%)
B	35–39	39/156 (25.0%)
C	≥40	7/73 (9.6%)

From Penzias AS, et al. Successful use of gamete intrafallopian transfer does not reverse the age dependent decline in fertility in women over 40 years of age. *Obstet Gynecol* 1991;77:37–39. Reproduced with the permission of the American College of Obstetricians and Gynecologists.

Difference between A and B is not statistically significant ($p = .44$, χ^2 analysis). Differences between A and C, B and C, and (A + B) and C are statistically significant (each with $p = .003$, χ^2 analysis).

native GnRH, which makes the protein less susceptible to enzymatic attack, thus increasing the half-life and potency of the agonist.

When GnRH-a is first administered, the pituitary responds by releasing both luteinizing hormone (LH) and follicle-stimulating hormone (FSH) in a flare response to excitement of the GnRH receptors. However, continued administration over time causes GnRH receptor downregulation. This confers the pituitary with a paradoxical insensitivity to further GnRH stimulation. Continued administration results in pituitary desensitization, a fall in gonadotropin levels, and an absent midcycle LH surge. Without its normal tropic stimulation, the gonad becomes dormant. The effect can be maintained indefinitely but is reversed by halting administration. Thus, a pharmacologic yet reversible hypophysectomy can be achieved.

Human menopausal gonadotropins are drugs that contain equal concentrations of LH and FSH or contain purified FSH alone. Some stimulation protocols employing GnRH-a call for the initiation of hMG during the period of flare response. Thus, the release of native LH and FSH from the pituitary is supplemented by the LH and FSH of the hMG. Other stimulation protocols await the onset of pituitary desensitization before initiating hMG. Intramuscular injection of hMG is continued daily until follicular development is judged to be adequate by the practitioner, typically through serial transvaginal ultrasonography, and frequent serum estradiol (E_2) sampling.

Human chorionic gonadotropin (hCG) is then administered to mimic the native LH surge. This sequence of events leads to the resumption of meiosis I and the production of a mature metaphase II oocyte.

Finally, GnRH antagonists are compounds that directly inhibit the release of pituitary gonadotropins. Direct pituitary inhibition with antagonist is a distinct contrast to the mechanism of action of GnRH-a. The agonist must first subject the pituitary to a period of stimulation that is followed by desensitization and downregulation. However, antagonists do not cause release of pituitary hormone stores prior to suppression. The pituitary is blocked im-

TABLE 22-5. *Age-dependent outcome for GIFT in women age 40 and older (n = 59)*

Age	Initiated cycles	Transfers	Clinical pregnancies	Spontaneous abortions	Deliveries
40	28	25	3	0	3
41	25	11	2	0	2
42	15	9	0	0	0
43	23	11	0	0	0
44	15	10	2	2	0
45	11	4	0	0	0
46	4	3	0	0	0
47	1	0	0	0	0

From Penzias AS, et al. Successful use of gamete intrafallopian transfer does not reverse the age dependent decline in fertility in women over 40 years of age. *Obstet Gynecol* 1991;77:37–39. Reproduced with the permission of the American College of Obstetricians and Gynecologists.

mediately by antagonist molecules that occupy GnRH receptors but do not stimulate them. Early clinical experience with GnRH antagonists is promising and awaits further investigation.

Selection of one or more medications for COH is based on the patient's needs and the mechanism of action of the drugs to be employed. Each medication regimen also imparts a different set of risks and benefits that can be tailored to the situation at hand. In general, combinations of GnRH-a and hMG result in fewer cycle cancellations and larger numbers of oocytes at retrieval than regimens using hMG alone or in combination with clomiphene citrate.

The endpoint of COH for ART is retrieval of a moderate number of mature oocytes. If, for example, 12 oocytes are retrieved from the ovary, are fertilized in vitro, and yield 12 embryos, the physician can choose to return 3 or 4 of these embryos to the patient and cryopreserve the remaining embryos for transfer at a later date. Physician control of the number of gametes or embryos returned to the patient limits the risk of high-order gestation.

An oocyte retrieval for IVF and ZIFT is scheduled when several ovarian follicles measure at least 16 mm in diameter by ultrasound and are accompanied by serum E_2 levels commensurate with follicle maturity. A transvaginal ultrasound–guided oocyte retrieval is performed 32–36 hours after intramuscular administration of 10,000 IU hCG (Figs. 22-1 and 22-2). The follicle contents are examined under a dissecting microscope by an embryologist. If an egg is recovered, it is ordinarily surrounded by a protective mass of granulosa cells known as the cumulus oophorus and the corona radiata. The oocyte cumulus corona complex (OCCC) is transferred to a dish containing a special nutrient culture media. Many successful types of culture media are available commercially.

Semen specimens are collected following the oocyte retrieval and the semen volume, sperm concentration, motility, and morphology are determined after complete liquefaction. Motile sperm cells are culled from the ejaculate using one of several separation techniques. The motile sperm are reconcentrated in liquid culture media and a drop containing approximately 50,000 sperm is added to each dish containing an egg.

The dishes containing sperm and eggs are placed in an incubator where the process of fertilization will take place. The incubator temperature is set at 37°C. The air inside the incubator is humidified with water and supplemented with 5% CO_2. Approximately 18 hours after the sperm and eggs have been placed together in the incubator, they are examined under a microscope for evidence of fertilization. If a single sperm has succeeded in fertilizing an egg, two pronuclei are seen (Fig. 22-3). At this stage the fertilized egg may be referred to as a pre-embryo. The term "pre-embryo" refers to the fact that although fertilization has occurred, the maternal and pater-

TABLE 22-6. *Medications for controlled ovarian hyperstimulation*

Clomiphene citrate
Human menopausal gonadotropins (menotropins)
Human chorionic gonadotropin (hCG)
Gonadotropin-releasing hormone agonist
Gonadotropin-releasing hormone antagonist
Growth hormone

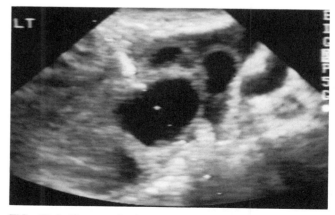

FIG. 22-1. Transvaginal ultrasound image of a stimulated ovary immediately prior to follicle puncture.

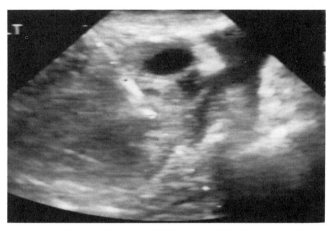

FIG. 22-2. The bright white reflection of the retrieval needle is evident within the collapsed ovarian follicle.

nal chromosomes have not yet fused. If more than one sperm has managed to enter the egg, three or more pronuclei are seen. Embryos that are fertilized by more than one sperm are not compatible with life and are not transferred back to the patient.

In the normal course of development, fertilization of an oocyte is followed by fusion of the maternal and paternal pronuclei (syngamy). The embryo begins as a single cell that divides in a process referred to as cleavage. A suitable number of embryos are transferred back to the patient 48–72 hours after egg retrieval. At the time of embryo transfer, each embryo comprises four to eight cells. The process of embryo transfer is accomplished by aspirating the embryos into a thin, flexible cannula, which is then inserted into the uterine cavity through the cervix.

Following embryo transfer, the luteal phase can be supported with the addition of exogenous progesterone or

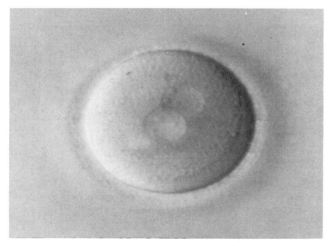

FIG. 22-3. A pre-embryo containing two pronuclei.

hCG. Progesterone support can be administered intramuscularly, with vaginal suppositories, or micronized in an oral capsule.

ASSISTED FERTILIZATION

While IVF is successful in treating a large number of infertility problems, its success hinges on entry of a single sperm into an oocyte. The fusion of male and female gametes ultimately requires sperm penetration through the cumulus oophorus and the zona pellucida.

Several conditions in men impede the normal process of fertilization, these include the presence of head-directed antisperm antibodies and, to varying degrees, low sperm concentrations, poor motility, and the absence of normally shaped sperm. When a barrier to fertilization exists, pregnancy through ordinary IVF cannot occur. In order to overcome sperm-related barriers to egg penetration, methods have been developed that bypass the normal fertilization sequence.

One method of assisted fertilization is the creation of a hole in the zona pellucida, a process called zona drilling or partial zona dissection. The goal of this technique is to exempt the sperm from the requirement of penetrating the zona on its own power. Once the zona is breached, the oocyte is placed in culture with sperm in the hopes that one will pass through the defect and fertilize the egg. Initially, although zona breaching procedures did facilitate fertilization, oocyte damage and polyspermic fertilization reduced the number of embryos available for transfer.

A variation of the zona drilling technique has been developed and is termed subzonal insemination (SUZI). In this technique, three to five motile sperm are injected beneath the zona pellucida but not into the cytoplasm of the oocyte itself. The basis for placing more than a single sperm underneath the zona is the otherwise low rate of fertilization in such cases. The techniques of zona breaching and SUZI appear about equal in efficacy in cases of low sperm concentrations.

When more than one sperm fertilizes an egg the resultant embryo has one or more additional sets of chromosomes, a condition incompatible with life. There have been preliminary attempts to restore multiply fertilized human eggs by removing one or more of the extra pronuclei prior to their fusion. In one study, six tripronuclear embryos were manipulated with successful removal of one pronucleus. All embryos subsequently underwent at least one cleavage division. However, the authors reported that in none of the tripronuclear eggs was it possible to definitely distinguish between the female and male pronuclei. Clearly, when removing a set of chromosomes, it is essential to remove one contributed by a sperm, thus leaving one maternal and one paternal set. Since the parental origin of a human pronucleus cannot be determined by its shape, size, or position within the oocyte, this technique remains experimental and is not used in clinical practice.

One obvious solution to the risk of polyspermic fertilization is to use a single sperm. However, subzonal insertion of a single sperm does not consistently result in fertilization. Recently, a technique for direct injection of a single sperm into the cytoplasm of an oocyte was applied to human eggs (Figs. 22-4 to 22-6). In this report, intracytoplasmic sperm injection (ICSI) was used to treat couples with infertility because of severely impaired sperm characteristics, and in whom standard IVF and SUZI had failed. Forty-seven oocytes were injected of which 38 remained intact after the procedure. Thirty-one oocytes became fertilized, 15 embryos were replaced in utero, and 3 deliveries resulted. In a larger follow-up study, this group of investigators performed 300 transvaginal oocyte retrievals in couples in which the male partner was the presumed cause of repeated failure to achieve conception by IVF or in which seminal parameters were unacceptable for conventional IVF. The efficacy of SUZI was compared to ICSI. Normal fertilization occurred in 18% of the oocytes treated by SUZI and in 44% after ICSI. Follow-up studies of the ICSI procedure in a number of centers around the world have confirmed the efficacy and reproducibility of the technique. This has largely led to the abandonment of zona drilling and SUZI and the expansion in the number of centers where ICSI is performed.

ASSISTED EMBRYO HATCHING

Whereas assisted fertilization may overcome problems of gamete union, assisted hatching refers to artificial thinning or breachment of the zona pellucida. During the normal course of embryo development, a stage is reached where the embryonic cells need to break out of the confines of the zona pellucida and make contact with the

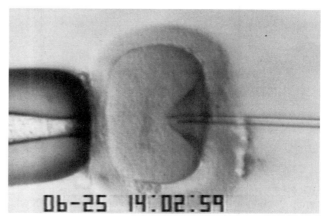

FIG. 22-5. The injection needle tents the surface of the oocyte just prior to penetration.

uterine surface. At that point, implantation can occur. Assisted hatching is a technique that enables an otherwise normal embryo that might have difficulty breaking through the zona pellucida to break out of its shell (Figs. 22-7 and 22-8). The technique has been applied successfully to human embryos.

The major question at this time is, whose embryos might benefit from assisted hatching? There are several proposed selection criteria for the assisted hatching technique: (1) patients with a uniformly thickened zona pellucida (>15 μm); (2) eggs retrieved from women <40 years old; (3) patients who have failed to achieve a pregnancy after several IVF cycles in which a sufficient number of quality embryos were generated and transferred. A recent study of 154 patients who had failed to achieve a pregnancy in three prior attempts showed a markedly higher pregnancy rate after assisted hatching, ie, 23.9% in the study group compared with only 7% of the controls, in women over 38 years of age. The authors concluded that in a selected group of patients (aged over 38 years,

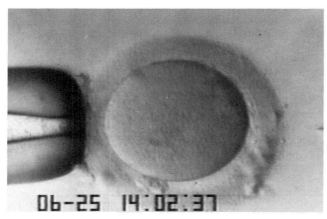

FIG. 22-4. A mature oocyte is held in place by gentle suction applied through the holding pipet at left, while a fine glass needle *(right)* containing a single sperm is brought into position.

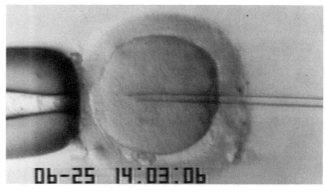

FIG. 22-6. The fine glass needle has entered the cytoplasm of the oocyte where the single sperm will be deposited.

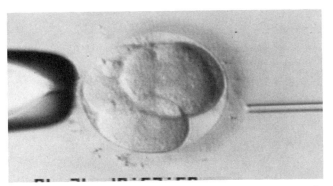

FIG. 22-7. A 4-cell embryo (3 cells visible) is held in place by gentle suction applied through the holding pipet at left while a fine glass pipet containing acid Tyrode's solution is brought into position next to the thickened zona pellucida.

who have failed to conceive in at least three previous IVF attempts) assisted hatching significantly increases the chances for pregnancy after embryo transfer.

The process of assisted hatching can be accomplished in one of several ways. The zona pellucida can be breached mechanically by taking a finely sharpened glass pipette and skewering the zona. Alternatively, a small area of the zona can be chemically dissolved with the use of an acid Tyrode's solution. Recently, another method has been introduced using laser technology. Unlike most laser beams, which produce intense heat at the point of contact, the argon fluoride excimer laser, in the deep ultraviolet region of the spectrum at 193 nm, can produce well-defined alterations in the zona pellucida without detectable heating or structural damage to the surrounding tissue.

PREIMPLANTATION GENETIC DIAGNOSIS

In vitro fertilization does not influence the risk of parental transmission of a heritable disease to their off-spring. Current diagnostic strategies include antenatal parental testing followed by preconception counseling and prenatal genetic diagnosis. Embryo biopsy prior to transfer and implantation seeks to identify unaffected embryos such that the developing fetus will not be affected by the disease.

Embryo biopsy refers to the microsurgical removal of one or more cells from a developing embryo prior to its transfer into the uterus (Fig. 22-9). In human IVF, embryos are routinely returned to the patient between 48 and 72 hours after the oocytes are first incubated with sperm. This roughly correlates with the transfer of embryos between the four-cell and eight-cell stages. Each embryonic cell theoretically should contain identical chromosomal and genetic information.

The ability of embryos to survive the process of blastomere removal, implant following manipulation, develop normally, and result in a healthy live-born is well established in both small experimental animals and farm animals. The major limiting factor in the application of these techniques to human embryos was our inability to make reliable genetic diagnoses from single cells. The development of methods including the polymerase chain reaction (PCR) and fluorescent in situ hybridization (FISH) now have made this possible.

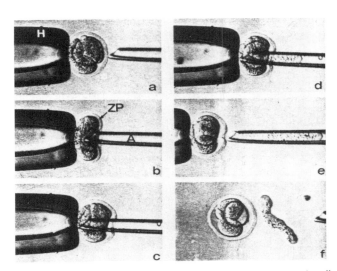

FIG. 22-9. Biopsy of a single blastomere from a 4-cell mouse embryo. **A:** The embryo is held in place by gentle suction applied through the holding pipet at left (H). **B:** The aspiration pipet (A) is pushed through the zona pellucida (ZP). **C:** The zona has been punctured and the aspiration pipet is inside the embryo. **D:** One blastomere is gently drawn into the aspiration pipet. **E:** The aspiration pipet containing a single blastomere is removed from the embryo. **F:** The single blastomere is released into the medium. (From Wilton LJ, Trounson AO. Biopsy of preimplantation mouse embryos: development of micrimanipulated embryos and proliferation of single blastomeres in vitro. *Biol Reprod* 1989;40:145–152. Reproduced with permission.)

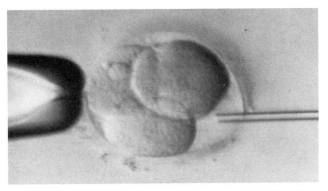

FIG. 22-8. A small section of the zona pellucida has been chemically dissolved by local application of acid Tyrode's solution.

Early studies in human embryos established that preimplantation development in vitro is not adversely affected by biopsy at the eight-cell stage. Other data confirms that biopsy at approximately the eight-cell stage is more successful and therefore preferable to biopsy at the two- or four-cell stage.

The first human live births following embryo biopsy were reported in 2 couples at risk of transmitting an X chromosome-linked recessive condition. Embryo biopsy of a single cell at the six- to eight-cell stage was performed in each case. Because this condition affects only males, embryonic gender determination was carried out by PCR of a Y chromosome-specific gene sequence. The major drawback to PCR amplification of a single sequence in single cells is the risk of losing the target DNA during processing. For example, the absence of Y chromosome-specific gene sequences could represent either an embryo containing only X chromosomes or the failure to amplify Y material that was indeed present. The addition of an internal control, however, can safeguard against this type of misdiagnosis. Since all normal human embryos contain an X chromosome as well, detection of X chromosome-specific sequences following amplification confirms that DNA was recovered from the target cell. In such cases, the absence of Y chromosome-specific sequences confirms that the embryo is female.

In the case of an X chromosome-linked recessive condition, a live birth has been reported after PCR amplification of DNA from both the X and Y chromosomes. DNA amplification now has been successfully applied to the preimplantation diagnosis of cystic fibrosis caused by the δ F508 deletion and Tay-Sachs disease.

As is the case with any diagnostic test, there are limitations to diagnosis by direct DNA amplification. For example, the δ F508 deletion is the most common cause of cystic fibrosis but it is not the only mutation responsible for the disease. Spontaneous mutations or variants may not be detected during PCR for preimplantation diagnosis of a single cell and therefore lead to the errant assumption that the embryo in question is unaffected. Therefore, a thorough understanding of the genetic basis of the disease in question is absolutely required before attempting to make a diagnosis by preimplantation genetic testing.

Another technique which allows rapid identification of individual chromosomes is fluorescent in situ hybridization (FISH). Simultaneous hybridization of fluorescent X chromosome- and Y chromosome-specific probes with single blastomeres has been successfully achieved. The recent development of chromosome specific probes allows the geneticist to count the number of chromosomes present. This may enable the identification of chromosomal abnormalities such as trisomy 13, 18, and 21. In experimental situations, short sequence probes with multicolored fluorescence targeted to specific chromosome regions have been used to detect structural chromosome abnormalities including translocations. Further studies are needed before the FISH technique can be employed clinically.

The chief feature common to both PCR and FISH is the rapidity with which a diagnosis can be achieved. A window of 6–8 hours from cell capture to diagnosis is necessary because it is desirable to transfer these embryos back to the patient on the day of biopsy. While biopsied mouse embryos have been successfully frozen, thawed, and transferred, this has not yet been attempted in humans. The chief difference is that human embryo biopsy is performed most successfully at the eight-cell stage, when cryopreservation is least likely to be successful.

EGG DONATION

Until recently, there was one absolute biological barrier to conception through IVF, ie, the loss of ovarian function. Patients who had undergone the surgical removal of their ovaries or experienced natural menopause were unable to participate in this technology because they could not bring the necessary gamete to the process. This barrier was lifted when a group at the University of Southern California demonstrated that young, fertile women who undergo ovarian stimulation and oocyte retrieval can successfully donate their eggs to women who lack ovarian function.

The process of oocyte donation requires artificial hormonal preparation of the recipient's uterus (Fig. 22-10). The construction of a receptive uterine lining is accomplished by the sequential administration of estrogen and progesterone in a specially designed protocol. The men-

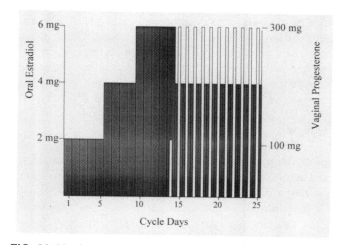

FIG. 22-10. A regimen for artificial hormonal preparation of a recipient's uterus prior to ovum donation. Sequential administration of oral estradiol *(dark bars)* and vaginal progesterone suppositories *(white bars)* create a receptive endometrium. In this scheme, embryo transfer occurs on cycle day 18.

strual cycle of the egg donor is synchronized to the artificial hormonal preparation of the recipient's uterus by using a GnRH agonist. The egg that is retrieved from the donor is fertilized with the sperm of the recipient's husband. The resulting embryos are then transferred to the recipient. Since there is no corpus luteum on the recipient's ovary, hormonal supplementation with both estrogen and progesterone is continued until the end of the first trimester. By the end of the first trimester, the placenta ordinarily has achieved full, pregnancy-sustaining hormone production. Premature discontinuation of hormonal supplementation, however, can result in the loss of the pregnancy.

At first, egg donation was applied to younger women with ovarian failure ranging in age from the mid-20s to the early-40s. However, it soon became apparent that egg donation could be implemented in menopausal women throughout their 40s and into their 50s. Isolated reports of women in their 60s delivering children as a result of egg donation have generated significant controversy. Detractors of the process suggest that parenthood was not meant to occur in older women after menopause. Advocates of egg donation, however, point to the fact that men who father children in their 50s and 60s receive little public attention. It is interesting to note that advancing maternal age does not appear to diminish the success of egg donation.

UTERINE SURROGACY

Patients who have functional ovaries but lack a uterus can achieve motherhood through the process of uterine surrogacy. Women who have had their uterus surgically removed, such as those with cervical or endometrial cancer, and those born without a uterus (Mayer–Rokitansky–Kuster–Hauser syndrome), can undergo ovarian stimulation and have their eggs retrieved. Other patients who can be considered for uterine surrogacy are those with a medical condition that is an absolute contraindication to pregnancy but who otherwise can function normally. The eggs of these women can be fertilized with their husbands' sperm and result in the production of embryos.

Following a process nearly identical to the uterine preparation of a recipient of donated eggs, a female volunteer can offer herself as a surrogate for those without a uterus. This volunteer has no direct genetic relationship to the child. The biological parents are the woman who provided the eggs and her husband who provided the sperm.

A number of psychological and ethical issues surround the process of uterine surrogacy. It is important to ensure that each of the participants thoroughly understands the procedure and provides consent, and to affirm that no one is being coerced or exploited in the process.

SUGGESTED READING

Assisted Reproductive Technologies

Balmaceda JP, Alam V, Roszjtein D, Ord T, Snell K, Asch RH. Embryo implantation rates in oocyte donation: a prospective comparison of tubal versus uterine transfers. *Fertil Steril* 1992;57:362–365.

Catt KJ, Dufau ML. Gonadotropic hormones: biosynthesis, secretion, receptors, and actions. In: Yen SSC, Jaffe RB, eds. *Reproductive Endocrinology*. 3rd ed. Philadelphia: WB Saunders, 1991;105–55.

Cohen J, Alikani M, Malter HE, Adler A, Talansky Be, Rosenwaks Z. Partial zona dissection or subzonal wperm insertion: microsurgical fertilization alternatives based on evaluation of sperm and embryo morphology. *Fertil Steril* 1991;56:696–706.

Fluker MR, Zouves CG, Bebbington MW. A prospective randomized comparison of zygote intrafallopian transfer and in vitro fertilization-embryo transfer for nontubal factor infertility. *Fertil Steril* 1993;60:515–519.

Garrisi GJ, Talansky BE, Grunfeld L, Sapira V, Navot D, Gordon JW. Clinical evaluation of three approaches to micromanipulation assisted fertilization. *Fertil Steril* 1990;54:671–677.

Gordon JW, Grunfeld L, Garrisi GJ, Novot D, Laufer N. Successful microsurgical removal of a pronucleus from tripronuclear human zygotes. *Fertil Steril* 1989;52:367–372.

Kruger TF, Menkveld R, Stander FS, Lombard CJ, van der Merwe JP, van Zyl JA, Smith K. Sperm morphologic features as a prognostic factor in in vitro fertilization. *Fertil Steril* 1986;46:1118–1123.

Laufer N. Fertilization of human oocytes by sperm from infertile males after zona pellucida drilling. *Fertil Steril* 1988;50:68–73.

Laufer N, Palanker D, Shufaro Y, Safran A, Simon A, Lewis A. The efficacy and safety of zona pellucida drilling by a 193-nm excimer laser. *Fertil Steril* 1993;59:889–895.

Palanker D, Ohad S, Lewis A, Simon A, Shenkar J, Penchas S, Laufer N. Technique for celular microsurgery using the 193-nm excimer laser. *Lasers Surg Med* 1991;11:580–586.

Palermo G, Joris H, Devroey P, Van Steirteghem AC. Pregnancies after intracytoplasmic injection of single spermatozoon into an oocyte. *Lancet* 1992;340:17–18.

Palermo G, Joris H, Derde MP, Camus M, Devroey P, Van Steirteghem A. Sperm characteristics and outcome of human assisted fertilization by subzonal insemination and intracytoplasmic sperm injection. *Fertil Steril* 1993;59:826–853.

Penzias AS, Thompson IE, Alper MM, Oskowitz SP, Berger MJ. Successful use of gamete intrafallopian transfer does not reverse the age dependent decline in fertility in women over 40 years of age. *Obstet Gynecol* 1991; 77:37–39.

Penzias AS. Luteal phase support. *Semin Reprod Endocrinol* 1995;13:32–38.

Society for Assisted Reproductive Technology, American Society for Reproductive Medicine. Assisted reproductive technology in the United States and Canada: 1993 results generated from the American Society for Reproductive Medicine/Society for Assisted Reproductive Technology registry. *Fertil Steril* 1995;64:13–21.

Stein A, Rufas O, Amit S, Avrech O, Pinkas H, Ovadia J, Fisch B. Assisted harching by partial zona dissection of human pre-embryos in patients with recurrent implantation failure after in vitro fertilization. *Fertil Steril* 1995;63:838–841.

Tanbo T, Dale PO, Abyholm T. Assisted fertilization in infertile women with patent fallopian tubes. A comparison of in-vitro fertilization, gamete intra-fallopian transfer and tubal embryo stage transfer. *Hum Reprod* 1990; 5:266–270.

Tournaye H, Devroey P, Camus M, Valkenburg M, Bollen N, Van Steirteghem AC. Zygote intrafallopian transfer in vitro fertilization and embryo transfer for the treatment of male-factor infertility: a prospective randomized trial. *Fertil Steril* 1992;58:344–350.

van der Merwe JP, Kruger TF, Swart Y, Lombard CJ. The role of oocyte maturity in the treatment of infertility because of teratozoospermia and normozoospermia with gamete intrafallopian transfer. *Fertil Steril* 1992;58: 581–586.

Genetic Diagnosis

Gibbons WE, Gitlin SA, Lanzendorf SE, Kaurmann RA, Slotnick RN, Hodgen GD. Preimplantation genetic diagnosis for Tay-Sachs disease:

Successful pregnancy after pre-embryo biopsy and gene amplification by polymerase chain reaction. *Fertil Steril* 1995;63:723–728.

Griffin DK, Wilton LJ, Handyside AH, Winston RM, Delhanty JD. Dual fluorescent in situ hybridization for simultaneous detection of X and Y chromosome-specific probes for the sexing of human preimplantation embryonic nuclei. *Hum Genet* 1992;89:18–22.

Grifo JA, Tang YX, Cohan J, Gilbert F, Sanyal MK, Rosenwaks Z. Pregnancy after embryo biopsy and coamplification of DNA from X and Y chromosomes. *JAMA* 1992;268:727–729.

Handyside AH, Kontogianni EH, Hardy K, Winston RM. Pregnancies from biopsied human preimplantation embryos sexed by Y-specific DNA amplification. *Nature* 1990;344:768–770.

Handyside AH, Lesko JG, Rarin JJ, Winston RM, Hughes MR. Birth of a normal girl after in vitro fertilization and preimplantation diagnostic testing for cystic fibrosis. *N Engl J Med* 1992;327:905–909.

Hardy K, Martin KL, Leese HJ, Winston RM, Handyside AH. Human preimplantation development in vitro is not adversely affected by biopsy at the 8-cell stage. *Hum Reprod* 1990;5:708–714.

Navidi W, Arnheim N. Using PCR in preimplantation genetic disease diagnosis. *Hum Reprod* 1991;6:836–849.

Tarin JJ, Conaghan J, Winston RM, Handyside AH. Human embryo biopsy on the 2nd day after insemination for preimplantation diagnosis: removal of a quarter of embryo retards cleavage. *Fertil Steril* 1992;58:970–976.

Tarin JJ, Handyside AH. Embryo biopsy strategies for preimplantation diagnosis. *Fertil Steril* 1993;59:943–952.

Wilton LJ, Shaw JM, Trounson AO. Successful single-cell biopsy and cryopreservation of preimplantation mouse embryos. *Fertil Steril* 1989;51:513–517.

Wilton LJ, Trounson AO. Biopsy of preimplantation mouse embryos: development of micrimanipulated embryos and proliferation of single blastomeres in vitro. *Biol Reprod* 1989;40:145–152.

Egg Donation

Sauer MV, Paulson RJ, Macaso TM, Francis MM, Lobo RA. Oocyte and pre-embryo donation to women with ovarian failure: an extended clinical trial. *Fertil Steril* 1991;55:39–43.

Saure MV, Stein AL, Paulson RJ, Moyer DL. Endometrial responses to various hormone replacement regimens in ovarian failure patients preparing for embryo donation. *Int J Gynaecol Obstet* 1991;35:61–68.

Sauer MV, diDonato P, Nola VF, Paulson RJ. Failure to comply with hormone replacement may jeopardize pregnancies in functionally agonadal women: a series report. *J Assist Reprod Genet* 1994;11:49–51.

Sauer MV, Paulson RJ, Lobo RA. Reversing the natural decline in human fertility. An extended clinical trial of oocyte donation to women of advanced reproductive age. *JAMA* 1992;268:1275–1279.

Sauer MV, Paulson RJ, Lobo RA. Pregnancy after age 50: application of oocyte donation to women after natural menopause. *Lancet* 1993;341:321–323.

Sauer MV, Paulson RJ, Ary BA, Lobo RA. Three hundred cycles of oocyte donation at the University of Southern California: assessing the effect of age and infertility diagnosis on pregnancy and implantation rates. *J Assist Reprod Genet* 1994;11:92–96.

Sauer MV, Paulson RJ. Demographic differences between younger and older recipients seeking oocyte donation. *J Assist Reprod Genet* 1992;9:400–404.

Clinical Reproductive Medicine,
Edited by Bryan D. Cowan and David B. Seifer
Lippincott-Raven Publishers, Philadelphia © 1997

CHAPTER 23

Gonadotropin-Releasing Hormone Analogs

John D. Isaacs, Jr.

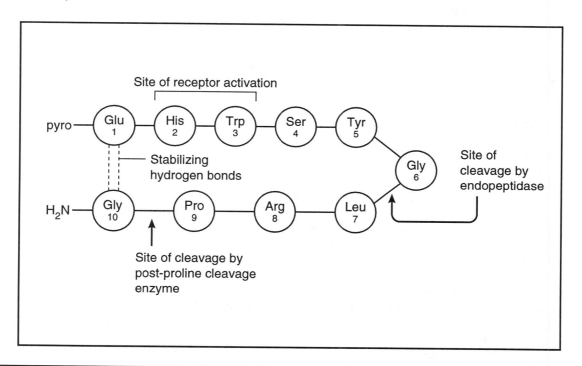

Molecular Characterization of GnRH
  Native GnRH
  Receptor Interaction
  Gonadotropin Responses to GnRH
Analog Development

GnRH Agonists
GnRH Antagonists
Clinical Applications
Suggested Reading

J. D. Isaacs, Jr.: Division of Reproductive Endocrinology, Department of Obstetrics and Gynecology, University of Mississippi Medical Center, Jackson MS 39216-4505

Gonadotropin-releasing hormone (GnRH) was isolated and synthesized simultaneously by Andrew Schally and Roger Guillemin in 1971. These investigators shared the 1977 Nobel Prize for this remarkable accomplishment. In the years that followed, chemical modification of the naturally occurring GnRH molecule resulted in analogs with agonistic or antagonistic actions depending on the unique alterations of the analog. Initially, investigators anticipated that GnRH agonists would be used as fertility-enhancing agents and GnRH antagonists would prove useful as contraceptives. However, today most clinical applications of GnRH agonists utilize inhibitory rather than stimulatory actions of the preparations.

MOLECULAR CHARACTERIZATION OF GnRH

Native GnRH

The gene encoding for GnRH is composed of four exons located on the short arm of chromosome 8. Translation results in a 92-amino-acid precursor protein for GnRH (pre-pro GnRH). Posttranslational processing produces the decapeptide known as GnRH and a 56-amino-acid peptide known as GnRH-associated peptide (GAP) (Fig. 23-1). The biological significance of GAP remains to be elucidated. GnRH is a highly conserved molecule and virtually all mammals have the same 10 amino acid sequence.

Endogenous GnRH molecules assume a hairpin configuration (Fig. 23-2). The native GnRH molecule can undergo major conformational changes from a linear to a highly folded form. The formation of a β-type II turn at Gly^6-Leu^7 results in a configuration that has a high affinity for GnRH receptors. The formation of hydrogen bonds between the pyrrolidone carbonyl residue at position 1 and the glycine amide group at position 10 stabilize this configuration. Close apposition of amino acids at the terminal positions is important in the binding of GnRH to its membrane receptor. In addition, this hairpin configura-

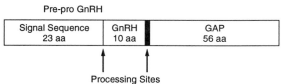

FIG. 23-1. Posttranslational processing of the prohormone by the GnRH neurons of the median eminence yields the decapeptide GnRH.

tion makes amino acids five, six, and seven especially vulnerable to degradation by pituitary endopeptidases. Another pituitary enzyme, carboxyl amide peptidase (post–proline cleavage enzyme), further inactivates native GnRH by cleaving the bonds between amino acids 9 and 10. These pituitary peptidases are largely responsible for the short 2- to 4-minute half-life of GnRH.

Receptor Interaction

Activation of the gonadotropes of the anterior pituitary following binding of GnRH to GnRH receptors in the cell membrane appears to be dependent on the three N-terminal residues of the ligand. Following GnRH binding to gonadotrope receptors, the ligand–receptor complex undergoes aggregation and initiates extracellular calcium mobilization. This calcium influx ultimately and rapidly leads to a release (exocytosis) of secretory granules containing luteinizing hormone (LH) and follicle-stimulating hormone (FSH). Calmodulin, an intracellular calcium receptor molecule, mediates the effect of calcium on gonadotropin release. GnRH binding also activates protein kinase C through the initiation of a cascade involving phospholipase C, diacylglycerol, and inositol 1,4,5-phosphate. This slow pathway leads to cytosolic protein phosphorylation and an increase in new gonadotropin synthesis (Fig. 23-3).

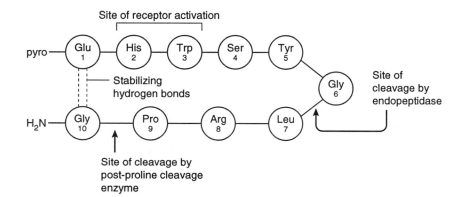

FIG. 23-2. The "hairpin" configuration of the native GnRH molecule results in susceptibility to cleavage by endopeptidases at the 6 position.

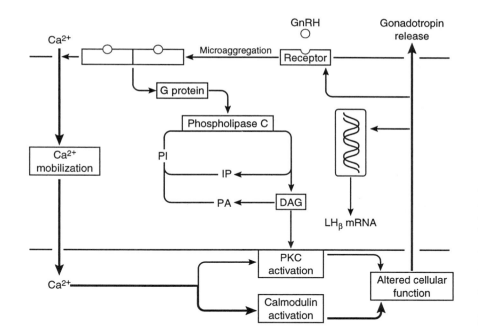

FIG. 23-3. GnRH interaction with its receptor results in calcium mobilization and activation of a phospholipase C–type enzyme. The influx of calcium activates calmodulin and results in the release of gonadotropins. Calcium acts in concert with the products of the phospholipase C pathway to alter biosynthesis of gonadotropins (gene expression). LH_β denotes the β subunit of luteinizing hormone. PI, phosphatidylinositol; IP, inositol phosphate; and PA, phosphatidic acid.

Gonadotropin Responses to GnRH

Pulsatile release of GnRH by the hypothalamus was first demonstrated in the late 1970s by Ernst Knobil. In the Rhesus monkey ablation of GnRH producing neurons in the hypothalamus inhibits spontaneous secretion of FSH and LH. Gonadotropin release could be restored only by a pulsatile infusion of GnRH. Physiologic release of FSH and LH only occurred when GnRH was administered at hourly intervals. Pulses given more frequently, less frequently, or as a continuous infusion resulted in abnormalities or suppression of gonadotropin secretion.

The paradoxical suppression of gonadotropins produced by continuous GnRH or its agonistic analogs results in hypogonadotropic hypogonadism. Two possible mechanisms have been proposed to explain this phenomenon. *Desensitization* refers to an uncoupling of the activated GnRH receptor binding complex from intracellular events normally initiated after receptor binding. *Downregulation* refers to a decrease in the number of available GnRH receptors on the pituitary gonadotroph. The precise mechanisms governing desensitization and downregulation are yet to be fully elucidated, but these concepts help explain the state of hypogonadotropic hypogonadism that accompanies long-term administration of GnRH or its agonistic analogs.

ANALOG DEVELOPMENT

GnRH Agonists

The native GnRH molecule has a half-life of 2–4 minutes due to proteolytic cleavage by endogenous pituitary peptidases. GnRH agonists more potent than the native molecule can be produced by stabilizing the analog against enzymatic attack, increasing serum protein binding or enhancing ligand affinity for the receptor. Analogs with synthetic D-amino acids at position 6 or modifications of the carboxy terminal Gly^{10} are more resistant to proteolysis (Table 23-1). Through these

TABLE 23-1. *GnRH analogs*

	1	2	3	4	5	6	7	8	9	10
Native GnRH	Glu	His	Trp	Ser	Tyr	Gly	Leu	Arg	Pro	Gly-NH₂
Agonists										
Leuprolide						D-Leu				NH-Ethylamide
Buserelin						D-Ser				NH-Ethylamide
Nafarelin						D-Nal(2)				
Goserelin						D-Ser				Aza-Gly
Antagonists										
Detirelix	N-Ac-D-Nal(2)	D-pC¹phe	D-Trp			D-hArg(Et₂)				D-Ala
Antide	N-Ac-Nal(2)	4ClDphe	D₃Pal		Lys/Nic	D-Lys(Nic)		Lys(iPr)⁸		D-Ala

modifications, GnRH agonists with prolonged half-lives and a resultant enhancement of biopotency have been developed (Table 23-2).

When potent GnRH agonists are administered, gonadotropin responses occur in two phases (Fig. 23-4). The first phase is a brief stimulatory phase with gonadotropin release and ovarian stimulation. Typically, this phase lasts 3–10 days and is often referred to as the "flare" effect. This is followed by a downregulation phase and occurs when the pituitary can no longer respond to GnRH. This "downregulated" phase is sustained for the pharmacologic duration of the agonist and represents the most important clinical application for GnRH agonist administration today.

GnRH Antagonists

Amino acids 2 and 3 of native GnRH are involved in the stimulus–response coupling of the receptor. Therefore, initial attempts at antagonist synthesis were focused on modifications at positions 2 and 3. Remarkable increases in potency result from the replacement of His[2] with D-amino acids. These early, first-generation GnRH antagonists were effective in vitro and, at high doses, in in vivo antiovulatory assays. Unfortunately, there were side effects that limited clinical use of these first-generation agents. A number of second-generation GnRH antagonists were synthesized with an emphasis on enhancement of potency with a simultaneous reduction of side effects. One of these compounds, Nal-Glu, showed particularly promising potency both in vitro and in vivo. However, local reactions in the form of transient erythema and induration continued to be a problem. Currently, a third generation of GnRH antagonists is advancing through clinical trials and appears to approach the desired combination of high potency and few side effects.

Some representative GnRH antagonists are shown in Table 23-1. GnRH antagonists exhibit a greater variety of

TABLE 23-2. *GnRH agonists in clinical use*

Agonist	Dosage	$t^{1/2}$	Route	Potency
Leuprolide	0.5–1.0 mg/day	3 hr	SC	15
	3.75–7.5 mg/month		IM	
Buserelin	900–1200 µg/day	3 hr	Nasal	20
	200–400 µg/day		SC	
Nafarelin	200 µg bid	4.5 hr	Nasal	100
Goserelin	3.6 mg/month	4 hr	SC pellet	100

structural modifications relative to GnRH agonists. Whereas most potent agonists contain only one or two modifications at positions 6 and 10, the antagonists have as many as 7 of the 10 amino acid residues replaced by novel amino acids. The only amino acids that have not been modified in GnRH antagonist synthesis are Ser[4] and Pro[9].

GnRH antagonists induce an immediate and profound suppression of pituitary gonadotropin secretion leading to a rapid induction of a hypogonadotropic hypogonadal state (see Fig. 23-4). There is no initial stimulation of gonadotropin secretion characteristic of the GnRH agonists. GnRH antagonists produce this effect through inhibition by classic receptor antagonism, preventing the release of LH/FSH from the gonadotrope. This produces nearly immediate cessation of gonadal steroidogenesis. These effects are a result of the high receptor affinity and prolonged duration of action of these agents.

CLINICAL APPLICATIONS

Initially, investigators anticipated that GnRH agonists would be used as fertility-enhancing agents and GnRH antagonists would prove useful as contraceptives. However, the ability of GnRH agonists to downregulate gonadotropin release has provided unanticipated clinical advantages of these drugs.

GnRH analogs produce hypogonadotropic hypogonadism with a decrement of ovarian sex steroid production when administered chronically. After suppression,

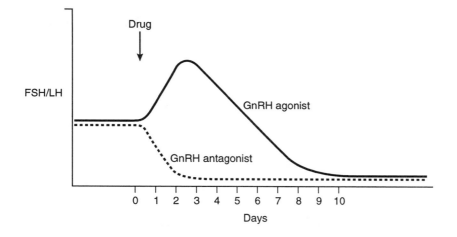

FIG. 23-4. Administration of GnRH agonist produces a biphasic response with an initial stimulatory ("flare") component lasting about 3 days followed by a rapid suppression of gonadotropin secretion. In contrast, GnRH antagonists rapidly induce a hypogonadotrophic state without producing an initial gonadotropin flare.

TABLE 23-3. *Reported therapeutic applications of GnRH analogs*

Hormone-dependent cancer (men and women)
Endometriosis
Uterine fibroids
Precocious puberty
Ovulation induction
Prevention of LH surge
Polycystic ovarian disease
Hirsutism
Pelvic pain
Cyclic affective mood disorders (premenstrual syndrome)
Dysfunctional uterine bleeding
Gonadal protection against chemotherapy
Adjunct to pelvic surgery

LH, luteinizing hormone.

TABLE 23-4. *Adverse effects of GnRH agonist therapy*

Symptom	% Reporting
Hot flushes	80
Vaginal bleeding	30
Headache	20
Depression/emotional lability	20
Insomnia	20
Vaginal dryness	30
Decreased libido	20

serum estradiol concentrations are similar to those seen after menopause (ie, approximately 20 pg/ml). Conditions commonly treated with GnRH agonists are listed in Table 23-3. With the exception of central precocious puberty, treatment of prepubertal or postmenopausal women with GnRH agonist therapy is rarely indicated. In addition, the usual precautions for potent agents that interact with the reproductive axis apply to these agents and they should not be administered to women who are pregnant or who have undiagnosed genital bleeding.

Treatment with GnRH agonists is typically begun during the luteal phase of the cycle. The luteal phase initiation of therapy dampens the flare effect (see Fig. 23-4). A unique disadvantage of the luteal phase initiation of therapy is that despite the use of sensitive pregnancy tests, some patients with very early pregnancies will escape detection prior to therapy. Additionally, the gonadotropin flare has been reported to induce transient functional cyst formation and even ovarian hyperstimulation.

The most commonly encountered adverse symptom of GnRH agonist treatment is hot flushes. These hot flushes usually occur 3–5 weeks after initiation of therapy, affect 80–100% of patients, and often decrease in frequency and intensity as therapy progresses. Amenorrhea occurs in roughly two thirds of women after a single bleeding episode that occurs 2–6 weeks beyond the initiation of therapy. Heavy vaginal bleeding has been observed in women with submucous fibroids. Headache occurs in approximately 20% of patients treated with GnRH agonists and is the most common reason for discontinuation of therapy. Depression is seen in 20% of patients and represents a potentially dangerous complication of therapy if not recognized. Additional adverse effects are usually minor and are detailed in Table 23-4.

An asymptomatic side effect that limits the duration of treatment with GnRH agonists is bone demineralization. After 6 months of treatment with GnRH agonists most women experience a reversible loss of bone density between 6% and 12%. This bone loss is a reflection of reduced estrogen levels. Treatment strategies to extend the duration of GnRH treatment beyond 6 months have been devised that involve an add-back regimen of sex steroids or biphosphates. These therapies reverse or slow the estrogen deprivation–induced bone loss.

SUGGESTED READING

Molecular Characterization of GnRH

Braden TD, Conn PM. GnRH and its mechanism of action. In: Leung PCK, Hsueh AJW, Friesen HG, eds. *Molecular Basis of Reproductive Endocrinology.* New York: Springer-Verlag, 1993;12–38.
Conn PM, Crowley WF Jr. Gonadotropin-releasing hormone and its analogues. *N Engl J Med 1991;*324:93–103.
Davidson JS, Flanagan CA, Becker II, Illing N, Sealfon SC, Millar RP. Molecular function of the gonadotropin-releasing hormone receptor: insights from site-directed mutagenesis. *Mol Cell Endocrinol* 1994;100:9–14.
Knobil E. The neuroendocrine control of the menstrual cycle. *Rec Prog Horm Res* 1980;36:53–88.
Schally AV, Arimura A, Kastin AJ, Matsuo H, Baba Y, Redding TW, et al. The gonadotropin-releasing hormone: one polypeptide regulates the secretion of luteinizing and follicle stimulating hormones. *Science* 1971;173:1036–1038.

Analog Development

Friedman AJ. The biochemistry, physiology, and pharmacology of gonadotropin releasing hormone (GnRH) and GnRH analogs. In: Barbieri RL, Friedman AJ, eds. *Gonadotropin Releasing Hormone Analogs. Applications in Gynecology.* New York: Elsevier, 1991;1–15.
Henzl MR, Polan ML. How GnRH agonists were discovered and developed. In: Polan ML, Henzl MR, eds. *Infertil Reprod Med Clin North Am* 1993;4:1–6.
Karten MJ, Rivier JE. Gonadotropin-releasing hormone analog design. Structure–function studies toward the development of agonists and antagonists: rationale and perspective. *Endocr Rev* 1986;7:44–66.

Clinical Applications

Barbieri RL. Gonadotropin-releasing hormone agonists: treatment of endometriosis. *Clin Obstet Gynecol* 1993;36:636–641.
Loy RA. The pharmacology and the potential applications of GnRH antagonists. *Curr Opin Obstet Gynecol* 1994;6:262–268.
Tan SL. Luteinizing hormone-releasing hormone agonists for ovarian stimulation in assisted reproduction. *Curr Opin Obstet Gynecol* 1994;6:166–172.
Van Leusden HAIM. Impact of different GnRH analogs in benign gynecological disorders related to their chemical structure, delivery systems and dose. *Gynecol Endocrinol* 1994;8:215–222.

Clinical Reproductive Medicine,
Edited by Bryan D. Cowan and David B. Seifer
Lippincott-Raven Publishers, Philadelphia © 1997

CHAPTER 24

Ovulation Induction:
Clomiphene Citrate and Menotropins

John D. Isaacs, Jr.

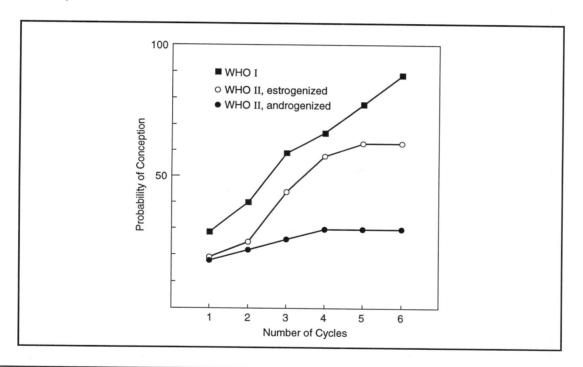

Patient Selection
Clomiphene Citrate
    Pharmacology and Physiology
    Mechanism of Action
    Clinical Use
    Monitoring Response to Therapy
    Complications
    Toxicity

Results of Treatment
Conclusion
Menotropins
    Evaluation
    Method of Treatment
    Complications
    Results of Treatment
Suggested Reading

D. Isaacs, Jr.: Division of Reproductive Endocrinology, Department of Obstetrics and Gynecology, University of Mississippi Medical Center, Jackson MS 39216-4505

Anovulation and oligo-ovulation are common causes of female infertility. The introduction of hormonal and chemical agents designed to produce ovulation in this group of patients represents one of the major advances in the field of reproductive endocrinology.

PATIENT SELECTION

Identification of patients who are proper candidates for ovulation induction relies on a thorough evaluation of ovulatory status. The diagnosis of ovulatory dysfunction is established by an absence of features that characterize the ovulatory menstrual cycle.

The menstrual history is the simplest and most important indicator of ovulation. Over 90% of women that have regular menses at intervals of 24–35 days will be ovulatory. Furthermore, ovulatory cycles are characterized by moliminal symptoms (premenstrual breast tenderness, bloating, dysmenorrhea, and *Mittelschmerz* or midcycle pain), and absence of these features suggests anovulation. Following ovulation, the ovarian follicle is transformed into the corpus luteum, which is responsible for progesterone secretion. Anovulation is characterized by a lack of progesterone secretion and can be diagnosed by a monophasic basal body temperature graph (progesterone is a thermogenic hormone), a serum progesterone level <3 ng/ml 5–10 days prior to the onset of menses, or an endometrial biopsy that does not show a secretory endometrium.

Ovulation dysfunction may be secondary to an underlying metabolic or hormonal disorder such as hyperprolactinemia, thyroid dysfunction, or androgen excess. These should be considered prior to the induction of ovulation to avoid missing a potentially treatable endocrine cause for the ovulatory disturbance. The majority of anovulatory or oligo-ovulatory women are euestrogenic (WHO Class II). Included in this group are patients with polycystic ovarian syndrome (PCOS) and those with subtle defects in hypothalamic-pituitary function. Serum gonadotropin determination will separate hypoestrogenic women into two groups. Women with elevated gonadotropins (WHO Class III) have ovarian failure and respond poorly to any attempts at induction of ovulation. This is in contrast to hypoestrogenic patients with hypothalamic-pituitary dysfunction and low to normal levels of serum gonadotropins (WHO Class I).

CLOMIPHENE CITRATE

First synthesized in 1956, clomiphene citrate is a nonsteroidal estrogen that acts as a potent contraceptive in animal models. When administered to women, however, clomiphene citrate produced marked ovarian enlargement, and its potential as a fertility-enhancing drug was soon realized. The initial clinical trials in 1960 reported induction of ovulation in 28 of 36 patients with amenorrhea, Stein–Leventhal syndrome, and dysfunctional uterine bleeding due to anovulation. Pregnancy occurred in a significant proportion of cases where infertility had been a complaint. Since gaining Food and Drug Administration approval for clinical use in 1967, clomiphene citrate has become the initial drug of choice for induction of ovulation in infertile patients with an ovulatory disturbance.

Pharmacology and Physiology

Clomiphene citrate is a triphenylethylene derivative and a member of the stilbene family (eg, diethylstilbestrol) of nonsteroidal agents (Fig. 24-1). Commercially available preparations contain a racemic mixture of the two stereochemical isomers of clomiphene citrate. Zuclomiphene citrate (the cis form) accounts for approximately 40% of the total mixture. Enclomiphene citrate (the trans form) makes up approximately 60% of most clomiphene citrate formulations.

Clomiphene is rapidly absorbed following oral ingestion and is secreted primarily in the feces. Only about 50% of the drug is secreted 5 days after oral administration and radiolabeled clomiphene citrate appears in stool up to 6 weeks following the last dose.

Mechanism of Action

The ability of clomiphene citrate to induce ovulation resides in its ability to function as an antiestrogen at the

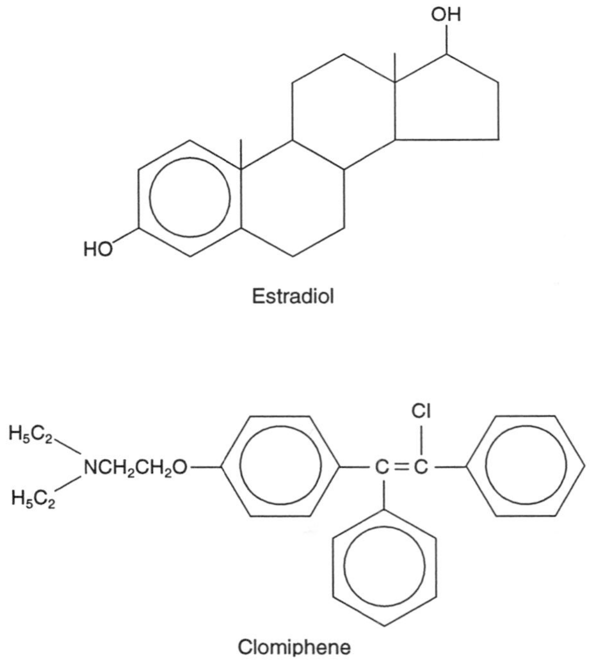

FIG. 24-1. Structure of clomiphene citrate compared to 17β-estradiol. The cis isomer is depicted.

level of the hypothalamus. Possible effects on the pituitary and ovary have also been postulated. The drug binds to hypothalamic estrogen receptors and blocks the negative feedback role usually exerted by estrogen. This action produces a transient elevation of serum gonadotropins. Specifically, clomiphene seems to produce an increase in gonadotropin-releasing hormone (GnRH) pulse frequency rather than amplitude (Table 24-1). This increased GnRH pulse frequency leads to elevated levels of follicle-stimulating hormone (FSH) and luteinizing hormone (LH) that induce follicular recruitment and ovarian estradiol production. Following discontinuation of the drug, rising estradiol levels negatively affect the hypothalamic release of GnRH, FSH, and LH levels decline just as in the late follicular phase of the normal menstrual cycle (Chapter 7).

Clinical Use

Clomiphene citrate is most appropriately used in the anovulatory patient with normogonadotropic, normoprolactinemic ovulatory dysfunction (WHO II). These patients may present with a history of oligo-ovulation or amenorrhea or with dysfunctional uterine bleeding. This includes patients with some or all of the features of the polycystic ovary syndrome. Clomiphene-responsive patients are usually well estrogenized as determined by progestin-induced withdrawal bleeding. Clomiphene citrate therapy is generally unsuccessful in patients who are hypoestrogenic (WHO I and WHO III).

There are few contraindications to the use of clomiphene citrate. Cystic ovarian enlargement due to pathologic changes or follicular cysts is generally viewed as a contraindication to treatment as a precaution against further ovarian enlargement. No evidence exists that clomiphene citrate is a human teratogen; however, pregnancy should always be excluded prior to the initiation of drugs in a new cycle. Because alterations in hepatic metabolism make the drug difficult to manage and potentially dangerous, significant hepatic dysfunction usually precludes the use of clomiphene.

TABLE 24-1. *Clomiphene citrate increases pulse frequency of LH and FSH, but not pulse amplitude*

	LH	FSH
Pulses/24 hr		
No clomiphene	10	12
Clomiphene	21*	15
Amplitude (mIU/ml)		
No clomiphene	4	2
Clomiphene	5	3

Modified from Kerin JF, et al. *J Clin Endocrinol Metab* 1985;61: 265–268.
*$p < 0.01$.

TABLE 24-2. *Dose-related response to clomiphene*

Dose (mg)	% Total ovulating	% Total pregnancies
50	52.1	52.8
100	21.9	20.7
150	12.3	9.8
200	6.9	8.8
250	4.9	6.2

From Gysler M, et al. *Fertil Steril* 1982;37:161.
Percentages indicate the proportion of all ovulations or pregnancies at each dose of clomiphene.

Clomiphene therapy is initiated at a dosage of 50 mg daily for 5 days beginning 3–5 days following the onset of spontaneous menstrual or progestin withdrawal bleeding. Ovulation generally occurs between days 14 and 19 of the cycle and may be inferred through the use of basal body temperature (BBT) graphs, urinary LH monitoring (to detect the preovulation LH surge), measurement of the serum progesterone concentration, or an endometrial biopsy. If the initial 50-mg dosage does not result in ovulation, in subsequent cycles it should be increased by 50 mg. Caution should be used when advancing the dosage above 150 mg as 53% of ovulatory cycles with clomiphene citrate occur at the 50-mg dose and 86% occur at a dosage of 150 mg or less (Table 24-2). The dosage of clomiphene should be increased only if the patient fails to ovulate, not because of a failure to conceive.

If the decision is made to increase the total dosage of clomiphene, two approaches may be taken. The total daily dose may be increased or the duration of therapy may be extended. Some patients who fail to respond to a dose of drug given over a 5-day period will respond to the same dose given over a longer time (e.g., 7 days). Once an ovulatory response is obtained, most conceptions will occur within the first 6 ovulatory cycles (Fig. 24-2).

Glucocorticoids are a useful adjunct in patients who fail to respond to clomiphene citrate. Dexamethasone or prednisone suppresses production of adrenal androgens and makes the ovarian hormonal milieu more conducive for follicular development and ovulation. Such adjunctive therapy has proven effective in women with PCOS or clinical evidence of hyperandrogenism. These powerful corticosteroids appear most effective for patients with elevated adrenal dehydroepiandrosterone sulfate (DHEAS). It is given orally as a single daily bedtime dose and is discontinued once pregnancy is confirmed.

Ovulation failure despite adequate follicular development with clomiphene citrate therapy may occur for reasons that are poorly understood. The apparent lack of the midcycle gonadotropin surge may be overcome by the administration of human chorionic gonadotropin (hCG) as an ovulatory trigger. Candidates for this form of therapy are most accurately detected when preovulatory ovarian ultrasonography detects a lead follicle with a mean di-

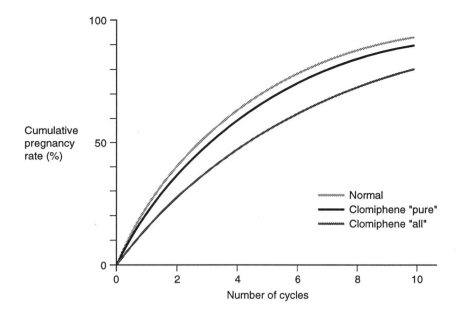

FIG. 24-2. Patients who ovulate with clomiphene have cumulative pregnancy rates similar to parous women discontinuing barrier contraception provided that other fertility factors are not present.

ameter of approximately 22–24 mm. Human chorionic gonadotropin is given as a 5000- to 10,000-IU intramuscular dose. Ultrasonography may be repeated at 2- to 3-day intervals to confirm ovulation.

Monitoring Response to Therapy

Prior to and immediately following institution of a new regimen of clomiphene citrate, the ovaries should be evaluated for evidence of enlargement. A bimanual pelvic exam will usually suffice for this purpose. Ultrasonography is useful in the evaluation of a palpably abnormal adnexa or for obese patients in whom a bimanual exam yields little useful information.

Ovulation should be confirmed initially with BBT records, documentation of the midcycle urinary LH surge, or by measurement of a luteal phase serum progesterone level. Clomiphene-induced cycles in which conception occurs are generally characterized by a midluteal progesterone concentration of 15 ng/ml or greater.

Ultrasound is a useful adjunct in patients who fail to respond to initial stepwise therapy with clomiphene citrate. It can distinguish women who demonstrate a complete lack of response to therapy from those who develop a dominant follicle but fail to ovulate. Ultrasonography also allows accurate timing of hCG administration.

Complications

Cystic enlargement of the ovaries following treatment with clomiphene citrate has been reported to occur in 5–11% of cycles (see Table 24-3). In most cases, the ovaries measure 5–9 cm and return to normal size in 2–4 weeks. Cyst formation does not appear to be a dose-related phenomenon and recurrent cyst formation occurs

only rarely in subsequent cycles at the same dose. If ovarian enlargement is detected at the beginning of the cycle, clomiphene citrate should be withheld until the cyst regresses. This will avoid the risk of further ovarian enlargement, torsion, and possible rupture.

Multiple gestations associated with clomiphene citrate are confined to an increase of the rate of dizygotic twin gestations from about 1% in the general population to about 5–7% in women who conceive after clomiphene citrate therapy. This is likely due to the recruitment of multiple follicles by the sustained early follicular gonadotropin levels seen in clomiphene citrate–treated cycles.

Toxicology

Hot flushes are reported in 11% of clomiphene citrate–treated cycles, presumably from its antiestrogenic properties (see Table 24-3). Visual symptoms (chiefly blurring, spots, or flashes) occur in approximately 1.5% of cycles and appear to be dose-related. The mechanism responsible is unknown but the effects are self-limited.

TABLE 24-3. *Complications of clomiphene citrate treatment*

Complication	Incidence (%)
Ovarian enlargement (>6 cm)	5–13
Abdominal discomfort	7
Twin gestation	5–7
Three or more fetuses	0.5
Hot flushes	11
Visual symptoms	1.5
Mood disturbances	<2
Vaginal dryness	<2
Breast tenderness	<2
Nausea and/or vomiting	<2

Other commonly reported side effects include mood changes, vaginal dryness, and breast tenderness.

Results of Treatment

Most authors have reported that approximately 80% of patients treated with clomiphene can be expected to ovulate and about 50% of these will conceive (Table 24-4). This discrepancy between ovulation and conception may be due to factors such as loss to follow-up present in many studies. Studies designed to minimize the influence of such factors through life table analysis have shown that patients who ovulate with clomiphene treatment have conception rates similar to those of ovulatory women who discontinue barrier contraceptives (see Fig. 24-2).

In an analysis of outcome in 2369 pregnancies resulting from treatment with clomiphene citrate, the incidence of spontaneous abortion (19.2%), stillbirth (1.1%), ectopic pregnancy (1.2%), and congenital anomalies (2.4%) was not significantly increased above that observed in spontaneous conceptions. Additionally, in a group of 158 women who inadvertently received clomiphene during the 6 weeks following pregnancy, 8 (5.1%) had infants with congenital anomalies, a nonsignificant increase over the expected incidence in spontaneous conceptions. However, clomiphene citrate has been shown to produce a wide array of birth defects in the offspring of laboratory animals following administration of massive doses of the drug to pregnant animals during the period of organogenesis. Concerns about the delayed excretion of clomiphene citrate and its persistence in the circulation during the early stages of pregnancy have prompted careful scrutiny. To date, there is no evidence that clomiphene citrate administered during the follicular phase leads to an increase in the incidence of congenital anomalies. Termination of pregnancy is not recommended following inadvertent early gestational exposure to clomiphene.

Conclusion

Clomiphene citrate is a highly effective, relatively safe agent for the treatment of normogonadotropic, normoprolactinemic ovulatory dysfunction. Patients who do not respond may be candidates for therapy with agents such as menotropins.

TABLE 24-4. *Ovulation and uncorrected pregnancy rates following clomiphene therapy (7 studies)*

N	Ovulation %	Pregnancy %
5152	72	35

Modified from Hammond MG. *Fertil Steril* 1984;42:499–507.

MENOTROPINS

Induction of ovulation using gonadotropins extracted from human cadaveric pituitary glands was reported in 1958. By 1962, a pregnancy resulting from ovulation induction with gonadotropins derived from the urine of postmenopausal women (menotropins) was reported. The relative ease with which gonadotropins could be extracted from urine and the relative scarcity of human pituitary glands led to the development of human menopausal gonadotropin (hMG) as the major commercially available preparation. Over 30 years after its introduction, hMG remains at the forefront of treatment for ovulatory dysfunction and infertility.

Currently, in the United States, two preparations of gonadotropins are commercially available. Human menopausal gonadotropins (Pergonal, Humegon) are available as a lyophilized powder containing 75 or 150 IU each of FSH and LH as well as nonspecific urinary proteins. Recently, a purified preparation of FSH (Metrodin) has been introduced that contains 75 IU of FSH and <0.1 IU of LH as well as nonspecific urinary proteins. Clinical trials of ultrapurified FSH and recombinant FSH are currently in progress. These agents offer the advantage of subcutaneous administration and increased availability.

Evaluation

Patients who are candidates for therapy with hMG can be divided into two broad categories: those with ovulatory dysfunction resistant to clomiphene and those with other indications for menotropin therapy. The ovulatory dysfunction group includes women who are normoestrogenic (WHO II) as well as those with hypogonadotropic, hypoestrogenic (WHO I) anovulation. Other indications for menotropins include the empiric treatment of unexplained infertility, superovulation for assisted reproductive technologies, poor-quality cervical mucus, and luteal phase defects.

Prior to initiation of therapy with hMG, other factors impacting on fertility should be identified and treated. A semen analysis is obtained and uterotubal abnormalities excluded by hysterosalpingogram or laparoscopy. Gonadotropin therapy is not appropriate for women with ovarian failure and a serum FSH should be measured in patients who are hypoestrogenic. Patients considering treatment with menotropins should be advised of the likelihood of multifetal gestation, risk of ovarian hyperstimulation, and they must be able to comply with the rigid demands of monitoring. Menotropins should not be administered to patients with preexisting ovarian enlargement or in the presence of an ongoing gestation.

Method of Treatment

Treatment is typically begun on cycle day 3 (spontaneous or progestin-induced) consisting of daily intramuscular injection of 75–150 IU of hMG. After 3–5 days of treatment, the ovarian response is evaluated with a morning serum estradiol determination and ovarian ultrasound imaging. The estradiol level provides a marker of the ovarian biochemical response to FSH. It typically doubles every 2–3 days in response to hMG. If an appropriate rise occurs in the serum estradiol concentration, the same dosage is maintained and monitoring is repeated every 1–3 days. In the absence of an appropriate increase in estradiol levels, the dose of hMG is increased by 50–100% and estradiol levels are repeated every 3–5 days until an appropriate response occurs.

Ovarian ultrasound imaging provides a visual assessment of follicular growth and development. Follicular growth usually occurs at a rate of 1–3 mm/day. Ultrasound is especially helpful in monitoring follicular proliferation in patients prone to hyperstimulation (i.e., PCOS) to allow titration of hMG dose accordingly.

When one or more follicles reach a mean diameter of 16 mm or greater (Fig. 24-3) and the serum estradiol is within the appropriate preovulatory range of 500–1500 pg/ml (200–250 pg/ml/follicle), an intramuscular injection of hCG (5000–10,000 IU) is given. Ovulation typically occurs 36 to 40 hours after hCG. Intercourse, intrauterine insemination, or oocyte recovery can be planned accordingly. A single preovulatory injection of 10,000 U of hCG will usually provide adequate support for the corpus luteum throughout the luteal phase. Additional luteal support is not routinely required, but if doses of hCG less than 10,000 U are used, luteal support may

be required, especially in patients with hypogonadotropic hypogonadism or who have received GnRH agonist to prevent a premature LH surge.

Ovulation should be documented in each hMG cycle with a serum progesterone level drawn 8–10 days after the hCG injection. Ovarian enlargement is common and strenuous physical activity and intercourse should be discouraged beginning approximately 5 days after hCG to avoid the possibility of ovarian trauma or torsion. Patients should report any excessive pelvic pain or rapid weight gain that occurs during this time as these may indicate impending ovarian hyperstimulation.

If pregnancy does not occur, treatment may be administered in successive cycles. Drug requirements and ovarian response are relatively constant from one cycle to the next and previous results help to guide further therapy.

Complications

Ovarian hyperstimulation syndrome (OHS) is the most frequent complication following ovulation induction with menotropins. This syndrome is characterized by ovarian enlargement, third-space fluid accumulation, variable degrees of electrolyte disturbance, and hypovolemia. It has been estimated to occur in some form in half of all hMG cycles. Patients at increased risk develop multiple small follicles following a relatively short exposure to hMG. Circulating levels of estradiol reflect the total contribution of the entire follicular pool and appear to be a better predictor of OHS than ultrasonographic parameters. When estradiol levels exceed 2000–4000 pg/ml on the day of hCG administration, OHS is more likely to occur.

The etiology of OHS has been difficult to define precisely (Fig. 24-4). This syndrome occurs exclusively in association with supraphysiologic levels of gonadotropins and is triggered by administration of hCG. Cycles in which hCG is withheld do not result in OHS no matter how extreme the ovarian stimulation has been. The major expressions of OHS are a result of increased capillary permeability. Hormonally responsive substances such as plasma renin-like activity (PRA) have been identified as possible mediators. Morbidity is generally due to hemoconcentration and a resulting hypercoagulable state that leads to stroke and venous embolism.

OHS is classified as mild, moderate, or severe (Table 24-5) and the specific treatment is directed by the severity of hyperstimulation present. Mild OHS occurs most frequently and is characterized by ovarian enlargement up to 8 cm in the absence of significant clinical symptoms. Hospitalization may be required for significant pain, excessive nausea and vomiting, electrolyte disturbances, or hemoconcentration. Pain control can be provided with prostaglandin synthetase inhibitors, and

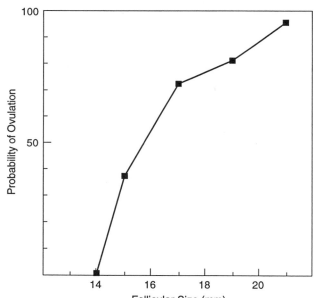

FIG. 24-3. Incidence of ovulation based on follicular size on the day of human chorionic gonadotropin (hCG) administration during human menopausal gonadotropin (hMG) therapy. Modified from Silverberg KM. *Fertil Steril* 1991;56:296.

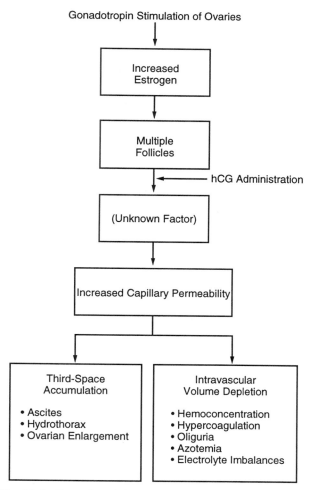

Gonadotropin Stimulation of Ovaries

Increased Estrogen

Multiple Follicles

← hCG Administration

(Unknown Factor)

Increased Capillary Permeability

Third-Space Accumulation
• Ascites
• Hydrothorax
• Ovarian Enlargement

Intravascular Volume Depletion
• Hemoconcentration
• Hypercoagulation
• Oliguria
• Azotemia
• Electrolyte Imbalances

FIG. 24-4. Genesis of human menopausal gonadotropin (hMG)–mediated ovarian hypostimulation syndrome (OHS); hMG induces increased estrogen and multiple follicles. Human chorionic gonadotropin purportedly produces an unknown factor that increases capillary permeability. Third-space accumulation of fluid and intravascular volume depletion are the clinical consequences of these responses.

antiemetics may help decrease nausea and vomiting. Progression to severe OHS may occur, especially if the cycle results in conception.

Severe OHS is a potentially life-threatening condition characterized by ascites, pleural effusion, electrolyte abnormalities, and marked hemoconcentration. Patients with severe OHS should be hospitalized and aggressively

TABLE 24-5. *Classifying OHS*

Classification	Incidence (%)	Ovarian enlargement	Pain	Ascites/hydrothorax
Mild	8–56	Yes (5–8 cm)	No	No
Moderate	1–7	Yes (8–12 cm)	Yes	No
Severe	<1–2	Yes (<12 cm)	Yes	Yes

From Cowan BD. *Female Patient* 1991;16:37–44.

treated. Intravenous crystalloid solution should be administered at an initial rate of 150–200 cm³/hr until hemodilution and diuresis occur. Intravascular volume expansion with colloid solutions (mannitol, albumin, Hespan) provides an increase in intravascular colloid pressure, thereby promoting diuresis and decreasing hemoconcentration without the need for large volumes of crystalloid solution. Pulmonary capillary wedge pressure monitoring is a valuable adjunct in patients who require intensive therapy. Paracentesis or thoracentesis will relieve abdominal distension, dyspnea, or cardiac compromise and will often promote a dramatic diuresis as well.

Multifetal pregnancy (MFP) occurs in up to 30% of hMG-stimulated cycles as a result of the induction of multiple follicles and multiple ovulations. The incidence of MFP has remained constant since the advent of sonographic monitoring as has the widespread adoption of guidelines advocating that hCG be withheld if more than three to five mature follicles are present. If this devastating complication should occur, patients should be advised that selective reduction of pregnancies with three or more fetuses to a twin or singleton gestation is available. This often provides the only opportunity to avoid catastrophic complications associated with these pregnancies.

Spontaneous abortion occurs in 12–29% of hMG conceptions. This is higher than the rate observed after spontaneous conceptions. The reasons for this difference are not clear but may include the closer scrutiny of early pregnancy in infertility patients, the higher average age of patients, or subtle defects of the luteal phase. The rate of congenital anomalies is not increased in hMG-stimulated conceptions and long-term follow-up studies reveal normal growth and development in these children.

In recent years, concerns have arisen that the use of ovulation-inducing drugs might lead to an increase in a woman's subsequent risk for the development of ovarian cancer later in life. These concerns are based on observations that a protective effect against the development of ovarian cancer appears to be conferred by conditions in which ovulation is suppressed such as the use of oral contraceptives, pregnancy, or lactation. Additionally, epidemiologic reports of a slightly increased risk for the development of ovarian cancer among infertile women have been ascribed to the use of fertility drugs. These observations emphasize the importance of judicious use of ovulation induction drugs and the continued scrutiny of this therapy.

Results of Treatment

Induction of ovulation is successful in >90% of menotropin-stimulated cycles. Pregnancy rates vary according to etiology of the ovulatory dysfunction, age of the patient, and the presence of co-existing infertility

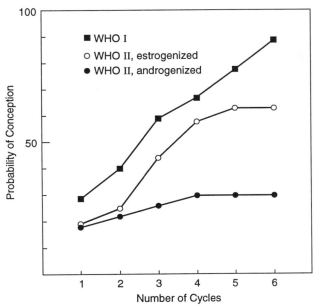

FIG. 24-5. Results of menotropin therapy based on type of ovulatory defect. Modified from Fluker MR, et al. *Obstet Gynecol* 1994;84:189–196.

factors. In general, WHO I patients have the best prognosis with pregnancy rates of approximately 25% per cycle and approaching 80% after four cycles of treatment (Fig. 24-5). WHO II patients represent a heterogeneous population and pregnancy rates are affected by the presence of factors affecting ovulation such as hyperandrogenism. In general, these patients can expect per-cycle pregnancy rates of 5–20% with approximately 30–60% of patients conceiving after four cycles of treatment. Pregnancy rates are lower in women over 35 and in those with elevated levels of FSH present on cycle day 3.

Menotropins remain a valuable agent for the induction of ovulation in modern infertility practice. Careful monitoring of ovarian response will reduce the incidence of ovarian hyperstimulation and maximize pregnancy rates. Multifetal pregnancy remains an unpreventable complication of menotropin therapy and patients should be counseled accordingly. The development of recombinant forms of gonadotropins may increase ease of administration and purity of these drugs.

SUGGESTED READING

Clomiphene

Adashi EY. Clomiphene citrate-initiated ovulation: a clinical update. *Semin Reprod Endocrinol* 1986;4:255–276.
Adashi EY. Clomiphene citrate: mechanism(s) and site(s) of action—a hypothesis revisited. *Fertil Steril* 1984;42:331–344.
Glasier AF, Irvine DS, Wickings EJ, Hillier SG, Baird DT. A comparison of the effects on follicular development between clomiphene citrate, its two separate isomers and spontaneous cycles. *Hum Reprod* 1989;4:252–256.
Gysler M, March CM, Mishell DR Jr, Bailey EJ. A decade's experience with an individualized clomiphene treatment regimen including its effect on the postcoital test. *Fertil Steril* 1982;37:161.
Hammond MG. Monitoring techniques for improved pregnancy rates during clomiphene ovulation induction. *Fertil Steril* 1984;42:499–507.
Kerin JF, Liu JH, Phillipou G, Yen SSC. Evidence for a hypothalamic site of action of clomiphene citrate in women. *J Clin Endocrinol Metab* 1985;61:265–268.
Lobo RA, Paul W, March CM, Granger L, Kletzky OA. Clomiphene and dexamethasone in women unresponsive to clomiphene alone. *Obstet Gynecol* 1982;60:497–501.
Rossing MA, Daling JR, Weiss NS, Moore DE, Seif SG. Ovarian tumors in a cohort of infertile women. *N Engl J Med* 1994;331:771–776.
Wu CH, Winkel CA. The effect of therapy initiation day on clomiphene citrate therapy. *Fertil Steril* 1989;52:564–568.

Menotropins

American Fertility Society. Induction of ovulation with human menopausal gonadotropins. *Guideline for Practice*, 1993.
Ben-Rafael Z, Dor J, Mashiach S. Blankstein J, Lunenfeld B, Serr DM. Abortion rate in pregnancies following ovulation induced by human menopausal gonadotropin–human chorionic gonadotropin. *Fertil Steril* 1983;39:157–161.
Cowan BD. Ovarian hyperstimulation syndrome. *The Female Patient* 1991;16:37–44.
Diamond MP, Wentz AC. Ovulation induction with human menopausal gonadotropins. *Obstet Gynecol Surv* 1986;41:480–490.
Dor J, Itzkowic DJ, Mashiach S, Lunenfeld B, Serr DM. Cumulative conception rates following gonadotropin therapy. *Am J Obstet Gynecol* 1980;136:102–105.
Flucker MR, Urman B, Mackinnon M, Barrow SR, Pride SM, Yuen BH. Exogenous gonadotropin therapy in World Health Organization groups II and II ovulatory disorders. *Obstet Gynecol* 1994;83:189–196.
Pearlstone AC, Fournet N, Gambone JC, Pang SC, Buyalos RP. Ovulation induction in women aged 40 and older: the importance of basal follicle-stimulating hormone level and chronological age. *Fertil Steril* 1992;58:674–679.
Shoham Z, Balen A, Patel A, Jacobs HS. Results of ovulation induction using human menopausal gonadotropin or purified follicle-stimulating hormone in hypogonadotropic hypogonadism patients. *Fertil Steril* 1991;56:1048–1053.
Silverberg KM, Olive DL, Burns WN, Johnson JC, Groff TR, Schenken RS. Follicular size at the time of human chorionic gonadotropin administration predicts ovulation outcome in human menopausal gonadotropin-stimulated cycles. *Fertil Steril* 1991;56:296–300.
Whittemore AS, Harris R, Intyre J. Collaborative Ovarian Cancer Group. Characteristics relating to ovarian cancer risk: collaborative analysis of 12 US case-control studies. II. Invasive epithelial ovarian cancers in white women. *Am J Epidemiol* 1992;136:1184–1203.

Clinical Reproductive Medicine,
Edited by Bryan D. Cowan and David B. Seifer
Lippincott-Raven Publishers, Philadelphia © 1997

CHAPTER 25

Recurrent Pregnancy Loss

Michael J. Gast

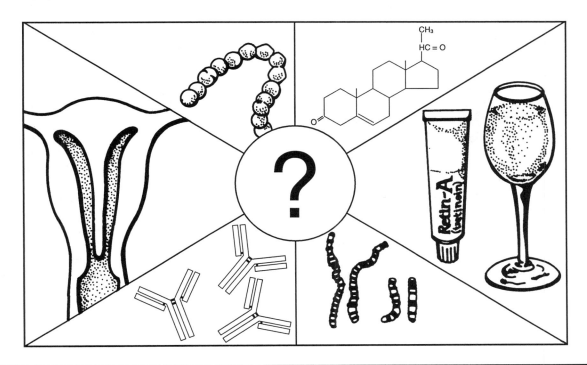

Clinical History
    Documentation of Pregnancy Loss
    Incidence of Pregnancy Loss
    Genetic Component of Pregnancy Loss
Causes of Recurrent Pregnancy Loss
    Uterine Anomalies
    Acquired Defects of the Uterus
    Chromosomal Rearrangements
    Progesterone Deficiency
    Systemic Disease

Infectious Causes
Immunologic Infertility
Pharmacologic and Environmental Toxins
Other Caveats
Evaluation and Therapy of Recurrent Pregnancy Loss
Counseling and Follow-up
Conclusions
Suggested Reading

M. J. Gast: Department of Obstetrics and Gynecology, Washington University School of Medicine, Phoenixville, PA 19460

Early pregnancy loss is one of the most common events that can befall the reproductive-aged woman. Early pregnancy loss (miscarriage) is quite common, occurring in at least 20% of all clinical pregnancies, and it may occur in up to 60% of fertilization events. The incidence of recurrent pregnancy loss (the loss of more than two pregnancies) is in the range of 1–3%.

CLINICAL HISTORY

Patients who have lost two or more early pregnancies often present to the gynecologist seeking explanations for this problem. It is possible to provide a rapid and coherent evaluation of these patients and either identify a correctable etiology or reassure the patients that no serious ongoing problem exists and that their chances of a successful conception and the birth of a viable infant in subsequent pregnancies is high.

Postfertilization pregnancies can be divided clinically into two types. Aborted pregnancy can occur at any time from implantation until 20 weeks gestation. Viable pregnancies will become live-born children (or will be ongoing pregnancies beyond the 20-week limit, beyond which they are no longer considered to be abortions). Depending on the duration of pregnancy and the level of awareness of the patient, aborted pregnancies can be further subclassified as either clinical or unrecognized. Some women who become pregnant will lose the pregnancy within the first several days or even the first 1–2 weeks beyond the missed menstrual period. Oftentimes the patient will consider this to be a "late menses" and will not report the event. On occasion these patients will present with complaints of infertility. The flip side of this situation is also encountered; patients who present with a history of multiple pregnancy losses that are undocumented.

Documentation of Pregnancy Loss

The initial step in the recurrent pregnancy loss history is to ask the question, "Was this really a pregnancy?" It is important to carefully document all pregnancies in patients for whom you are caring, as well as in patients whose history of miscarriages you are reviewing. The four key criteria to establishing a high probability of pregnancy are (1) positive pregnancy test, (2) physical examination, (3) ultrasound, and (4) pathology reports.

Positive pregnancy tests are either urinary or serum-based. Urinary chorionic gonadotropin assays are quite sensitive and are capable of detecting urinary concentrations of gonadotropin as low as 50 IU/L. Serum tests reliably detect human chorionic gonadotropin (hCG) concentrations of 25 IU/L or lower.

Physical examination is ordinarily the least helpful evaluation of recurrent pregnancy loss. Increases in uterine size, descriptions of "tissue" passed by the patient,

and the description of cervical and vaginal change are suggestive but not necessarily descriptive of pregnancy. A history of a physician hearing a heartbeat with a Doppler instrument or noting the passage of placental tissue is helpful. Historical signs alone (e.g., *fatigue, nausea, breast soreness*) are inadequate documentation that a true pregnancy has occurred.

Ultrasound is extraordinarily helpful in the evaluation of pregnancy. The presence of progressively more complex placental and fetal structures can provide the physician with verification of pregnancy and the reassurance that the pregnancy is within the uterus and that a fetus is present. The timing of pregnancy losses can be confusing because clinical abortion can occur weeks after loss of fetal viability. Early sonographic imaging can also establish the age of fetal demise.

The best evidence for pregnancy loss is a pathology report demonstrating chorionic villi and/or the presence of fetal tissue.

Incidence of Pregnancy Loss

While "clinical" rates for miscarriage vary from 10% to 25% in most series of women with normal reproductive function, the true incidence of postfertilization loss may be considerably higher. Hertig and Rock allowed women to conceive and then performed hysterectomies in the conception cycle. Carefully dissecting the reproductive tract they were able to identify embryos in many of these patients. They found abnormal embryos within the fallopian tube and implanted on endometrium. These 10- to 20-day-old embryos had a 50% incidence of histologic abnormalities, the most common of which was absence of the embryonic disk. They concluded that the true rate of preimplantation pregnancy loss was as high as 50%. The rate of pregnancy loss in in vitro fertilization and infertility programs where monitoring of early pregnancy often begins at or around the time of menses is 15–30%.

Coulam et al. looked at the incidence of clinical abortion in 2400 women who were actively attempting to conceive. In women with no prior pregnancy losses, the incidence of abortion was 12.6%. For those with second pregnancies where the first pregnancy had been lost, the incidence was 16.6%; 37.5% of women who had two previous pregnancy losses experienced a loss in their third pregnancy. It is generally reported that women with two successive spontaneous abortions have a recurrence risk of 25–45%. The prognosis for a successful pregnancy is increased by 10–20% in women with at least one previous live birth.

Genetic Component of Pregnancy Loss

Chromosomal mistakes of a random variety are the most important contributor to all pregnancy losses. The frequency of chromosomal anomalies in abortuses and still-births when evaluated by trimester of pregnancy also demonstrates the importance of genetic integrity to the development and continuation of pregnancy. The frequency of chromosomal abnormalities in abortuses in the first trimester is generally felt to be 40–60% (Table 25-1). Among second-trimester spontaneous losses, the frequency of chromosomal anomalies is about 10%. Of stillborn fetuses in the third trimester, the incidence of major chromosomal anomalies is 5–10%, whereas the incidence among liveborns is generally <1%. On a smaller scale, the same phenomenon has been demonstrated for individual chromosomal abnormalities, such as Turner's syndrome or trisomy 21. Thus, the magnitude of the genetic aberration in the pregnancy likely determines the duration through which it may continue. This system of biologic "checks and balances" may in part be responsible for maintaining the low rate of life-threatening congenital abnormalities encountered in liveborns.

One set of investigators undertook genetic study of 447 abortuses. Over half of the aborted fetuses evaluated were chromosomally abnormal. Ten percent of all of the aborted fetuses in this study had a Turner's syndrome karyotype of 45,XO whereas 31% had primary autosomal trisomies. The remainder had a variety of other chromosomal abnormalities including triploidy (2%), mosaicisms (1%), and structural rearrangements such as deletions and translocations (2.5%). Other studies demonstrate differing percentages, but there is general agreement that the trisomic abortus is the most common cause for chance pregnancy loss.

Trisomy is the most commonly encountered genetic abnormality in aborted pregnancies with gross structural genetic change, in general; it is detected in about 30% of all such gestations. Trisomies from all autosomes except 1 and 17 have been identified in aborted material. About one third of trisomies from spontaneously aborted fetuses represent trisomy 16. The risk of a repeat pregnancy affected by a trisomy is 2–5%; these women may be offered

early prenatal diagnosis in subsequent pregnancies. The monosomy 45,XO acccounts for the genetic defect in about 10% of chromosomally affected fetuses and seems to be due to the loss of a sex chromosome at zygote formation. Errors in meiosis or from double fertilization of a single ovum cause triploidy in about 8% of abortions with chromosomal abnormalities. Tetraploidy accounts for about 3% of the chromosomal abnormalities in abortions. Roughly 3% of chromosomal abnormalities in abortions are due to rearrangements such as primary translocations and inversions, but these anomalies are the most common structural rearrangement encountered in repetitive abortions. Inversions, which occur when one chromosome breaks at two points and the broken segment turns on its axis before recombining, exist in 0.1% of females and 0.1% of male partners experiencing repetitive abortions.

CAUSES OF RECURRENT PREGNANCY LOSS

Our understanding of the biochemical and physiologic events responsible for the maintenance of early pregnancy is not adequate to explain most recurrent losses. In all likelihood, the overwhelming majority of spontaneous pregnancy losses are the result of random (chance) genetic events in the sperm, ovum, or early embryo. Another important cause is likely to be very early (before 2 weeks postconception) mechanical or hormonal events that interrupt otherwise genetically normal pregnancies. When one of the definable causes of recurrent pregnancy loss is found, however, identification and treatment or appropriate counseling of the couple will be extremely rewarding. Possible etiologies include anatomic abnormalities of the uterus; genetic defects in the parents; endocrine dysfunctions; infection; autoimmune disease; alloimmune disorders; and environmental factors (Table 25-2).

Uterine Anomalies

Anatomic defects of the uterus make up one of the largest definable categories of recurrent loss etiologies. Although there is general agreement that some of these abnormalities contribute to the general pool of recurrent loss patients, estimates of the incidence of these defects

TABLE 25-1. *Cytogenetic analysis of spontaneous abortion specimens[a]*

	Percentage of total analyzed		
	Kaji (1980)	Sankraranarayanan (1982)	Simpson (1986)
Euploid	46	49.7	54
Autosomal trisomy	31	27	22
Monosomy X	10	9	9
Triploidy	7	8	8
Tetraploidy	2	3	3
Structural anomaly	3	2	2
Mosaics	—	1	1.3

[a]Approximately 50% of abortion specimens are cytogenetically abnormal, with trisomies as a group accounting for the majority of abnormalities. Monosomy X is the single most common cause of miscarriage.

TABLE 25-2. *Causes of recurrent pregnancy loss*

Cause	Incidence (%)
Uterine abnormalities	10
Endocrine abnormalities (ovarian/placental, thyroid)	30
Chromosomal abnormalities in the parents	5
Infections of the cervix and the uterus	<1
Abnormalities in immune status	5
Unknown causes	50

and their importance in any individual pregnancy are the source of extended and often acrimonious debate in the gynecologic community. A variety of uterine anomalies (both congenital and acquired) may contribute to recurrent pregnancy loss (Table 25-3). Although the etiologies for such losses secondary to mechanical factors remain uncertain, it is likely that the absence of appropriate blood supply to the endometrium and myometrium, the mechanical effects of compression, or failure to expand of the uterine cavity are among the primary reasons for such losses.

Anomalies that have been associated with excessive pregnancy wastage include the presence of a large fibromuscular septum within a single uterus and uterine fibroids. The septate uterus is the most likely to cause recurrent pregnancy losses with abortion rates between 40% and 80%. Losses from the unicornuate uterus may be as high as 10–30% but decrease with subsequent pregnancies. Arcuate deformities of the uterus do not contribute significantly to recurrent pregnancy loss. Failed Mullerian fusion (didelphis and the bicornuate uterus) has an outcome similar to that of the unicornuate uterus. It is important to recognize that in addition to spontaneous pregnancy losses, the incidence of fetal malpositions, preterm labor, preterm rupture of the membranes (all of which lead to premature delivery) are higher than expected in patients with congenital uterine anomalies.

An interesting congenital anomaly of the uterus is that caused by in utero exposure to the estrogenic stilbene, diethylstilbestrol (DES). During the 1940s, 1950s, and 1960s, many women were treated with this drug for a history of first-trimester pregnancy losses. The drug was also used as treatment for vaginal bleeding in early pregnancy. The daughters of women treated with DES were later found to have a variety of reproductive tract problems including adenocarcinoma of the vagina and a characteristic pattern of reproductive tract problems including cervical hoods and T-shaped uterine cavities. The T shape was caused by enlargement of the fibromuscular bundles of the upper uterine cavity. The pregnancy implications of DES exposure vary widely. The increased risk for spontaneous abortion is approximately twofold among DES daughters. Similarly, the risk for preterm labor and ectopic pregnancy were three- and eightfold higher in this population of young women, respectively. It has been our experience that the more severe the hysterographic defect in uterine integrity the more likely these women are to suffer from infertility or recurrent pregnancy loss. The use of DES in pregnancy was discontinued in the mid-1960s and we will soon no longer see women exposed to the drug in utero in our gynecologic practices.

Acquired Defects of the Uterus

The acquired Mullerian defects that contribute to recurrent pregnancy loss are often underemphasized. Asherman's syndrome and uterine myomas (fibroids) are the source of a significant number of recurrent abortions. Complete or partial obliteration of the uterine cavity can have profound effects on distendability, implantation site, and blood supply in the uterus during nidation and early pregnancy. Women with significant intrauterine synechiae have clinical pregnancy loss rates varying from 25% to 80%. After hysteroscopic resection of these adhesions, the loss rates vary from 15% to 30% (i.e., in line with the expected miscarriage rates in a normal patient population). The most common source for Asherman's syndrome in the United States is vigorous sharp and/or repeated curettage following a spontaneous pregnancy loss. Infection is a common concomitant (if not obligatory) condition.

Submucosal uterine myomas can contribute to infertility as well as recurrent pregnancy loss. Between 10% and 30% of all or women have fibroid tumors of the uterus and the frequency is probably higher among African-Americans. Myomas can occur in a variety of locations and sizes, but those associated with recurrent pregnancy loss are most likely to be very large submucosal myomas distorting the cavity of the uterus. The presence of multiple myomas and intercavitary myomas produce spontaneous pregnancy loss rates varying from 20% to 80%. In addition, they have been associated with prematurity and premature rupture of the membranes. Large myomas can also interfere with the delivery process, making caesarean section difficult and providing significant dystocia if they are present in the lower uterine segment.

Cervical incompetence classically results in second- or third-trimester losses, though effacement can occur in the first trimester. Cervical trauma, such as cone biopsy, forced cervical dilatation, or an operative obstetric procedure, may precede cervical incompetence. DES exposure has also been implicated.

Chromosomal Rearrangements

Chromosomal rearrangements in the prospective parents are an important identifiable cause of recurrent pregnancy loss. The incidence of chromosomal rearrangements found in couples experiencing recurrent loss varies

TABLE 25-3. *Uterine defects leading to recurrent pregnancy loss*

Defect	Probability of loss
Congenital	
Diethylstilbestrol exposure in utero	High
Cervical incompetence	High
Fibromuscular septum	Moderate
Unicornuate uterus	Low
Uterus didelphys	Low
Bicornuate uterus	Low
Acquired	
Myomata uteri	Moderate
Asherman's syndrome	Moderate

from less than 2% to as high as 10% depending on the series (and more important, the center) at which the evaluation has occurred.

Among the random pregnancy loss patients, 40–50% of the patients have trisomies and 25–35% have sex chromosomal anomalies. Triploidy, another random chromosomal event, also contributes significantly. Recurrent losses, on the other hand, tend to be characterized by an extremely high percentage (>80%) of translocations. Thus, the pattern is one of random chromosomal mistakes in the normal population but inherited errors among people with recurrent pregnancy loss.

Translocation losses can occur from either maternal or paternal sources. Translocations may be reciprocal or Robertsonian. In about 4% of couples experiencing at least two abortions, one of the partners will have a balanced translocation. When a large series of cytogenetic investigations of couples with recurrent pregnancy losses are evaluated, it becomes evident that there is no preponderance of translocations transmitted by either the mother or the father. Chromosomal karyotyping of couples with recurrent pregnancy loss, although expensive, is a valuable way to identify those couples with chromosomal problems and provide precise risk estimates for continued recurrent losses and for the conception of chromosomally abnormal viable pregnancies. Karyotyping of the products of conception in a miscarriage may be cost-effective in the context of two previous losses.

Progesterone Deficiency

Progesterone is a critical hormone for the maintenance of early pregnancy. Secretory maturation of the endometrium is a progesterone- dependent phenomenon. Defects in the hormone's production or failure of the uterus to respond to circulating progesterone are associated with recurrent pregnancy loss. The incidence of luteal phase endometrial inadequacy (as determined by endometrial biopsy) in patients with recurrent spontaneous pregnancy loss has been reported variously from 10% to 60%.

The progesterone production critical to pregnancy begins during the luteal phase of the conception cycle. Concentrations of serum midluteal progesterone range from 10 to 20 ng/ml in normal cycles. In women with values below 10 ng/ml there is a significant incidence of failure of maturation of the uterine lining. Such failure is demonstrated by an "out-of-phase" endometrial biopsy. Luteal phase endometrial biopsies may be performed either in the midluteal time frame (about 7 days before anticipated menses) or in the late luteal phase (1 or 2 days prior to menses). Although disagreement exists about the most appropriate time to perform biopsy evaluation, it is generally agreed that the endometrial maturation (characterized by the criterion of Hertig and Noyes) must be greater than 48–72 hours in two different menstrual cycles to confirm luteal phase defect.

A second aspect of hormonally (progesterone) mediated pregnancy loss may be the phenomenon of premature corpus luteum failure during the early weeks of pregnancy. Progesterone levels should be 15–30 ng/ml in very early pregnancy; they eventually rise to 100–300 ng/ml by term. Caspo demonstrated that the corpus luteum is integral to maintenance of early pregnancy up to at least 7–8 weeks of gestation. Placental progesterone production begins at about the eighth week of gestation.

Several authors have demonstrated individual patients and occasionally small groups of patients with progesterone deficits in the presence of viable pregnancies. They have corrected these with the use of a variety of progesterone supplements and successfully achieved live births. Conclusive evidence of this problem as a cause of recurrent loss is lacking, however, and prospective randomized trials of both decreased progesterone levels in early viable pregnancy and treatment of such pregnancies with replacement hormone may never be accomplished due to the scarcity of such patients and the unwillingness of a woman with the problem to forego some form of therapy.

Systemic Disease

Systemic diseases can produce recurrent pregnancy loss. In general, systemic diseases of nonimmune origin are only associated with recurrent pregnancy loss when clinically evident.

Diabetes is the classic disorder that has been associated with recurrent pregnancy loss. When evaluating pregnancies by White's classification, women with class B, C, and higher diabetes have marginally higher incidences of pregnancy loss. However, when such loss is studied prospectively and correlated with diabetic control, it is evident that the poorer the blood sugar control in the diabetic, the greater the likelihood of pregnancy loss. Patients with hypothyroidism have a two- to threefold increased incidence of pregnancy loss, although the numbers of patients who conceive while significantly hypothyroid is small. There are few data on early pregnancy outcomes in women with active hyperthyroidism. Pregnancy loss in the patient with adrenal disease is also uncertain. Pregnancy is rare in patients with Cushing's disease because of menstrual abnormalities and high-level serum androgens. However, there is no evidence that patients with Cushing's disease who conceive have a higher incidence of pregnancy loss. Patients with Addison's disease seem to have a normal incidence of pregnancy loss and customarily only develop serious problems (usually related to mineralocorticoid and cortisol deficiency) in late pregnancy.

Infectious Causes

Bacterial colonizations with *Mycoplasma, Toxoplasma, Listeria,* group B *Streptococcus* (GBS), and

Chlamydia have been suggested as possible abortifacients. The prevalence of these organisms in pregnant women varies by the population under study. The recovery rate of mycoplasma and/or ureaplasma in sexually active women can exceed 50%. Vaginal colonization of GBS occurs in anywhere from 5% to 41% of pregnant women. The prevalence of *Chlamydia* in pregnant women has been reported from 2% to as high as 37%.

Although several organisms have been implicated as potential causes of spontaneous abortions, there is no good evidence to suggest an infectious etiology for *recurrent* pregnancy losses. Many of these organisms can be isolated from women with no history of spontaneous abortions. Data for recurrent pregnancy loss are inconclusive and therapy based on strictly scientific grounds is thus problematic.

Immunologic Infertility

Immunologic causes of recurrent pregnancy loss represent the newest and potentially most exciting area of diagnosis and treatment in this field. As a prelude to what follows, however, one must remember that much of the data regarding the true incidence of immunologic recurrent pregnancy loss are controversial. The techniques that are used to evaluate the problem are not perfect and may not represent the best method of diagnosis. Therapies for immunologic recurrent pregnancy loss are still in their seminal stages and none have yet conclusively demonstrated outcomes better than standard management of such pregnancies. Thus said, immunologic recurrent pregnancy loss may be divided into two categories:

1. Autoimmune pregnancy loss includes pregnancy losses associated with antiphospholipid syndromes. These may be detected by testing antinuclear, anticardiolipin, or a variety of antiphospholipid antibodies. Lupus anticoagulant, which may or may not be associated with the syndrome of systemic lupus erythematosus, may also be evaluated.
2. Alloimmune origins of pregnancy loss include maternal nonrecognition of paternal antigens, increased similarities of maternal and paternal antigen patterns, and paternal antigenic rejection. A variety of tools are currently used in the immunologic evaluation of alloimmune pregnancy loss. They include HLA sharing, evaluation of maternal blocking factor activity, mixed lymphocyte reactivity measurements, maternal antipaternal antibody determinations, and trophoblast antigen testing.

Pharmacologic and Environmental Toxins

Much of the literature regarding potential pharmacologic and environmental toxins is retrospective and contains methodologic flaws. However, several agents are believed to cause an increase in miscarriage and/or fetal anomalies. Pharmacologic agents known to increase the risk of pregnancy loss or fetal anomaly include mifepriston (RU-486), aminopterin, alcohol, isotretinoin (Accutane). Mifepriston is a progesterone antagonist. Aminopterin is a folic acid antagonist. Both agents have been used to induce termination of pregnancy. Fetuses not aborted following RU-486 exposure may suffer from malformations of the heart, brain, and ear. Infants not aborted after aminopterin also suffer from structural and functional anomalies. There is no risk if these drugs are used preconception. Isotretinoin (Accutane), a vitamin A congener used in the treatment of cystic acne, has been shown to increase pregnancy loss in animal models, and its oral and topical use are contraindicated in early pregnancy.

Alcohol is a known human teratogen that, either through direct action or secondary nutritional consequences of chronic excessive use, results in a pattern of defects known as "fetal alcohol syndrome." Even moderate alcohol use in the first trimester has been linked by epidemiologic evaluation to a 2.3-fold relative risk increase in spontaneous pregnancy loss. Smoking during pregnancy also appears to increase the risk of miscarriage in a dose–response fashion. Any adverse pregnancy outcome associated with radiation depends on the dose absorbed, the rate of exposure, and the gestational age at the time of exposure. Radiation at doses associated with diagnostic studies has not been shown to have an adverse effect on viable first- trimester pregnancy. Only therapeutic or accidental cytotoxic doses are known to affect the fetus.

Other Caveats

In addition to the classical sources of recurrent pregnancy loss, a variety of other factors must be considered. Spontaneous first-trimester pregnancy losses increase in the women beyond age 30 and are markedly increased after age 40. Stein et al. have demonstrated this association between maternal age and spontaneous abortion. The increase in incidence of spontaneous pregnancy losses beyond age 35 is in large measure accounted for by the increase in chromosomally abnormal abortions in this age group. There is, however, a small independent increase in the incidence of euploidic abortions as patients pass age 30. Couples should take this into consideration when they are given a prognosis for successful outcome of future pregnancies. Concurrent infertility is also relatively common among patients presenting with recurrent pregnancy loss.

EVALUATION AND THERAPY OF RECURRENT PREGNANCY LOSS

It is reasonable to begin the workup of the recurrent aborter after two spontaneous losses. The basic workup begins with a careful history (including a family history) for both members of the couple and an evaluation of medical records. A careful physical examination is part of every gynecologic patient's evaluation. Radiologic evaluation should include a hysterosalpingogram for evaluation of reproductive tract internal integrity. Laboratory examination includes midluteal progesterone levels and evaluation of early pregnancy progesterone levels. An endometrial biopsy is also helpful in the late luteal phase for evaluation of these patients. Chromosomal analyses of the parents is helpful.

The recurrent pregnancy loss work-up may be performed rapidly and directly (Table 25-4). Patients may be advised to use barrier contraception until the evaluation is complete. Immediately following presentation, the performance of a hysterosalpingogram, midluteal progesterone levels, endometrial biopsies, and blood chromosomes, as well as evaluation for systemic diseases involving the thyroid, the pancreas, and immunologic systems, should all be performed. Immunologic evaluation is generally deferred until other more classical etiologies of recurrent pregnancy loss have been ruled out.

The patient's reproductive and gynecologic history, laboratory, imaging, and physical or surgical findings play an important role in the counseling process of laying out the alternatives for treatment of repetitive pregnancy loss. The process of informing the patient about the physical and emotional costs of the therapeutic options and their likelihood of success can be meshed with the desires of the couple for treatment. Therapy is directed at an identified cause (Table 25-5).

COUNSELING AND FOLLOW-UP

The prognosis for subsequent normal pregnancy will depend on the etiology of recurrent pregnancy loss. Only in couples with genetic etiologies will overall prognosis of having a normal child fall below 50%. With anatomic factors, endocrine factors, and especially with unknown etiologies, success rates are around 70%. Canadian investigators have demonstrated that if followed in the long term, 80% of patients presenting with an initial diagnosis of recurrent pregnancy loss will have at least one viable child regardless of the etiology (or the workup or correction) of any existing deficiencies.

TABLE 25-4. *Basic evaluation for recurrent pregnancy loss*

History and physical examination
Hysterosalpingogram (or hysteroscopy) to exclude uterine anomalies
Hormonal evaluation of the woman (progesterone, thyroid, glucose)
Endometrial biopsy for luteal dysfunction
Chromosome studies of both the man and the woman for balanced translocation
Immunologic studies of both the man and woman

TABLE 25-5. *Proposed therapies for recurrent pregnancy loss*

Couples with demonstrated chromosomal abnormalities should receive genetic counseling. Decisions should be made depending on the risk of further problems in subsequent pregnancies.
Uterine abnormalities may be treated surgically, particularly by operative hysteroscopy.
Endocrine abnormalities can be treated by ovulation induction with gonadotropins (Pergonal or Metrodin), clomiphene, or progesterone supplementation. Thyroid problems or diabetes should be treated specifically.
Immunologic causes can be treated with heparin, aspirin, prednisone, or a combination of these. More sophisticated, investigational therapies include paternal or donor antigen exposure.
Cessation of alcohol and tobacco use.
Couples with a workup yielding no obvious cause of losses should be reassured regarding prognosis. Discussion of empiric therapies may include progesterone supplementation, low-dose aspirin, or heparin.

CONCLUSIONS

The odds of losing a pregnancy in the first trimester are about 1 in 6. Careful history and pathologic proof of pregnancy losses are essential to making the diagnosis prior to initiating a workup. A workup should be initiated after two to three pregnancy losses, but this may be mitigated by the clinical circumstances (eg, patient's age). The evaluation of recurrent pregnancy loss should be done before another pregnancy begins and is often extended into the early stages of the pregnancy itself. Couples should be counseled carefully and reassured that the overwhelming majority of couples with unexplained recurrent losses will eventually have a normal baby.

SUGGESTED READING

Brent RL, Beckman DA. The contribution of environmental teratogens to embryonic and fetal loss. *Clin Obstet Gynecol* 1994;37:646.

Coulam CB, ed. Recurrent pregnancy loss. *Clin Obstet Gynecol* 1986;29:4.

Coulam CB, Clark DA, Collins J, Scott JR, Schlesselman JJ. A worldwide collaborative observational study and meta-analysis on allogenic leukocyte immunotherapy for recurrent spontaneous abortion. *Am J Reprod Immunol* 1994;23:55.

Dodson MG, Gast MJ. Early pregnancy. In: Dodson MG, ed. *Transvaginal Ultrasound.* New York: Churchill-Livingstone, 1995;187.

Faulk WP, Coulam CB, McIntyre JA. Recurrent pregnancy loss. In: Seibel MM, ed. *Infertility: A Comprehensive Text.* East Norwalk, CT: Appleton and Lange, 1990;273.

Gilchrist DM, Livingston JE, Hulburt JA, Wilson RD. Recurrent spontaneous pregnancy loss. *J Reprod Med* 1991;36:3.

Giudice LC. The endocrinology of recurrent spontaneous abortion. In: Brody SA, Ueland K, eds. *Endocrine Disorders in Pregnancy.* Norwalk, CT: Appleton and Lange, 1989;467.

Mowbray JF, Liddell H, Underwood JL, Gibbings C, Reginald PW, Beard RW. Controlled trial of treatment of recurrent spontaneous abortion by immunization with paternal cells. *Lancet* 1985;1:941.

O'Shea DL, Gast MJ. Recurrent pregnancy loss. In: Jacobs AJ, Gast MJ, eds. *Practical Gynecology.* Norwalk, CT: Appleton and Lange, 1994;308.

Palifka JE, Friedman JM. Environmental toxins and recurrent pregnancy loss. *Clin North Am 1991;*2:1.

Reece EA, Gabrielli S, Cullen MT, Zheng XZ, Hobbins JC, Harris E. Recurrent adverse pregnancy outcome and antiphospholipid antibodies. *Am J Obstet Gynecol* 1990;162:1.

Scott JR, Branch DW. Potential alloimmune factors and immunotherapy in recurrent miscarriage. *Clin Obstet Gynecol* 1994;37:761.

Scott JR, Rate NS, Branch DW. Immunologic aspects of recurrent abortion and fetal death. *Obstet Gynecol* 1987;70:4.

Speroff L, Glass RH, Kase NG. Recurrent early pregnancy losses. In: *Clinical Gynecologic Endocrinology and Infertility*. Baltimore: Williams and Wilkins, 1994;841.

Yazigi RA, Saunders EK, Gast MJ. Hormonal therapy during early pregnancy. *Contemp Ob/Gyn* 1991;l36:61.

Clinical Reproductive Medicine,
Edited by Bryan D. Cowan and David B. Seifer
Lippincott-Raven Publishers, Philadelphia © 1997

CHAPTER 26

Reproductive Immunology

William A. Bennett

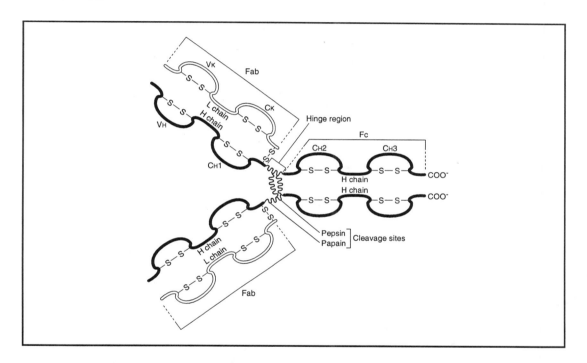

Basic Concepts in Immunology
  Effector Cells of the Immune Response
  Antigens and the Immune Response
  Major Histocompatibility Complex
  Structure and Function of Antibodies
  Cytokines and the Immune Response
Immunology of Pregnancy
  Selective Antigen Expression
  Trophoblast Resistance to Immune Effector Cells
  Immunosuppression by Pregnancy-Associated Factors
  Enhanced Trophoblast Function
Immunologic Mechanisms of Abortion
  Suppressor Cell Deficiency

Induction of Trophoblast Antigen Expression
  Antiphospholipid Antibodies
Immunologic Infertility
  Antisperm Antibodies and Infertility
  Male Sperm Autoimmunity
  Etiology of Sperm Antibodies
  Testing for Sperm Antibodies
  Autoimmunity in the Female
Contraceptive Vaccines
  Antizona Pellucida Vaccine Development
  Antisperm Antigen Vaccines
Summary
Suggested Reading

W. A. Bennett: Department of Obstetrics and Gynecolgy, University of Mississippi Medical Center, Jackson MS 39216-4505

Reproductive immunology is a rapidly expanding field that significantly affects human reproduction. Major topics in this field include (1) mechanisms responsible for the survival of the "fetal allograft"; (2) immunologic causes of early pregnancy loss; (3) antisperm antibodies and their relationship to infertility; and (4) development of contraceptive vaccines based on antibodies to gamete antigens or reproductive hormones.

BASIC CONCEPTS IN IMMUNOLOGY

Before considering some of the major problems addressed in the field of reproductive immunology, a basic understanding of the immune system is necessary. Molecules that evoke immune responses and react with antibodies are referred to as *antigens*. The various antigens are recognized by *lymphocytes*, each possessing cell surface receptors that can recognize a specific antigen configuration. The two major groups of lymphocytes are the *B lymphocytes* (bone marrow–derived lymphocytes or B cells) and the *T lymphocytes* (thymus-dependent lymphocytes or T cells).

Effector Cells of the Immune Response

Lymphocytes are characterized by centrally located round nuclei, the lack of specific granules, and basophilic cytoplasm with free ribosomes. The morphologic similarity of the different subsets of lymphocytes has led to the use of monoclonal antibodies to cell surface markers to distinguish the different lymphocyte subclasses (Table 26-1).

The initial T-cell marker was identified following the observation that subpopulations of human lymphocytes bind sheep red blood cells, forming rosettes. It was determined that the sheep red blood cells bind to a 55-kd glycoprotein on the lymphocyte surface, an antigen termed CD2. Mature T cells express CD2 along with another surface antigen called CD3. Additional subsets of T cells have been identified and characterized using monoclonal antibodies to other cell surface antigens. CD4 (57-kd surface protein) can be detected on 50–65% of peripheral T cells, whereas CD8 (32-kd glycoprotein) is found on 25–35% of T lymphocytes. The CD4+ T cells recognize antigens presented in association with major histocompatibility class II molecules (see "Major Histocompatibility Complex"). CD8+ T cells recognized antigen associated with major histocompatibility complex (MHC) class I molecules (HLA-A, HLA-B, and HLA-C antigens). The CD4+ cells can also be subdivided based on their reaction to antibodies generated to surface antigens 2_H4 and 2_B4 and serum from patients with juvenile rheumatoid arthritis (JRA). One subset of CD4+ cells (2_B4+, 2_H4-, JRA-) are referred to as *helper-induced T cells*. These cells induce B cells to produce antibodies and proliferate in response to soluble antigen. Helper T cells do not proliferate in response to mitogen (concanavalin A, ConA) or autologous cells (mixed lymphocyte reaction, MLC). Another set of CD4+ T cells are the *suppressor-inducer T cells*, which are 2_B4-, 2_H4+, and JRA+. These cells proliferate in response to mitogen and autologous cells but do not respond to soluble antigens. They induce CD8+ T cells which suppress antibody production by B cells.

B cells are the antibody-producing cells of the immune system and can be identified by the presence of immunoglobulin on their surface. These cells comprise 5–15% of the peripheral blood lymphocytes. Under the combined effects of antigen, T-cell products (lymphokines), and accessory cells, B cells differentiate into *plasma cells*, the cells responsible for antibody production. B cells express a complement receptor (CR-2) and receptors for the Epstein–Barr virus and the Fc portion of IgG. Another commonly used marker for B cells is CD20, a 35-kd phosphoprotein. Plasma cells are larger than lymphocytes, no longer bear surface immunoglobulin, and are terminally differentiated.

Null cells are a subset of peripheral blood lymphocytes that lack the surface markers for either T or B cells. The greatest portion of these cells are *natural killer (NK) cells* that possess both complement C3 and Fc receptors. These cells are large granular lymphocytes that express nonspecific killing activity against a number of tumor cell lines.

TABLE 26-1. *Classification of human lymphocytes*

Class	Marker	Subsets	Restrictions	Functions
T cells	1. CD4+	a. Helper-inducer	MHC class II	Stimulate B cells to produce Ab, induce CD8+ CTL cells
		b. Suppressor-inducer	MHC class II	Induce CD8+ suppressor T cells to suppress Ab production by B cells
	2. CD8+	a. Suppressor	MHC class I	Inhibit Ab production by B cells
		b. Cytotoxic cells	MHC class I	Lyse antigen-bearing cells
NK cells	1. NKH1+	a. CD2+, NKH1+, CD3-, CD4-, CD8-		
	2. CD2+	b. CD2+, NKH1+, CD3+, CD4-, CD8+		
		c. CD2+, NKH1+, CD3+, CD4-, CD8-	Non-MHC- restricted	Kill tumor cell lines, exhibit antimicrobial activity
B cells	Smlg-+	—	Antigen-specific	Differentiate into AB-producing Smlg-plasma cells or memory B cells

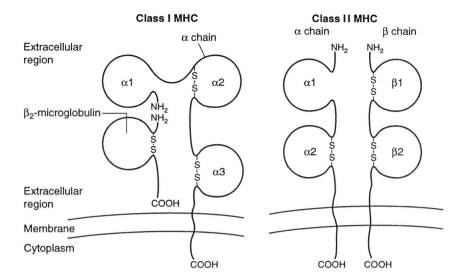

FIG. 26-1. Structure of class I and class II MHC molecules.

Natural killer cells lack the CD3 T-cell receptor and do not depend on the T-cell antigen receptor for recognition of their targets. These cells express the CD2 surface marker and can be identified by a 200-kd glycoprotein surface antigen referred to as NKH1.

Monocytes are large mononuclear cells that compose 3–8% of peripheral blood leukocytes. They have increased cytoplasm in comparison to other lymphocytes and have an eccentric and oval-shaped nucleus. Monocytes possess lysosomes that appear as vacuoles in the cytoplasm and contain degradative enzymes. They are derived from promonocytes, rapidly dividing cells of bone marrow origin. Upon entry to the peripheral blood system, these cells are referred to as monocytes. When these cells migrate to the tissues they undergo additional changes and are known as *macrophages*. Macrophages present antigen to lymphocytes and serve as effector cells mounting responses to microorganisms and neoplastic cells. Macrophages possess receptors for antibody and complement that increase their ability to phagocytize organisms coated with these materials. They also possess receptors for certain lymphokines, such as migration inhibitor factor (MIF) and interferon-γ (IFNγ). Macrophages produce several soluble factors that mediate the immune response, including interleukin-1 (IL-1) and tumor necrosis factor (TNF).

Antigens and the Immune Response

An *antigen* can be broadly defined as any substance that elicits an immune response. Such an immune response involves reaction with T cells and B cells to induce formation of antibody and sensitized lymphocytes. Under the appropriate conditions, a wide range of molecules can produce an immune response, and in abnormal states the body can mount immune attacks against self antigens.

Major Histocompatibility Complex

A critical feature of the immune system is its ability to discriminate between self and nonself antigens. This discrimination is accomplished by molecules of the *major histocompatibility complex* (MHC) (Figure 26-1). Both self and nonself antigens are recognized by T cells only when presented in association with MHC antigens. Helper T cells (CD4+) recognize antigens in conjunction with class II molecules, whereas cytotoxic T cells (CD8+) recognize antigens associated with class I antigens. During embryogenesis, a process termed *T-cell education* occurs during which T cells that recognize "self" antigens in combination with MHC molecules are eliminated. Those T cells that recognize foreign antigens are selected for survival.

The antigens encoded by the MHC are referred to as the *human leukocyte antigens* (HLA) and the genes that encode them fall into two major categories. Classes I and II MHC antigens are cell surface glycoproteins that are members of the immunoglobulin supergene family (Table 26-2). These molecules can be further classified on the basis of their structure, tissue distribution, and function.

Class I MHC molecules include the HLA-A, -B, and -C molecules. The heavy or α chain (44 kd) is a polymorphic

TABLE 26-2. *Comparison of class I and class II major histocompatibility antigens*

Properties	Class I	Class II
Antigens included	HLA -A, -B, -C	HLA -D, -DR, -DQ, -DP
Tissue distribution type	Virtually every cell, particularly B	Restricted to immune cells and macrophages
Functions	Present processed antigen fragments to CD8+ T cells	Present processed antigen fragments to CD4+ T cells

glycoprotein determined by genes in the HLA complex on chromosome 6. It is noncovalently linked to a non-polymorphic 12-kd protein, β_2-microglobulin, determined by a gene on chromosome 15. The entire class I molecule is anchored in the cell membrane by the 44-kd α chain (Fig. 26-1). Class I molecules are present on all nucleated cells and play a critical role in the immune response. Antigens must be presented in association with a class I molecule to be recognized by cytotoxic T cells (CD8+) (Fig. 26-2). This requirement is called *HLA restriction*. Following recognition, the cytotoxic T cell kills the target cell expressing the presented antigen. For example, in transplant rejection, foreign class I molecules are recognized by the host CD8 T lymphocytes during graft rejection.

Class II MHC molecules are heterodimers consisting of an α (34 kd) and β (29 kd) glycoprotein in noncovalent association (see Fig. 26-1). The HLA-DR, DQ, and DP genetic loci determine the class II antigens. Class II molecules have a limited cellular distribution, existing only on immunocompetent cells, B cells, antigen-presenting cells (macrophages and dendritic cells), and activated T cells. Some cell types that do not normally express class II molecules (resting T cells, endothelial cells, thyroid cells) can be induced to express them. Class II molecules function in the presentation of processed antigenic peptide fragments to helper T cells (CD8+) during initiation of the immune response (see Fig. 26-2). In transplantation immunity, class II molecules that have bound antigenic peptides on the host cells elicit a response from the ingrafted donor T cells resulting in a graft-versus-host reaction.

In summary, the HLA system contains a number of genes that are crucial to the initiation, regulation, and suc-cessful completion of an immune response. It is composed of the HLA-A, B, and C genes that encode the class I molecules and the HLA-DR, DQ, and DP subregions that encode the class II HLA molecules. These molecules are responsible for the presentation of foreign antigens to cytotoxic and helper T cells, which play critical roles in the immune response to foreign antigens and microorganisms.

Structure and Function of Antibodies

Antibodies are a heterogeneous group of serum proteins called *immunoglobulins*. They are produced by differentiated B cells termed plasma cells. Five different classes of immunoglobulins have been identified in human serum including IgG, IgM, IgA, IgD, and IgE. The clonal selection theory of antibody production states that one plasma cell produces only one specific antibody. Immunoglobulin monomers are comprised of two identical heavy chains and two identical light chains (Fig. 26-3). Each light chain is bound to a heavy chain by disulfide bonds (S-S) and the heavy chains are also attached by one or more of these bonds. Human immunoglobulins may appear as monomers (forms of IgG, IgA1, IgA2, and IgD), dimers (IgA), or pentamers (IgM). The amino acid sequence and disulfide binding patterns of the molecules contribute to their structure.

There are five general classes of immunoglobulins and each class contains its own specific heavy chain (Table 26-3). *IgG* is the principal serum immunoglobulin and is the final antibody produced following antigenic challenge. IgG is not produced by the fetus but crosses the placenta resulting in maternal antibodies in the newborn. Antibodies of the IgG class coat microorganisms, toxins,

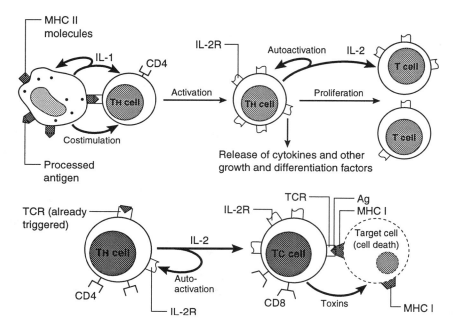

FIG. 26-2. Processing of antigen by CD4+ and CD8+ lymphocytes. CD4+ cells recognize foreign antigens when they are expressed in association with class II molecules.

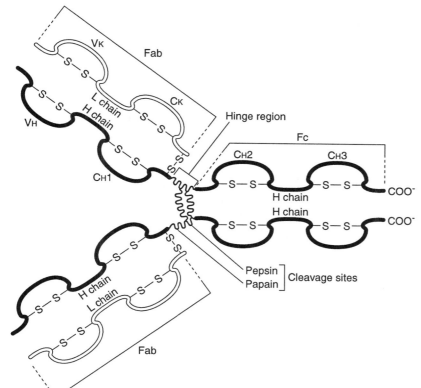

FIG. 26-3. Structure of human immunoglobulin. Human immunoglobulin consists of two heavy chains linked by disulfide bonds to two light chains.

and viruses and make them susceptible to phagocytosis or neutralization.

IgA is the predominant immunoglobulin in body secretions and is released as a dimer by localized plasma cells. Detectable levels can be identified in saliva, tears, colostrum, respiratory and gastrointestinal tracts, vaginal secretions, and the prostate. IgA can bind with a polypeptide (secretory piece) produced by the local epithelial cells. This allows IgA to be resistant to proteolytic digestion and permits active transport across the mucosal epithelium by endocytosis. Functions of IgA in the immune response include neutralization of viruses and bacteria preventing their attachment to mucosal surfaces.

IgM is a pentamer isolated primarily in serum where it makes up 10% of all immunoglobulins. IgM is highly efficient in agglutinating bacteria and red blood cells. IgM

is the initial immunoglobulin produced in response to antigen stimulation. IgM-producing cells do not become memory cells; therefore, additional challenges with the same antigen do not produce more IgM antibody than the initial response. The majority of B cells have IgM and IgD on their surface.

Monomeric *IgD* occurs in the serum in low levels and in relatively high concentrations in umbilical cord blood. Plasma cells with the ability to produce IgD have been isolated in the tonsils and adenoids but are very rare in other lymphoid tissues. The role of IgD in the human immune response is not known.

IgE is found in trace amounts in human serum, composing 0.004% of the total immunoglobulins. IgE binds to mast cells and basophils. IgE plays a primary role in the immune reactions in hay fever, extrinsic asthma, wheal-and-flare reactions, and anaphylaxis. Plasma cells

TABLE 26-3. *Classification and properties of human immunoglobulins*

Property	IgG	IgA	IgM	IgD	IgE
Molecular weight (kd)	160	170–340	970	184	188
Serum concentration (mg/dl)	1250	279	120	0.3–30.0	0.002–0.200
% Carbohydrate	3	8	12	13	12
Light chain	k, λ	k, λ	K, λ	k, λ	k, λ
Heavy chain	1λ, 2λ, 3λ, 4λ	α1, α2	μ	δ	ξ
J chain	No	In dimer	Yes	No	No
Serum half-life (days)	23	6	5	3	2.5

that produce IgE are found in the tonsils, adenoids, and mucosa of the gastrointestinal and respiratory tracts.

Cytokines and the Immune Response

Cytokines are an important group of peptide mediators that regulate immunologic, inflammatory, and reparative host responses. Cytokines produced by lymphocytes have been termed lymphokines, whereas those of macrophage origin are called monokines. An additional system of nomenclature refers to cytokines as interleukins, with regard to the ability of these soluble factors to communicate between different populations of leukocytes. Cytokines are usually present in very low levels in serum and normally act either in a paracrine (locally near the producing cells) or autocrine fashion (on the producing cells) rather than on distant target cells. With the exception of some transformed cell lines, normal resting cells must be activated to produce cytokines. Cytokines exert their regulatory effects by increasing or decreasing cell proliferation, altering cell differentiation, or changing differentiated functions. Cytokines share a number of common features that include (1) *ambiguity*—cytokines tend to have multiple target cells and actions; (2) *redundancy*—several cytokines may elicit the same response; (3) *synergism/antagonism*—exposure of cells to two or more cytokines at a time may lead to different responses; (4) *cytokine cascade*—a cytokine may increase or decrease the production of another cytokine; and (5) *receptor transmodulation*—a cytokine may increase or decrease the expression of receptors for another cytokine. Table 26-4 gives a brief description of the cytokines that regulate the afferent and efferent phases of the immune response.

Interleukins

Interleukin-1 (IL-1) is a cytokine produced primarily in response to inflammation, injury, immunologic challenge, or infection. Two distinct genes exist for IL-1, coding for proteins termed IL-1α and IL-1β, respectively. Although both forms of IL-1 have a molecular weight of approximately 17 kd, they only share approximately 26% amino acid homology. A third member of the IL-1 gene family is the IL-1 receptor antagonist (IL-1RA).

IL-1 is produced by a wide range of cell types including macrophages, smooth muscle cells, endothelial cells, neutrophils, fibroblasts, T-cell clones, astrocytes, dendritic cells, and keratinocytes. Macrophages can be stimulated to produce IL-1 by agents that activate lymphocytes, acting through either direct contact between the cells (controlled by class II MHC molecules) or the production of lymphokines such as TNF, colony-stimulating factor (CSF), or γ-IFN. IL-1 acts on target cells through high-affinity membrane receptors on the target cells. These receptors are downregulated by internalization after binding of IL-1. IL-1 stimulates the proliferation of T lymphocytes by increasing the production of lymphokines such as IL-2 and augments the expression of IL-2 receptors on T cells. IL-1 also enhances the ability of antigen-presenting cells to stimulate T-cell-dependent immune responses. In addition to these effects on T cells, IL-1 can stimulate B-cell proliferation, surface immunoglobulin receptor expression, and antibody production.

IL-1 is a potent inducer of hypotension and shock and can be lethal in animals. Intravenous administration of IL-1 in animals leads to an increase in body temperature as a result of elevated levels of prostaglandin E_2 (PGE-2).

TABLE 26-4. *Characteristics and functions of the various cytokines involved in the immune response*

Cytokine	Molecular weight	Primary source	Principal activity
IL-1	17,500	Macrophages	Inflammatory, hematopoietic
IL-2	15,500	T lymphocytes, LGL	T- and B-cell growth factor
IL-3	14,000–28,000	T lymphocytes	Hematopoietic growth factor
IL-4	20,000	Th cells	T- and B-cell growth factor
IL-5	18,000	Th cells	Stimulates B cells, eosinophils
IL-6	22,000–30,000	Fibroblasts	Growth factor for B cells and polyclonal Ig synthesis
IL-7	25,000	Stromal cells	Generates pre-B and -T cells, lymphocyte growth factor
IL-8	8,800	Macrophages	Chemoattracts neutrophils and T lymphocytes
IL-9	30,000–40,000	T_H2 T cells	Promotion of mast cell proliferation
IL-10	18,000	T_H2 T cells	Inhibits macrophage activity and T_H1 cytokine production
IL-11	23,000	Stromal fibroblasts	Stimulates erythropoiesis, early hematopoiesis, and neuronal differentiation
IL-12	75,000	Activated macrophage	Modulates NK cell function, stimulates TH, cell responses
IL-13	10,000	T_{H2} T cells	Upregulates MHC class II expression, induces B-cell proliferation
G-CSF	18,000–20,000	Monocytes	Myeloid growth factor
M-CSF	18,000–26,000	Monocytes	Macrophage growth factor
GM-CSF	14,000–38,000	T cells	Monomyelocytic growth factor
IFNα	18,000–20,000	Leukocytes	IFNα, IFNβ, and IFNγ (1) stimulate macrophages and NK cells and (2) induce cell membrane antigens
IFNβ	25,000	Fibroblasts	
IFNγ	20,000–25,000	T cells and NK cells	
TNFα	17,000	Macrophages and others	Inflammatory, immunoenhancing, tumoricidal
TNFβ	18,000	T lymphocytes	
TGFβ	25,000	Platelets, bone, etc.	Fibroplasia and immunosuppression

In humans, administration of an IL-1 receptor antagonist reduces death rates in patients with septic shock syndrome.

Interleukin-2 (IL-2) is a 15,400-kd peptide produced by activated lymphocytes. It stimulates proliferation and lymphokine production by B cells, T cells, and NK cells. The biological effects of IL-2 are mediated through its binding to specific receptors present on target cells. The high-affinity receptor for IL-2 comprises three subunits: (1) 55-kd α chain (IL-2Rα, Tac, p55), (2) 70- to 75-kd β chain (IL-2Rβ, p70–75), and (3) 64-kdγ chain (IL-2Rγ, p64). Antigen presentation is required to activate lymphocytes to maximally respond to IL-2. This IL-2-responsive state of the activated T cell is the result of expression of high-affinity IL-2 receptors. The binding of IL-2 to its high-affinity cellular receptor promotes the rapid clonal expansion of the effector T-cell population originally activated by antigen. This is followed by a decline in IL-2 synthesis and receptor expression resulting in a termination of the T-cell response.

In addition to T cells, other lymphoid cells respond to IL-2. B cells activated by antigen or mitogen bear high-affinity IL-2R, though at lower levels than activated T cells. IL-2 also supports B-cell growth, initiates immunoglobulin G (IgG) secretion, and induces J-chain synthesis leading to the assembly and secretion of IgM. NK cells also constitutively express receptors for IL-2 (IL-2Rβ), proliferate in response to high doses of IL-2, and exhibit enhanced cytolytic activity.

Culture of normal resting T cells in high concentrations of IL-2 results in the expansion of a class of lymphoid cells with enhanced cytotoxic activity against tumor cells. These lymphokine-activated killer (LAK) cells are under investigation as potential tools for adaptive immunotherapy.

The biological significance of the IL-2/IL-2R system can be illustrated by various clinical syndromes and animal models. T cells from patients with adult T-cell leukemia/lymphoma syndrome display high levels of IL-2Rα. Mice who are deficient in IL-2 production exhibit normal thymocyte and peripheral T-cell development and become severely immunocompromised during further maturation. Mice with a genetic defect in the region cloning for IL-2R are characterized by severely impaired cell-mediated and humoral immune responses. Thus, the IL-2/IL-2R system plays a critical role in normal immune function.

Interleukin-3 (IL-3) is a 14- to 28-kd polypeptide produced by activated T cells. It promotes the growth of multilineage colonies such as marrow colonies derived from a single stem cell containing granulocytes, monocytes, erythrocytes, and megakaryocytes at different stages of differentiation.

IL-3 has been cited to act as a link between the immune system and the hematopoietic system responsible for the generation of phagocytic and granulocytic cells that mediate defense and repair. IL-3 and other cytokines released during the stress response increase blood cell production and modulate the types of cells produced. This stress response involves acceleration of normal hematopoietic mechanisms and the overriding of normal processes that regulate the proportions of the different cell types produced.

Interleukin-4 (IL-4) is a 20-kd peptide produced by T-helper cells and mast cells. It stimulates the proliferation of B cells which have been previously activated by T-cell-dependent or independent antigens. IL-4 acts with IL-2 to stimulate B-cell growth and regulates immunoglobulin isotype expression, increasing IgE and decreasing some forms of IgG production by activated B cells. It also acts on non-lymphoid cells serving as a T-cell mitogen and as a growth factor for mast cells. Along with CSF, IL-4 stimulates the growth of hematopoietic precursors and induces the differentiation of mature myeloid cells. Finally, IL-4 stimulates the cytocidal function of macrophages and increases the expression of class II MHC antigens on macrophages and B cells. IL-4 binds to high-affinity receptors that are expressed in low numbers on virtually every cell type tested, including T and B lymphocytes, monocytes, granulocytes, fibroblasts, epithelial and endothelial cells.

IL-4 also plays an important role in the function of the T_H2 subclass of T cells. Recent studies with murine helper CD4+ T-cell clones have indicated the present of two cell types on the basis on their pattern of cytokine synthesis: (1) T-helper$_1$ (T_H1) cells secrete IL-2, IFNγ, and TNFα; and (2) T-helper$_2$ (T_H2) cells secrete IL-4, IL-5, and IL-10. Both types of cells secrete cytokines such as GM-CSF and IL-3. Human CD4+ T-cell clones have been found to exhibit T_H1- or T_H2-like cytokine production profiles. T_H1 and T_H2 cells are thought to differentiate from a common precursor pool controlled by cytokines from lymphocytes or accessory cells. IFNγ and IL-12 promote differentiation of precursors into T_H1 cells, while IL-4 induces differentiation into the T_H2 subclass. T_H1 cells induce macrophage activation, resulting in delayed-type hypersensitivity responses and the killing of intracellular parasites. T_H2 cells control humoral responses including the production of IgE and eosinophils. These two cell networks exert regulatory influences on each other. For example, IFNγ suppresses IL-4-induced B-cell activation, whereas IL-4 inhibits IL-2-induced T- and B-lymphocyte proliferation. IFNγ also inhibits T_H2 proliferation, whereas IL-4 and IL-10 inhibit cytokine production by T_H1 cells.

From these studies it is apparent that IL-4 plays an important role in immune responses to foreign antigens, especially as it applies to humoral immune responses.

Interleukin-5 (IL-5) is a glycoprotein produced by T lymphocytes with a molecular weight of 40–45 kd. Nearly half of the secreted IL-5 consists of carbohydrate.

IL-5 is the principal cytokine-mediating eosinophilia, a condition characteristic of a limited number of disease states, especially parasitic infections and allergy. Eosinophils are present in low numbers in normal individuals but can increase independently of the number of neutrophils. IL-3 and G-CSF are also involved in the induction of IL-5-responsive eosinophil precursor cells.

Interleukin-6 (IL-6) (22–30 kd) exhibits a variety of biological effects on multiple cell types. It is produced by T and B cells, monocytes, endothelial cells, epithelial cells, and fibroblasts. A number of stimuli induce the production of IL-6 including TNF, IL-1, platelet-derived growth factor, antigens, mitogens, and bacterial endotoxin. IL-6 enhances the ability of activated B cells to secrete immunoglobulins. It acts as a T-cell- activating factor or T-cell costimulant. IL-6 augments the proliferation of thymocytes and T cells stimulated with phytohemagglutinin (PHA) through IL-2-dependent and independent pathways and enhances IL-2 production and the expression of the high-affinity IL-2 receptor.

IL-6 acts on activated B cells to induce IgM, IgG, and IgA production. Anti-IL-6 antibody inhibits IL-4-driven IgE production, suggesting that endogenous IL-6 plays an obligatory role in the IL-4- dependent induction of IgE. In addition to antigenic stimulation, additional signals such as IL-2 are required for B cells to acquire IL-6 responsiveness.

IL-6 also plays a number of important roles in T-cell activation, growth, and differentiation. These include (1)induction of the IL-2 receptor, (2) promotion of growth of T cells stimulated with PHA, (3) induction of thymocyte proliferation, (4) enhancement of thymocyte proliferation in response to IL-4, and (5) synergism with IL-1 and IL-6 to induce IL-2 production and IL-2Ra expression.

IL-6 can induce a variety of acute phase proteins by hepatocytes including fibrinogen, α_1-antichymotryspin, and α_1-acid glycoprotein. Serum levels of IL-6 positively correlate with C-reactive proteins and fever in patients with burns. An increase in IL-6 has been observed prior to elevations in C-reactive protein in patients undergoing surgical operations, supporting a causal role of IL-6 in acute phase responses.

Increasing experimental evidence suggests that deregulated production of IL-6 is involved in a variety of diseases including inflammation, autoimmune diseases, and malignancies. Abnormal elevations in IL-6 have been noted in a number of disease states including cardiac myxoma, pulmonary tuberculosis, Cattleman's disease, and rheumatoid arthritis. The critical role of IL-6 in T-cell activation suggests that overproduction of IL-6 may play a critical role in autoimmune diseases.

Interleukin-7 (IL-7) (25 kd) is produced by stromal cells of the bone marrow. Its primary role is to stimulate proliferation and maturation of T- and B-cell progenitors. IL-7 also has been cited to have hematopoietic properties through the stimulation of myeloid precursors and megakaryocytes to produce colony-forming units and platelets.

Interleukin-8 (IL-8) has been primarily characterized as a neutrophil-associated protein. Although first isolated from stimulated leukocytes, IL-8 can be produced by a wide variety of cell types in response to other cytokines. Fibroblasts, endothelial cells, epithelial cells, smooth muscle cells, and a variety of more specialized cell types can produce IL-8 in response to the primary cytokines IL-1 and TNFα. It can also be produced by neutrophils and under some conditions can be considered as an autocrine chemotactic factor. After bacterial infection, IL-6 and IL-8 are efficiently produced by peripheral blood monocytes, whereas fibroblasts exhibit similar responses during viral infections. Endogenous IL-1 from monocytes can efficiently stimulate the release of the secondary cytokines IL-6 and IL-8.

High-affinity receptors for IL-8 have been identified on the surface of human neutrophils that bind IL-8 but not IL-1 or TNFα. Lower levels of receptor expression have also been noted on various leukocytes, including T cells and monocyte cell lines. Lymphocyte migration induced by IL-8 is specifically inhibited by Ca^{2+} channel antagonists. Interleukin-8 (IL-8) also activates kinases resulting in protein phosphorylation. IL-8 stimulates neutrophil migration and phagocytosis. The predominant effect of IL-8 injection in humans is neutrophil accumulating in proximity to dermal blood vessels. Clinically, IL-8 was first demonstrated in skin lesions of psoriasis patients. IL-8 may play a role in hyperproliferation and chemotaxis of keratinocytes. Cytokines, hormones, cyclooxygenase products, antioxidants, and immunosuppressive agents can promote a negative feedback for IL-8 production.

Interleukin-9 (IL-9) is a 30- to 40-kd glycoprotein produced by T_H2 lymphocytes. This cytokine was initially characterized based on its synergism with IL-3 or IL-4 in the promotion of mast cell proliferation. IL-9 has subsequently been described as a T_H2 factor that interacts with other cytokines to influence mast cell responses and T-cell oncogenesis.

In vitro responsiveness to IL-9 is not a characteristic of a defined T-cell population but is gradually acquired by the maintenance of cells in long-term culture. This process resembles certain types of malignant transformation. In humans, an association has been cited between dysregulated IL-9 expression and lymphoid malignancies such as Hodgkin's and large cell anaplastic lymphomas. In addition, an association has been suggested between IL-9 production and the mucosal mast cell hyperplasia induced by worm infections, especially in cases where IL-3 and IL-4 secretion is limited.

Interleukin-10 (IL-10) is a cytokine first discovered as a result of studies examining a factor produced by T_H2 cells, which inhibited the formation of T_H1 cells. This cytokine inhibits macrophage functions, including antigen presentation to T_H1 cells, cytokine synthesis, and microbial activities. IL-10 generally enhances or stimulates mast cells and B cells. IL-10 inhibits cytokine production in cultures of T_H1 cells, antigen-presenting cells, and antigen.

IL-10 inhibits the synthesis of several cytokines normally secreted by both human and mouse monocytes/macrophages in response to lipopolysaccharide (LPS). These cytokines include GM-CSF, IL-1, TNF, IL-6, IL-8, and IL-12. IFNγ and IL-10 are antagonistic, with each inhibiting the synthesis of the other. IL-10 also inhibits expression of MHC class II antigens on certain class of monocytes and macrophages. IL-10 enhances the proliferation of mast cells in synergy with other cytokines such as IL-3 or IL-4. IL-10 induces the differentiation of human B cells and synergizes with TGFβ to induce IgA production.

During pregnancy the maternal immune response shows enhanced antibody responses but reduced DHT (T_H1-like) reactions. This may be associated with the observation that IL-10 and other T_H2 cytokines are expressed constitutively at high levels in placental tissues. IL-10 messenger RNA (mRNA) has been localized by in situ hybridization to the maternal–fetal interface. Local T_H2 responses may be important to protect the fetus from the known damaging effects of NK cells and T_H1-like responses. A less desirable side effect of this local T_H2 bias may be a systemic inhibition of the mother's immune system, resulting in increased susceptibility to intracellular pathogens.

In summary, IL-10 appears to have a variety of functions, particularly those involving the inhibition of macrophage activation and function. The in vivo production of IL-10 is often associated with T_H2-like responses and suppression of cell-mediated immunity. IL-10 can be deleterious in situations when a cell-mediated response is appropriate, such as during infections with intracellular pathogens. In contrast, IL-10 may have advantageous effects in situations such as autoimmune disease, transplantation, and pregnancy where T_H1 responses would cause extensive tissue damage via cell-mediated immune responses.

Interleukin-11 (IL-11) was originally isolated from bone marrow–derived stromal fibroblasts. Characterization of IL-11 was based on its mitogenic activity on an IL-2-dependent mouse plasmacytoma cell line. IL-11 is a multifunctional cytokine whose effects include the following: (1) it synergizes with IL-3, GM-CSF, and stem cell factor to stimulate proliferation; (2) it acts in concert with IL-2 to stimulate synthesis of type I acute phase proteins; (3) it suppresses adipogenesis and lipoprotein lipase activity in murine preadipocytes; (4) it induces in vitro formation of osteoclasts in culture and enhances bone resorption; (5) it stimulates neuronal differentiation; (6) it enhances megakaryocyte maturation and increases platelet numbers in normal and splenectomized mice; and (7) it accelerates the recovery of the peripheral blood leukocytes, mainly neutrophils and platelets, in transplant mice.

Many of the biological activities of IL-11 overlap with those of IL-6. IL-11 and IL-6 utilize different ligand-binding subunits but share a common signal transduction protein, sp130. In general, IL-6 has a much broader spectrum of activities than IL-11, and its potency in mediating erythropoiesis, early hematopoiesis, neuronal differentiation, and osteoclastogenesis varies.

Interleukin-12 (IL-12) is a 75-kd heterodimeric cytokine formed by disulfide-linked subunits of 35 and 40 kd, respectively. The primary cellular source of IL-12 is the activated macrophage. IL-12 receptor expression is limited to activated T and NK cells through which IL-12 modulates their cytolytic and proliferative activities. IL-12 is a potent inducer of IFNγ and to a lesser extent TNFα production in peripheral blood mononuclear cells. IL-12 directs naive T-helper cells toward a T_H1 pattern of cytokine release.

Studies of IL-12 action found it to be a potent mediator of in-vitro NK function. Effects which are attributed to IL-12 include: 1) generation of LAK cell activity, 2) enhancement of the spontaneous lytic activity of NK cells, 3) inhibition of IL-2-driven NK proliferation, 4) upregulation of a variety of cell surface molecules on NK cells, 5) enhanced binding of these cells, and 6) enhanced NK secretion of IFNγ and TNFα. Studies have shown that IL-12 induces proliferation and enhances cytotoxicity in both naive and memory T-cells. IL-12 also may play a crucial role in the development of a T_H1 type immune response, directing T-cells to produce more IFNγ and less IL-4.

Interleukin-13 (IL-13) is a cytokine produced by activated T_H2 cells in the mouse and human. It is produced by the T_H2 lymphocyte subset, which also expresses mRNA for IL-3, IL-4, GM-CSF, and IL-10. Functionally, IL-13 induces changes in human monocyte morphology and the phenotype of monocytes and B lymphocytes by upregulating MHC class II expression and inducing low-affinity receptors for IgE. IL-13 also induces B-cell proliferation and IgE isotype switching. This cytokine also may act as a mediator of inflammatory and immune responses, by suppressing inflammatory cytokine release in response to IFNγ or LPS.

Interferons

Another class of cytokines is the interferons (IFNs), which are a large family of secreted proteins with antiviral activity. Interferons are produced by most cells in response to viral infection or other related stimuli. Type I IFNs are induced by viral infection or double-stranded RNA, and are characterized by their stability at acidic pH (pH = 2.0). IFNα is a subspecies of antigenically similar peptides. The amino acid sequences of these peptides are about 80% homologous to each other. IFNβ is the major interferon synthesized by non-leukocytic cells (fibroblasts) but can be produced by leukocytes. IFNβ exhibits only 30% homology with IFNα. Type II or γ interferon (IFNγ) is produced during immune reactions by antigen-, mitogen-, or lectin-stimulated T lymphocytes or by large granular lymphocytes (LGLs) with NK activity.

In addition to antiviral activity, IFNs have potent cellular effects. They suppress cell proliferation and either inhibit or enhance cell differentiation, depending on the cell type and level of IFN. IFNs also play important roles in normal host defense by exerting effects on macrophages, T and B lymphocytes, and LGLs with NK activity. IFNs increase the bactericidal and tumoricidal capabilities of macrophages and enhance their accessory cell functions. They possess macrophage-activating factor (MAF) and monocyte migratory inhibitory factor (MIF) activities. IFNγ and, to a lesser degree, IFNα and IFNβ maintain the expression of class II antigen on the surface of macrophages as well as other cell types. This aids in the induction of antigen-specific, T-cell-mediated immune responses that require presentation of antigen by an accessory cell to a T-helper cell.

Humoral Immune Response

When effector cells of the immune system encounter a foreign antigen, a cellular immune response or a humoral immune response occurs. Both of these immune responses depend on specific classes of lymphocytes. The pathway for antibody production involves a variety of cell types: an antigen-presenting cell, the CD4+ helper-inducer T cell, the CD4+ suppressor-inducer T cell, and the B cell which differentiates into the antibody-producing plasma cell (Fig. 26-4). The three steps leading to the production of antibodies are the *activation* of the virgin or memory B cell, *proliferation* (clonal expansion) of participating cells, and *differentiation* of antibody-producing plasma cells. Before B-cell activation and antibody production can occur, antibody on the B-cell surface must recognize an antigen either in soluble form or attached to the surface of a macrophage. In most instances, antigen alone will not trigger B-cell activation. Cooperation from helper-inducer T cells and macrophage-derived IL-1 is required. Once antigen is presented in association with

MHC molecules, the helper-inducer T cells become activated, proliferate, and differentiate. These cells produce the cytokines IL-4, IL-5, and IL-6 which induce B-cell proliferation and differentiation into antibody-producing plasma cells or memory cells.

Suppressor T cells also play an important role in controlling antibody production and preventing autoimmune disease. Activation of suppressor-inducer T cells induces the formation of CD8+ suppressor cells. These cells produce suppressive factors that inhibit antibody production by B cells. A second challenge from the same antigen will result in a response involving many more antigen-reactive T cells and B cells.

Cell-Mediated Immunity

Antigen presentation to T cells occurs by a different mechanism than antigen presentation to B cells. Presentation of antigen to the B cell is not restricted by the MHC complex. In contrast, T cells cannot recognize native antigen; instead it must first be processed by an antigen-presenting cell and then presented in association with MHC class I or class II molecules (Fig. 26-5). Only processed peptides, not intact antigens, are necessary for presentation to T cells. Once activated, the T cells help the B cells to produce antibody.

T-cell activation results in the transcription, translation, and expression of various gene products that are important in the immune response. One of the key steps in this process is the secretion of IL-2 and the expression of its membrane receptor. The stimulation of this receptor by secreted IL-2 leads to T-cell proliferation. In addition to B and T cells, other effector cells, such as macrophages and NK cells, play important roles in the immune response to foreign antigens.

Activated macrophages mount the primary immune response to various microorganisms such as *Mycobacterium tuberculosis*, *Listeria monocytogenes*, *Toxoplasma*

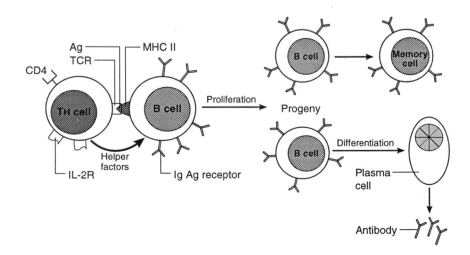

FIG. 26-4. The humoral immune response. B-cell activation requires an encounter between a B cell and native antigen in addition to stimulation from an activated helper-inducer T cell.

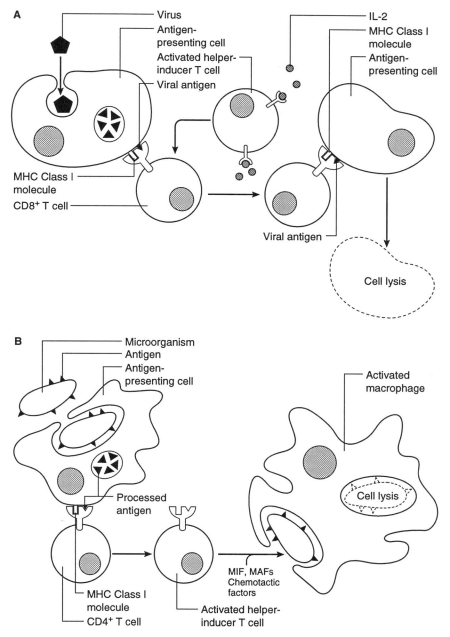

FIG. 26-5. The cellular immune response. T-cell activation requires processing of antigen by an antigen-presenting cell followed by expression of the antigen in association with an MHC class I (CD8+ suppressor T cell, **A**) or class II (CD4+ helper-inducer cells, **B**) molecule.

gondii, and *Leishmania.* In this effector pathway, the macrophage ingests the microorganism, processes the antigen, and presents the antigen in association with MHC class II molecules to the CD4+ helper T cells. Following an additional presentation of the identical antigens by another macrophage, the activated T cells are stimulated to produce and secrete chemotactic factors that attract more macrophages as well as granulocytes and lymphocytes to the reaction site. Macrophage function is altered by macrophage-activating factors such as

IFNγ, granulocyte-macrophage colony-stimulating factor (GM-CSF), IL-3, and IL-4 secreted by the sensitized T cells. Localization of macrophages is mediated by the action of MIF. The enhancement of macrophage killing activity occurs in a non-specific fashion.

NK cells destroy tumor cells and microorganisms. They do not require prior sensitization and their cytolytic activity is not MHC- restricted. NK cells secrete IL-1 and in response to IL-2 become super killers capable of lysing more cells than regular NK cells, termed lymphokine-ac-

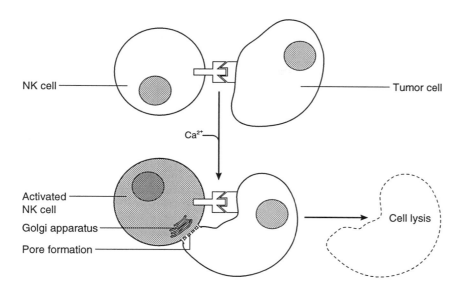

FIG. 26-6. Natural killer (NK) cell response. NK cells elicit non-MHC restricted killing activity.

tivated killer (LAK) cells. The lymphokine IL-3 is produced by sensitized T cells and causes the NK cells to secrete interferon, which functions in an autocrine manner to enhance NK cell activity. NK cells attach to their target cells by a receptor in a Ca^{2+}-independent step (Fig. 26-6). However, once NK cells are activated, they require Ca^{2+} ions for lysis. A subset of cytotoxic T cells has been identified that can kill cells in a method similar to that of NK cells without prior sensitization or MHC restriction.

To summarize, the human immune system includes a number of different cell types (several classes of lymphocytes, NK cells, macrophages) that act in an integrated fashion to respond to foreign microorganisms, antigenic molecules, and tumor cells. Discrimination between self and nonself antigens is accomplished by molecules of the major histocompatibility complex. In the humoral immune response, differentiated B lymphocytes (plasma cells) produce immunoglobulins that play important roles in the neutralization of bacteria and viruses. Cellular immune responses involve the activation of T lymphocytes and the subsequent production of a variety of cellular regulators termed cytokines. These nonrestricted regulators of immune function increase the killing activity of cytotoxic T cells, macrophages, and NK cells. They also enhance antibody production by B lymphocytes. When viewed in light of the aggressive nature of the human immune response, the maternal acceptance of the antigenically distinct fetus is truly remarkable. In the next section, we will examine some of the theories purported to explain the immunologic survival of the fetal allograft.

IMMUNOLOGY OF PREGNANCY

The immunologic survival of the fetus remains one of the unsolved mysteries in reproductive biology. Many of the theories purported to explain the so-called "enigma of the fetal allograft" emphasize the role of the fetal trophoblast. In humans, this tissue forms a continuous interface separating maternal blood and tissue from the developing fetus. Major proposals cited to explain the acceptance of the fetus by the maternal immune system include (1) selective antigen expression by the trophoblast (*invisibility*), (2) resistance of the trophoblast to effector cell lysis (*invulnerability*), (3) suppression of the maternal immune response (systemically or locally) by pregnancy-associated factors (*self-defense*), and (4) trophoblast stimulation by products of maternal effector cells (cytokines and growth factors, *immunotropism*). A combination of some or all of these protective mechanisms is likely required to ensure the immunologic protection of the fetus.

Selective Antigen Expression

This theory proposes that lysis of trophoblast by maternal anti-paternal HLA cytotoxic cells and cytotoxic antibodies is prevented by the failure of these cells to express MHC antigens with paternally derived allotypic determinants. Several lines of experimental evidence support this hypothesis and indicate that different populations of human trophoblast express varying levels of MHC expression. No normal trophoblast population constitutively expresses classical HLA antigens at the maternal–fetal interface. A novel class I MHC molecule, HLA-G, has been reported. Trophoblast HLA-G was initially detected in cloned choriocarcinoma cells, termed *chorionic cytotrophoblast,* and first-trimester cytotrophoblasts. Because only five isoforms of HLA-G (37–39 kd, pI 4.5–5.5) were detected in each of 13 individuals, HLA-G was described as exhibiting restricted polymorphism.

Syncytiotrophoblast contains low to undetectable levels of class I HLA-mRNA. These findings indicate that the trophoblast layer that is continuously exposed to maternal cytotoxic cells and antibodies possesses a highly effective protective mechanism to avoid recognition.

A second pattern of trophoblast antigen expression has been noted in villous cytotrophoblast cells. These cells lie directly beneath the syncytial layer and are not exposed to maternal blood or decidua. Although these cells do not express class I MHC antigens, they do contain class I mRNA. These cells are prominent in first-trimester placentas but are uncommon in term tissues.

A third subpopulation of trophoblast is the extravillous cytotrophoblast that proliferates and migrates to the decidua. This cell type exhibits class I antigens and contains class I mRNA. Substitution of a nonclassical class I antigen, HLA-G, for classical HLA-A, -B, and -C appears to be a special feature of extravillous cytotrophoblast cells that reside in or near the decidua.

The contribution of HLA-G to the immunotolerance of pregnancy is not fully understood. It has been proposed that the limited polymorphism exhibited by HLA-G restricts antigen presentation by its transcript. This unique trophoblast antigen may also prevent responses of decidual NK cells to otherwise class I–negative trophoblast (missing self hypothesis).

Trophoblast Resistance to Immune Effector Cells

Another important concept in pregnancy immunology is the resistance of the trophoblast to lysis by certain maternal effector cells. In transplanted organs, T cells with cytotoxic markers accumulate within the graft. This is not the case with the fetal allograft, as lymphocytes in the decidua contain only a small portion of cells with cytotoxicity.

Analysis of leukocyte populations in early human decidua has revealed that the predominant cell type is an unusual large granular lymphocyte-like mononuclear cell, known as the endometrial granulocyte. These cells are positive for one NK marker (NKH-1) but negative for others. This cell population is present at low levels in the nonpregnant cycling uterus until the secretory phase; then they increase dramatically. Thus, the implantation and postimplantation human decidua contains a large number of cells with morphologic and phenotypic characteristics of NK cells. While human trophoblast cells have been generally shown to be resistant to NK killing, the presence of NK-like cells is a consistent feature of the early decidua.

The general consensus of trophoblast vulnerability to maternal effector cells is that for NK cells to lyse trophoblast, they must become highly activated, a state that depends on high local levels of IL-2. Thus, the potential for trophoblast killing in vitro seems to exist but would require the activation of the potential NK effectors to increase lytic activity by high levels of IL-2. The central question that remains to be resolved is the likelihood that such high levels of IL-2 would be found in the implantation area.

Immunosuppression by Pregnancy-Associated Factors

Another hypothesis that has been proposed to explain the immunologic acceptance of the semiallogenic fetus is that of local immunoregulation by decidual or trophoblast-derived products. These factors are proposed to create a zone of immunoprotection at the maternal–fetal interface while not compromising systemic immune responses. One of the most widely reported of these observations is that of immunosuppressive factors produced by decidual suppressor cells (Fig. 26-7). In humans and mice, the suppressive activity appears to be present during successful pregnancy and declines near term. The sol-

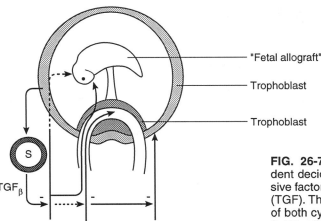

TGF$_\beta$

T cells   Non-T effectors

FIG. 26-7. Decidual suppressor cells. Trophoblast-dependent decidual suppressor cells produce an immunosuppressive factor chemically related to transforming growth factor–β (TGF). This suppressive factor interferes with IL-2 activation of both cytotoxic T cells and lymphokine-activated killer cells (LAK cells).

uble suppressor factor produced by these suppressor cells acts by blocking the action of IL-2 and displays significant homology with TGFβ.

A number of lines of experimental evidence support the hypothesis that the human trophoblast secretes immunoregulatory macromolecules. The pregnant mouse placenta contains ConA-binding glycoproteins that are located in the membrane and are released in soluble form. Mixed lymphocyte reactions performed in the presence of placental extracts syngenic to the responding cells results in a low secondary MLR with a concomitant generation of suppressor cells. Media from dispersed 8- to 10-week placenta markedly suppress mitogen-stimulated lymphocyte proliferation. A similar suppression was observed in the mixed lymphocyte reaction. This supernatant was able to reduce the NK activity against K562 target cells. The suppressive factor(s) in cultures of dispersed human placenta do not affect expression of the IL-2 receptor and do not affect IL-2 production by activated T cells. Collagenase-dispersed murine placental cells block target cell lysis by NK, LAK, and cytotoxic T cell-type killer cells.

In domestic animals, maternal recognition of pregnancy is maintained by trophoblast-derived factors. The proteins responsible for these responses were originally termed ovine and bovine trophoblast protein–1 (oTP-1 and bTP-1, respectively) and have recently been reclassified as τ-interferon (IFN-τ). These proteins have molecular weights of approximately 17–22 kd and isoelectric points ranging from 5.3 to 5.7. Some of the features of IFN-τ are as follows: (1) it is produced between days 12 and 21 of gestation; (2) it originates in the trophoblast; (3) it is taken up by surface and upper uterine gland epithelium; (4) it stimulates protein secretion by ovine endometrial explant cultures; and (5) it has antiluteolytic functions. IFN-τ inhibits the pulsatile secretion of prostaglandin $F_{2\alpha}$ ($PGF_{2\alpha}$) by the uterus and allows for maintenance of the corpus luteum. In the sheep, IFN-τ is produced at a rate of more than 100 μg/embryo between days 15 and 17 of pregnancy, and exhibits potent antiviral activity. Massive induction of IFN-τ mRNA occurs on day 13 concurrent with the initiation of maternal recognition of pregnancy. This is associated with the morphologic transition of the sheep embryo from a spherical to an elongated form.

IFN-τ or a related cytokine is secreted by the human trophoblast. The derived nucleotide sequence of this IFN expresses high homology with that of sheep IFN-τ, and measurable mRNA levels were detected in syncytiotrophoblast and extravillous trophoblast during the first trimester of pregnancy and at term. Because of the high levels of expression in the migrating extravillous trophoblast, such as those that invade the uterine spiral arteries, it was proposed that this IFN may play an important role in protection against viral transmission from the mother to the fetus.

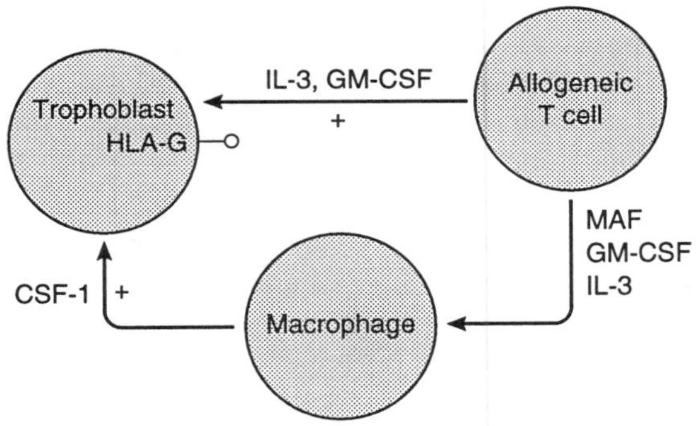

FIG. 26-8. The immunotropic hypothesis. This hypothesis states that maternal T cells, if properly primed, are capable of recognizing fetally derived class I antigens that are known to be expressed in the placenta. The release of cytokines is then proposed to stimulate placental growth and function.

Enhanced Trophoblast Function

Another hypothesis purported to explain the immunologic privilege of the trophoblast states that the recognition of foreign alloantigens on fetal trophoblast leads to lymphokine release that results in improved placental growth and function (Fig. 26-8). The initial event in this model is maternal T-cell recognition of class I antigens on the trophoblast. Activated T cells then release factors such as IL-3 and CSF-1 which influence trophoblast growth and function. Cytokines of the CSF family, including IL-3 and GM-CSF, have been shown to increase the chances of fetal survival when injected into abortion-prone mice. In contrast, IFNγ and IL-2 reportedly enhanced resorptions in these same murine models of spontaneous abortion. Both GM-CSF and CSF-1 increase ³H-thymidine uptake by murine trophoblast in culture, a response that has been attributed to endoreduplication and the formation of terminally differentiated trophoblast giant cells. The CSF-1 receptor has been localized to trophoblast cells in the murine placenta by in situ hybridization.

IMMUNOLOGIC MECHANISMS OF ABORTION

A number of immunologic mechanisms have been proposed as contributing factors to unexplained immunologic pregnancy wastage. These include (1) a deficiency of suppressor cells and associated immunosuppressive factors; (2) induction of polymorphic class I antigen expression on the trophoblast; and (3) antiphospholipid antibodies.

Suppressor Cell Deficiency

In mouse models of spontaneous abortion, decidual suppressor cell deficiency occurs prior to the onset of abortion. In humans, endometrial curettings of failed IVF pregnancies show a mononuclear infiltrate–deficient in suppressor cells similar to that noted in the mouse model. Suppressor cells are reduced in decidua of women with missed abortions. In addition, macrophage activation and function are enhanced in the decidua of women with spontaneous abortion as compared with those having elective abortions. These observations support the concept that a deficiency of suppressor cells and/or suppressor cell–derived factors may contribute to immunologic failures of early pregnancies.

Induction of Trophoblast Antigen Expression

Based on the theory of trophoblast invisibility, researchers have proposed that inappropriate trophoblast antigen expression could lead to the immunologic rejection of the fetal allograft. Upregulation of trophoblast antigens could result from the release of inflammatory cytokines (ie, IL-2, TNFα, IFNγ) subsequent to infection. This enhancement of MHC expression by fetal trophoblast could make them targets for rejection by classical cell-mediated immune responses. This concept of immunologic abortion is supported by animal studies reporting abortion following the administration of inflammatory cytokines. In addition, placental tissue obtained following spontaneous abortion is cited to express class II MHC antigens, a feature not characteristic of normal trophoblast.

Antiphospholipid Antibodies

Another factor that has been associated with spontaneous abortion is the presence of *antiphospholipid antibodies*. Antiphospholipid antibodies are autoantibodies that can be detected by standard tests for syphilis, lupus anticoagulant, or by an enzyme-linked immunosorbent assay for anticardiolipin antibody. The autoantibodies are associated with venous and arterial thrombosis, thrombocytopenia, and recurrent reproductive failure. Thrombosis occurs in 25–33% of patients with the lupus anticoagulant and in over 75% of patients with high levels of IgG anticardiolipin antibodies. The exact mechanism of pregnancy loss in these women remains unknown but may involve placental vessel thrombosis and subsequent placental insufficiency. Retrospective studies have demonstrated an association between the presence of lupus anticoagulant, α-anticardiolipin antibodies, and recurrent fetal loss.

From these different studies, it appears that at least a portion of presently unexplained human pregnancy loss may be related to immunologic factors. Further research is needed to define the significance of decidual suppressor cells and suppressor factors to the success of the fetal allograft. In addition to serving as a contributing factor to spontaneous pregnancy loss, immunologic events may also be associated with human infertility.

IMMUNOLOGIC INFERTILITY

Human infertility is a relatively common problem estimated to occur in 15% of married couples. In the male, the principal cause is impaired sperm quality, commonly evaluated in terms of sperm count, motility, and morphology. Female infertility is associated with ovulation defects, obstructed fallopian tubes, and endometriosis. A recently recognized class of infertility is immunologic infertility, most often characterized by the presence of antibodies to sperm (AsAb) in one or both partners.

Antisperm Antibodies and Infertility

Antisperm antibodies (AsAb) present on human spermatozoa at ejaculation along with those transferred from other body fluids, such as female serum, can alter the behavior and fertility potential of motile sperm. The prevalence of AsAb has been cited to range from 0–2% in the general population to 20–25% in male partners of couples with unexplained infertility. Sites at which sperm antibodies may impair reproduction include spermatogenesis, sperm transport, gamete interaction, and embryo survival. AsAb in male serum and/or semen has been associated with a decrease of fertilization in vitro, particularly when 80% or more of the sperm are coated with antibody. AsAb reportedly impair sperm–egg interaction by interfering with sperm binding to the zona pellucida, penetration through the zona pellucida, and sperm–vitellus fusion. Studies with in vitro fertilization and embryo transfer (IVF-ET) have demonstrated poorer success rates for couples with sperm-associated AsAb. Tail-directed AsAb are associated with motility loss in the presence of complement, whereas head-directed antibodies impede gamete interaction primarily by inhibiting zona recognition. In general, head-directed antibodies may prevent or reduce fertilization, whereas tail-directed antibodies do not. In addition, IgG subclass binding is primarily to the sperm head, whereas IgA AsAb have preferential binding to the tail region and may influence motility.

One of the problems in evaluating AsAb is that immunity to sperm often is incomplete, resulting in a subfertile rather than an infertile state. Another complicating factor is variations in antibody levels between serum, reproductive tissues, and semen. Serum antibodies can be present whereas levels are undetectable in semen or the female reproductive tract. In addition, local immune responses to sperm occur in the absence of detectable systemic antibodies in men and women. Humoral AsAb do not necessarily impair fertility unless they are also present within the female reproductive tract and on the living sperm surface.

Male Sperm Autoimmunity

In the male, the blood–testis barrier formed by the tight junctions of the Sertoli cells provides immunologic protection of sperm antigens. This is accomplished by blocking testicular cells from coming in contact with the lymphoid tissue and preventing antibodies and most immunocompetent cells from entering the seminiferous tubules. There also appear to be immunoregulatory mechanisms in the testis that suppress autoimmune responses. The combined effect of these mechanisms has given rise to the concept of the testis as an immunologically privileged site.

Etiology of Sperm Antibodies

The presence of AsAb in men is correlated with conditions that disrupt the barrier between the male reproductive tract and the immune system. This may occur following vasectomy, testicular injury, mumps orchitis, and other genital tract infections. In fact, the "blood–testis" barrier is commonly compromised with the leakage of small quantities of sperm antigens. Some researchers have proposed that a type of immune tolerance is generated in the male due to recurrent leakage of sperm antigens. It has also been suggested that the activation of nonspecific T-suppressor cells in the epididymis and the presence of immunosuppressive factors in seminal plasma may regulate immunologic responses to sperm.

In women, the uterus possesses immunocompetent cells that phagocytose sperm and process their antigens for recognition. The general lack of immunity in the majority of individuals is surprising because coitus results in the inoculation of the female with millions of antigenically foreign cells. The formation of AsAb is influenced by a number of factors, including (1) flushing of sperm from the genital tract, (2) degradation of sperm antigens by extracellular enzymes, (3) phagocytosis of sperm by somatic cells and macrophages, (4) immunopotentiation by other foreign antigens in the genital tract, (5) paternal lymphocytes present in semen, and (6) seminal immunosuppressive factors.

Testing for Sperm Antibodies

In the clinical setting, a number of different tests have been used to detect the presence of AsAb in serum and reproductive tract secretions in both men and women. These include (1) immunofluorescence tests, (2) sperm agglutination tests, (3) sperm immobilization tests, (4) enzyme-linked assays (ELISAs), (5) cervical mucous slide inhibition test, and (6) immunobead technique. The tray agglutination (Friberg method), ELISA, and immunobead techniques have gained widespread acceptance and applications in the clinical evaluation of AsAb.

The Friberg method involves the mixing of small volumes of sperm and serum in microsyringes. Using this test, several patterns of agglutination can be observed including head–head, head–tail, and tail–tail patterns. This test is most frequently used in the detection of serum AsAb.

Both radioimmunoassays (RIAs) and ELISA tests have been used for measuring AsAb titers. These assays allow for the use of pooled frozen samples and can be performed as a qualitative or quantitative test. In addition, they are rapid and easily automated. While these techniques are highly quantitative, they are unable to indicate the location of binding for the AsAbs.

The immunobead technique utilizes suspensions of polyacrylamide beads (5–10 μm in diameter) to which antibody is attached. This rabbit antibody can be antihuman IgG, IgA, or IgM. When these beads are mixed with a sperm sample, binding occurs if the sperm cells are coated with antibody and the correct anti-immunoglobulin for the bead is chosen. The site of sperm binding also can be estimated, such as head, tail (midpiece), or tail (tip).

With the development of techniques allowing determination of the site of antibody interaction with sperm, attempts have been made to correlate this information with the mechanism of fertility reduction. Capacitation, the acrosome reaction, zona penetration, and fertilization are the sequential events necessary for human reproduction. Immunoglobulin on critical areas of the sperm surface may interfere with sperm penetration of heterologous ova targets and human IVF. It is thought that IgA antisperm antibodies attached to the sperm head are the most critical when considering immunoglobulin-mediated inhibition of sperm–ovum interactions. It is likely that the location of AsAb and the proportion of sperm associated with these antibodies may be important criteria in future evaluations of sperm quality.

In summary, AsAb can serve as a relative cause of infertility and may be present in as great as 20% of male partners in couples with unexplained fertility. Various clinical assay techniques are utilized for the detection of sperm-binding antibodies. Some of these techniques are highly quantitative (RIA, ELISA), whereas others permit detection of the site of sperm binding (Friberg agglutination test, immunobead techniques). Immunoglobulin on critical areas of the sperm surface may interfere with capacitation, the acrosome reaction, zona penetration, and fertilization. AsAb that bind to the sperm head are the most critical when considering immunoglobulin-mediated inhibition of sperm–ovum interaction. Finally, it is thought that the location of antibody binding and the proportion of sperm bound by these antibodies may be critical in future evaluations of sperm quality.

Autoimmunity in the Female

With the exception of autoimmune syndrome affecting ovarian theca and granulosa cells, there is no evidence the oocytes and the ovum serve as natural targets of immunologic attack. In contrast, the zona pellucida may protect the ovum and zygote from immunologic attack by the maternal immune system. There is interest, however, in the artificial generation of antizona immune reactions as potential contraceptive vaccines.

The immunologic relationship between mother and fetus has been implicated as a potential site for disruptions in normal human fertility and pregnancy. These findings have generated interest in the concept that artificial manipulation of this relationship could result in an efficient and safe means of contraception. The final section of this chapter will deal with current research directed at the development of a human contraceptive vaccine.

CONTRACEPTIVE VACCINES

The world's population continues to grow at a steadily increasing rate, currently by more than 220,000 per day. By the year 2000, the human population will reach 6.3 billion, double the number of 1960. It is estimated that 80% of these people live in third-world countries. These demographic statistics emphasize the need for new means of contraception. The methods of birth control presently available can be grouped as follows: (1) *hormonal*—oral pills, injectable steroids, and steroid-releasing implants; (2) *chemical*—spermicides; (3) *mechanical*—condoms, caps, intrauterine devices; (4) *surgical*—tubal ligation, vasectomy; and (5) *natural*—rhythm, withdrawal. Although these methods have found widespread acceptance in various parts of the world, this range of options is still inadequate to meet the widely different cultural, social, and religious demands existing in different cultures, particularly in third-world countries. In addition, many users are dissatisfied with the currently available methods due to annoying and uncomfortable side effects, unreliability, concerns about long-term safety, inconvenience, difficulties of storage and disposal, and irreversibility. A new approach to human contraception is the development of immunologic vaccines that will generate antibodies to gamete-associated antigens or reproductive hormones.

Major advantages of this mode of contraception include ease of administration, lack of use failure, long-lasting protection, low cost, and potential reversibility.

Several different criteria for the ideal antigen to be used in the development of a contraceptive vaccine have been proposed. First, the antigen should have a response confined to reproductive processes. It should be present in the circulation temporarily and/or at low concentrations. The formation of the immune complexes should not lead to autoimmune disease and the contraceptive effect should be reversible. Finally, the contraceptive effects should not cause danger to future offspring.

Three of the immunogens currently being evaluated are subunits of human chorionic gonadotropin (hCG), zona pellucida antigens, and sperm antigens. The preimplantation embryo produces and secretes hCG as early as 5 days postfertilization, stimulating the corpus luteum to maintain the production of progesterone needed for maintaining the uterine endometrium for embryo attachment and implantation. It travels by the maternal circulation from the embryonic trophoblast to the corpus luteum and therefore could be inactivated systemically by circulating antibodies.

Two main types of anti-hCG vaccines are currently being tested in clinical trials (Table 26-5). The first type, being tested by the Population Council in New York and the National Institute of Immunology (NII) in New Delhi, is based on the whole β subunit of the hormone (β-hCG). The other type of vaccine is being developed with the support of the World Health Organization (WHO) and relies on a synthetic peptide homologous to the carboxyl-terminal region of the β subunit of the hormone (β-hCG-CTP).

The vaccine being tested by the Population Council consists of β-hCG conjugated to tetanus toxoid (carrier molecule). Phase I clinical trials in human volunteers have demonstrated the immunogenicity of this preparation and no adverse side effects have been reported. The anti-hCG vaccine being tested by the NII is a heterospecies dimer with β-hCG associated with the α subunit of ovine luteinizing hormone conjugated to tetanus

TABLE 26-5. *Status of development of the primary anti-human chorionic gonadotropin (hCG) vaccines currently under evaluation in clinical trials with human subjects*

Institution	Immunogen	Trial status (completion)	Results
National Institute of Immunology, New Delhi	Pr-β hCG:TT	Phase I (1975)	Immunogenic
		Phase II (1976)	Ineffective
	HSD α-OLH:β-hCG:TT:DT	Phase I (1990)	Immunogenic
		Phase II (underway)	Effective
Population Council, New York	β-hCG:TT	Phase I (1990)	Immunogenic
		Phase II (underway)	
World Health Organization, Geneva	β-hCG-CTP:DT	Phase I (1988)	
		Phase II (underway)	Immunogenic

Pr-β-hCG:TT, natural β-hCG processed by passage over an anti-LH affinity column and conjugated to tetanus toxoid; HSD α-OLH:β-hCG:TT/DT, heterospecies dimer of natural ovine luteinizing hormone associated noncovalently with natural β-hCG and conjugated to tetanus toxoid and diphtherial toxoid; β-hCG:TT, natural β-hCG conjugated to tetanus toxoid; β-hCG-CTP:DT, synthetic peptide of the carboxy terminal 109–145 region of β-hCG conjugated to diphtheria toxoid.

toxoid and diphtheria toxoid carriers. This preparation has been utilized in both phase I and ongoing phase II clinical trials. The vaccine has been shown to be immunogenic and does not induce significant side effects. Investigators have reported that antibody titers above the estimated efficacy threshold were achieved by 80% of the women and one pregnancy has been reported in 1000 otherwise unprotected menstrual cycles in study participants. No evidence of menstrual cycle disturbances or anovulation were reported.

The WHO has been testing an anti-hCG vaccine based on the β-hCG-CTP since the mid-1970s. The ability to induce the production of adequate titers of antibodies capable of neutralizing the biological activity of hCG has been used as the principal criterion for the selection of the components used in the β-hCG-CTP vaccine. A 37-amino-acid peptide representing the 109–145 region of the molecule elicits neutralizing antibodies and is used in the β-hCG-CTP vaccine. Tetanus and diphtheria toxoids have been found to be the most potent carriers for the 109–145 peptide of β-hCG. The diphtheria toxoid was selected for the prototype β-hCG-CTP vaccine because this molecule is less likely to produce hypersensitivity reactions.

While vaccines against hCG hold promise for an effective and safe method of contraception, their application may be restricted due to their action as an early abortifacient rather than an antifertility treatment. Ideally, immunologic disruption of fertility should occur before fertilization.

Antizona Pellucida Vaccine Development

Fertilization (Chapter 15) involves extremely specific cell recognition events between the ovum and sperm that could be blocked by an antibody. The concept of a zona pellucida vaccine was based on studies concerning the influence of antiovarian antisera on mammalian IVF systems. Antiserum against ovarian tissue inhibited sperm binding to the zona pellucida and blocked fertilization. The responsible antigens are present in the zona pellucida. Antibodies against zona pellucida proteins block IVF in laboratory rodents by inhibiting sperm binding to the zona surface. Passive immunization against ovarian antigens in vivo can induce infertility in a number of species. A possible drawback to immunization against zona antigens is that antizona antibodies bind ovulated oocytes as well as those still in the follicles, resulting in prolonged infertility.

Ethical factors and limitations to the availability of human antigens prevent the collection of sufficient amounts of human zona for experimentation. Thus, the use of heterologous antigens is an essential element for development of a human contraceptive vaccine. Human and pig zona share common antigens that cross-react with common antibodies. Pig antibody binds to the outer surface of the human zona and inhibits subsequent fertilization of the ova. Therefore, a great deal of attention has focused on the biological and chemical characterization of antigens from the pig zona pellucida. The porcine zona pellucida is composed of multiple immunogens such as ZP-1 (82 kd), ZP-2 (61 kd), ZP-3 (55 kd), and ZP-4 (21 kd). The ZP-3 component possesses sperm receptor activity. Using this purified zona antigen in monkeys, high antibody titers and concurrent infertility have been achieved. These results encourage intensive research in the zona vaccine area and could lead to a much needed approach for fertility regulation in the human.

Antisperm Antigen Vaccines

As previously mentioned, antisperm antibodies can contribute to human infertility. Based on this, sperm-specific antigens have been sought as potential immunogens in contraceptive vaccines. Intact sperm can generate antibodies that induce infertility. However, this antigen preparation is not appropriate for a contraceptive vaccine because some antigens are shared with brain and kidney cells, erythrocytes, and lymphocytes. Therefore, only sperm-specific antigens are deemed appropriate vaccine immunogens.

Several sperm-specific enzymes have been purified to homogeneity and evaluated for immunoregulation of fertility. Antibodies to acrosin or hyaluronidase do not reduce fertility in females. In contrast, immunization with LDH-C4 reduces fertility in female rabbits, mice, and baboons. Other nonenzymatic antigens may also serve as effective immunogens for a contraceptive vaccine. The human sperm protein SP-10 is a differentiation antigen localized within the acrosomal vesicles of spermatids, with an intraacrosomal site in mature sperm, and appears to be testis specific. SP-10 is a useful marker for detecting immature germ cells in semen and for scoring the acrosome reaction. This protein has been designated as a "primary vaccine candidate" by a WHO task force on contraceptive vaccines due to its tissue specificity and evidence that antibody to SP-10 inhibits fertilization in the hamster egg penetration test. RSA-1 is another protein found on rabbit sperm that appears to be involved in sperm penetration of the zona pellucida. Antigens FA-1 and GA-1 are antigens derived from the rabbit sperm and murine testis, respectively, which also have been evaluated as potential immunogens for a contraceptive vaccine.

In summary, the gonadotropin hormone hCG, as well as specific sperm and zona pellucida antigens, may serve as potential immunogens for a contraceptive vaccine. Although a number of questions need to be resolved, it is very likely that immunologic contraception will play an important role in the future management of world population growth.

SUMMARY

Both immunology and reproductive biology are areas of intensive research and have experienced tremendous growth in recent years. As outlined in this chapter, the immune and reproductive systems interact in numerous ways, and disorders of one system often have serious effects on the function of the other. From this need for a better understanding of the relationships that govern these systems has sprung the field of reproductive immunology, which is presently seeking answers to many questions that impact human fertility and population control. Continued research in this field will likely provide solutions to many of the problems currently facing patients and physicians alike in the control and management of human reproduction.

SUGGESTED READING

Aboagye-Mathiesen G, Toth FD, Zdravkonic M, Ebbesen P. Human trophoblast interferons: production and possible roles in early pregnancy. *Early Pregn Biol Med* 1995;1:41.

Beer AE, Quebleman JF, Ayers JWI, Haines RF. Major histocompatibility complex antigens, maternal and paternal immune responses, and chronic habitual abortions in humans. *Am J Obstet Gynecol* 1981;141:987.

Beer AE, Simprini AE, Zhu X, Quebbeman JF. Pregnancy outcome in human couples with recurrent spontaneous abortions: 1) HLA antigen profiles; 2) HLA antigen sharing; 3) Female serum MLR blocking factors; and 4) Paternal leukocyte immunization. *Exp Clin Immunol Genet* 1985; 2:137.

Bell SC, Billington WD. Antifetal alloantibody in the pregnant female. *Immunol Rev* 1983;75:6.

Bronson R, Cooper G, Rosenfeld D. Sperm antibodies: their role in infertility. *Fertil Steril* 1984;42:171.

David J, Terhorst C, Fearon D, Carpenter CB, Robinson DR, Rocklin RE, Rosin FS, Fearon D, Piessens WF. Immunology. In: Rubenstein E, Federman DD, eds. *Scientific American Medicine.* 12th ed. New York: Scientific American, Inc., 1989;6.1–3.

Faulk WP, McIntyre JA. Immunological studies of human trophoblast; markers, subsets, and functions. *Immunol Rev* 1983;75:139

Faulk WP, Tempe A. Distribution of beta-2 microglobulin and HLA in chorionic villi of human placentae. *Nature* 1976;262:799.

Guilbert L, Robertson SA, Wegmann TG. The trophoblast as an integral component of a macrophage-cytokine network. *Immunol Cell Biol* 1993; 71:49.

Head JR, Drake BL, Zuckerman FA. Major histocompatibility antigens on trophoblast and their regulation: implications in the maternal–fetal relationship. *Am J Reprod Immunol* 1987;138:2481.

Hill JA. Immunological mechanisms of pregnancy maintenance and failure: a critique of theories and therapy. *Am J Reprod Immunol* 1990;22:33.

Jones WR, Bradley J, Judd SJ, et al. Phase I clinical trials of the World Health Organization birth control vaccine. *Lancet* 1988;1:1295.

Kirby DRS, Billington WD, James DA. Transplantation of eggs to the kidney and uterus of immune mice. *Transplantation* 1966;4:713.

Kovatz S, Main EK, Lilbrach C, Stubblebine M, Fisher SJ, DeMars R. A class I antigen, HLA-G, expressed in human trophoblasts. *Science* 1990; 248:220.

Lea RG, Underwood J, Flanders KC, Hirte H, Banwatt D, Finotto S, Ohno I, Daya S, Harley C, Michel M, Mobray JF, Clark DA. A subset of patients with recurrent spontaneous abortion is deficient in transforming growth factor beta-2 producing "suppressor cells" in uterine tissue near the placental attachment site. *Am J Reprod Immunol* 1995;34:52.

Lin H, Mossmann TR, Guilbert L, Tuntipopipat S, Wegmann TG. Synthesis of T-helper 2-type cytokines at the maternal–fetal interface. *J Immunol* 1993;151:4562.

McIntyre JA, Faulk WP, Verhulst SJ, Colliver J. Human trophoblast-lymphocyte cross-reactive (TLX) antigens define an alloantigen system. *Science* 1983;222:1135.

McIntyre JA, Faulk WP. Trophoblast antigens in normal and abnormal human pregnancy. *Clin Obstet Gynecol* 1986;29:976.

Mowbray JF, Gibbings C, Lindell H. Reginald DW, Underwood JC, Beard RW. Controlled trial of treatment of recurrent spontaneous abortion by immunization with paternal cells. *Lancet* 1985;1:941.

Nossal GJV. Current concepts: the basic components of the immune system. *N Engl J Med* 1987;316:1320.

Roitt I, ed. The basis of immunology. II. Specific acquired immunity. In: *Essential Immunology.* 6th ed. Oxford: Blackwell Scientific, 1989;44.

Saji F, Negoro T, Matsuzaki N, Koyama M, Kameda T, Tanizawa O. An immunoregulatory role of human trophoblasts. *Prog Clin Biol Res* 1989; 294:435.

Schwartz BD. The human major histocompatibility human leukocyte antigen (HLA) complex. In: Stites DP, ed. *Basic and Clinical Immunology.* 7th ed. East Norwalk, CT: Appleton and Lange, 1991;45.

Scott JR, Rote NS, Branch D. IV. Immunologic aspects of recurrent abortion and fetal death. *Obstet Gynecol* 1987;70:645.

Shulman S. Sperm antigens and autoantibodies: effects on fertility. *Am J Reprod Immunol Microbiol* 1986;10:82.

Simmons RL, Russel PS. The histocompatibility antigens of fertilized mouse eggs and trophoblast. *Ann NY Acad Sci* 1966;129:35.

Talwar GP, Singh O, Rao LV. An improved immunogen for antihuman chorionic gonadotropin vaccine eliciting antibodies reactive with a conformation native to the hormones without cross-reaction with human follicle stimulating hormone and human thyroid stimulating hormone. *J Reprod Immunol* 1988;14:203.

Clinical Reproductive Medicine,
Edited by Bryan D. Cowan and David B. Seifer
Lippincott-Raven Publishers, Philadelphia © 1997

CHAPTER 27

Molecular Technologies in Reproductive Medicine

Cecil A. Long

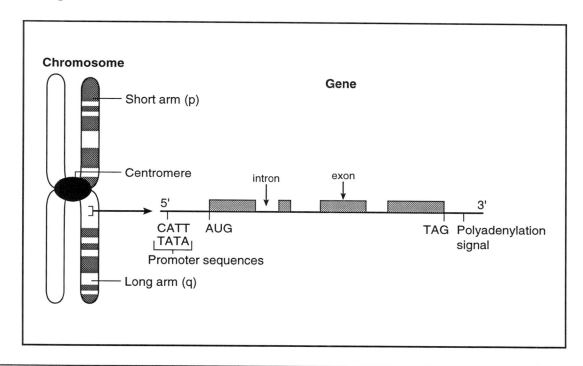

DNA
    Structure and Function
    Nature and Biological Role of Genes
    Gene Expression
Techniques of DNA and RNA Identification
    Restriction Endonucleases
    Gel Electrophoresis
    Blotting Techniques
    In Situ Hybridization
    Cloning Techniques
    Polymerase Chain Reaction
Identification of Genetic Errors and Differences
    Karyotyping

    Restriction Length Polymorphism
    Gene Error Identification
Current Applications of Molecular Techniques
    Prenatal Diagnosis
    Recurrent Pregnancy Loss
    Sexual Differentiation
    Congenital Adrenal Hyperplasia
Future Direction of the Molecular Biology
    Human Genome Project
    Genome Imprinting
    Recombinant Medication
    Gene Therapy
Suggested Reading

C. A. Long: Department of Obstetrics and Gynecology, ART Program at Birmingham, Birmingham, AL 35209

The practice of medicine has changed dramatically in the 1990s. Advances in medical science, similar to those that provided antibiotics, analgesics, and tissue prosthetics, have brought us to an era when diagnosis and even treatment have fallen within the scope of the new science of molecular biology. The ramifications of recombinant DNA technology have touched every discipline of medicine, yielding a more comprehensive understanding about disease etiology, development of more precise diagnostic tools, and advancement to more specific therapeutic modalities. This chapter will focus on recently developed molecular biology techniques as well as applications of these tools in the field of reproductive medicine.

Molecular biology, the study of the infrastructure and inner workings of cells and, particularly, of the proteins, enzymes, and nucleic acids that make cells work is beginning to open new doors in all fields of medicine. To keep pace with these changes, obstetrician-gynecologists now must become familiar with a variety of new terms such as clone, vector, and complimentary nucleic acid. This is less of a challenge for the recent medical school graduate for whom molecular biology has been an integral part of college and postgraduate education. Still, many physicians' knowledge of molecular biology extends no further than the works of Gregor Mendel with his blue and pink flowers and tall and short peas. Although that form of population genetics still has some relevance to the practice of medicine, the new biology more often involves concepts such as antibody recognition and nucleic acid sequencing.

DNA

Structure and Function

A basic knowledge of molecular genetics is essential for understanding and applying the tools of molecular biology. Central to this understanding are the molecules known as nucleic acids. One of the nucleic acids, deoxyribonucleic acid (DNA), is responsible for encoding all of the cellular protein responsible for human physical characteristics and bodily function. DNA molecules are divided into regions, called *genes,* and these genes control specific aspects of cellular chemistry.

The nucleic acids are made up of two distinct species in eukaryotes. DNA is the genetic backbone of the organism and RNA performs messenger and structural functions within the cell. Not only is ribonucleic acid (RNA) used to transmit messages from DNA to the cell structures that synthesize protein but, in addition, it acts as a platform on which those proteins may be synthesized.

There are two critical components of a DNA or RNA molecule. The first is called a nucleotide base. Four bases are found in DNA: adenine and cytosine (the purines), and guanine and thymine (the pyrimidines) (Fig. 27-1).

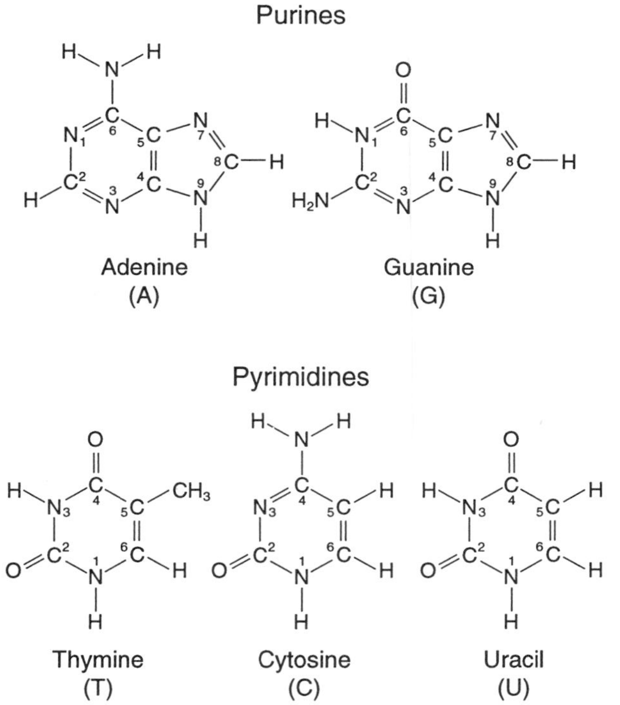

FIG. 27-1. Structural formulas for nucleotide bases.

Thymine is replaced in RNA by the nucleotide uracil. The four bases of DNA are often represented by the letters A, T, G, and C, respectively, whereas U is used to designate uracil. These bases establish the essence of a species and of the individual differences within members of the species. A major function of the nucleotide base is to encode the proteins of the cell. Three nucleotides in a precise order are known as a codon. Most codons correspond to one of the 20 amino acids (Table 27-1A, B). Several different codons may code for the same amino acid. Additionally, a few special codons do not code for any amino acid but act as termination markers that signal the end of synthesis of the protein chain.

The unique pattern of this four-letter genetic alphabet is responsible for the generation of all of the proteins and thus all of the events that occur in the human body. Just as important, the varying patterns of DNA base sequence

TABLE 27-1A. *Amino acids*

Glycine (Gly)	Lysine (Lys)
Alanine (Ala)	Arginine (Arg)
Valine (Val)	Asparagine (Ash)
Isoleucine (Ile)	Glutamine (Glu)
Leucine (Leu)	Cysteine (Cys)
Serine (Ser)	Methionine (Met)
Threonine (Thr)	Tryptophan (Trp)
Proline (Pro)	Phenylalanine (Phe)
Aspartic acid (Asp)	Tyrosine (Tyr)
Glutamic acid (Glu)	Histidine (His)

TABLE 27-1B. *The genetic code*

UUU	Phe	UCU	Ser	UAC	Tyr	UGU	Cys
UCG	Phe	UCC	Ser	UAC	Tyr	UGC	Cys
UUA	Leu	UCA	Ser	UAA	Stop	UGA	Stop
UUG	Leu	UCG	Ser	UAG	Stop	UGG	Trp
CUU	Leu	CCU	Pro	CAU	His	CGU	ARG
CUC	Leu	CCC	Pro	CAL	His	CGC	Arg
CUA	Leu	CCA	Pro	CAA	Gln	CGA	Arg
CUG	Leu	CCG	Pro	CAG	Gln	CGG	Arg
AUU	Ile	ACU	Thr	AAU	Asn	AGU	Ser
AUC	Ile	ACC	Thr	AAL	Asn	AGC	Ser
AUA	Ile	ACA	Thr	AAA	Lys	AGA	Agr
AUG	Met	ACG	Thr	AAG	Lys	AGG	Agr
GUU	Val	GCU	Ala	GAU	Asp	GGU	Gly
GUC	Val	GCC	Ala	GAC	Asp	GGC	Gly
GUA	Val	GCA	Ala	GAA	Glu	GGA	Gly
GUG	Val	GCG	Ala	GAG	Glu	GGG	Gly

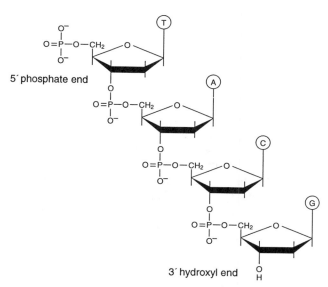

FIG. 27-2. Schematic of linkage of nucleotides for a single strand of DNA. A nucleotide is a unit composed of one base, one sugar, and one phosphate.

are also responsible for providing structure to the DNA molecules so that particular stretches of the molecules may be identified by the proteins and enzymes that are responsible for turning genes off and on.

The second component of the DNA or RNA molecule is a solid backbone of phosphate molecules attached to ribose or deoxyribose sugars. The attachment of these identical sugar/phosphate residues through a series of phosphodiester bonds is responsible for the strong strand-like structures that form DNA (Fig. 27-2). In a sense, they are the binders that make up the book's individual genes and chromosomes in humans and other eukaryotic species. Only special enzymes, known as DNA and RNA polymerases, and certain nuclease species are capable of interrupting this solid chain–like formation.

DNA consists of two strands of phosphodiester bonded chains which are linked together in the now famous "double helix" first postulated by Watson and Crick (Fig. 27-3). In one of the most important biological phenomenon we know of, these chains are held together by very weak thermal and pH-dependent hydrogen bonds in a very specific pattern. Thymine is always specifically paired with adenine and cytosine with guanine by the number and length of hydrogen bonds that stretch between the DNA helices. The fact that these bonds are specific and that they differ in length provides an always differing physical confirmation between unique segments of DNA. In this way, DNA is not merely a flat double helix but a structure that is bumpy or wavy, depending on the type of bond involved. These differences in landscape are what allows DNA-binding proteins, effector and repressor molecules to specifically bind only to carefully determined areas of the genetic material.

In addition, some areas of DNA are allowed to bind to *themselves* because of areas of palindromic sequences (reversed and complementary bases on a single strand of DNA). Palindromic sequences may function as sign

posts in the DNA double helix to further geographically identify start and stop and binding sites for the types of molecules that turn biological processes on and off. RNA molecules, such as transfer RNA, are provided binding specificity by the presence of palindromic and loop-like sequences.

Perhaps the most important aspect of the hydrogen bonds between the DNA strands is that they are incredibly easy to break and, similarly, to reform in a precise

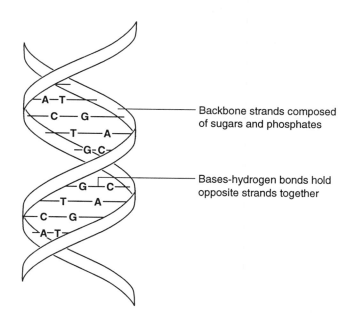

FIG. 27-3. "Double-helix" model postulated by Watson and Crick.

base-to-base reconfirmation. This allows the DNA molecule to unwrap, replicate itself, and then rewrap with the replicated DNA molecule. This process is central to the phenomenon of cell division.

Nature and Biological Role of Genes

Humans are organisms with eukaryotic cells. Eukaryotic cells have a true nucleus and, with the exception of DNA contained within mitochondria, all of the DNA is contained within the nucleus of the cell. In contrast, bacteria are prokaryotic cells and have no true nucleus. Chromosomes are packages of genetic material. DNA molecules are organized into functional segments along chromosomes termed genes. Genes are responsible for the generation of cellular protein products. Because of the evolutionary role of the genome, any organism's DNA must be viewed as a work in progress containing experiments in regulatory and protein function. Thus, genes may exist as single copies, as multiple copies on different chromosomes, as repeated copies on the same chromosome, and as inactive copies contiguous to or near the authentic (active) copy of the gene. In humans, there are 46 chromosomes arranged as 22 autosomal pairs and 2 sex chromosomes (X and Y). One copy of each of the 23 chromosomes is contributed by the mother and a second by the father. Hundreds of thousands of genes exist on each of the chromosomes.

Each gene consists of two categories of base sequences. The first, termed exons, are unique base sequences that will be transcribed directly into RNA and, after transport from nucleus to cytoplasm, translated into protein. Other sequences, called introns, seem to function in a structural or signal-producing sense and as spacers between actively translated portions of the gene. When one looks at the gene in a functional sense, the exons often correspond closely to functional units of the gene, such as specific binding sites, segments that direct protein transfer outside of the cell to membranes or to mito-

chondria, and structural segments that direct folding, carbohydrate binding, or secondary structure. The introns, which lie between these functional portions of the genetic material, may then serve the function of allowing "prefabricated" portions of the gene to be moved to other places in the genome during the evolutionary process in order to create different and more functional proteins from preexisting subunits rather than from scratch.

Another component to the gene is the presence of signals and markers within the gene that are recognized by the enzymes that regulate transcription of the gene into RNA. These warning, start, and stop signs have funny names, such as CATT and TATA boxes and polyadenylation segments, and are important yet structurally simple portions of an actively transcribed gene. Adding even more complexity to the gene are those areas upstream (called 58) and downstream (38), and within the introns of the gene, that bind proteins and nonprotein material serving to turn the gene on and off during different periods of development, cell life, or during the cell cycle. These effectors, repressors, inhibitors, derepressors, and so forth are important to the ordered function of the organism which contains the DNA and may be found anywhere from a very few bases away from the gene to thousands and even tens of thousands of base pairs distant. The complex structure of a typical gene may be seen in Fig. 27-4.

Gene Expression

Gene expression is the process of producing a protein from the information stored in DNA. This protein production process involves two specific events, transcription and translation. During transcription, an enzyme called RNA polymerase recognizes and binds a DNA nucleotide sequence near one end of the gene. As RNA polymerase moves down the DNA strand it creates an RNA chain by linking together ribonucleic acids floating free in the cell. The order of the nucleotides in the new chain is determined by complimentary base pairing.

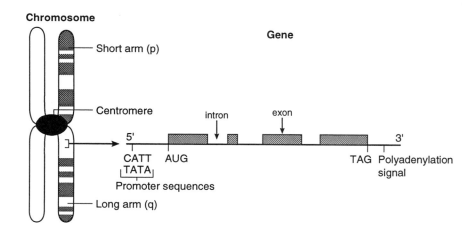

FIG. 27-4. Packaging of DNA. Chromosomes harbor DNA molecules. Banding techniques using fluorescent quinacrine (Q banding) or Giemsa (G banding), among others, permit specific identification of chromosomal segments. Regions of DNA molecules along chromosomes are organized and termed genes. Genes are divided into exons and introns.

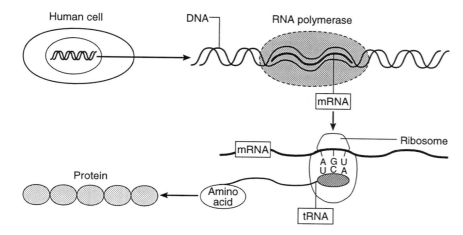

FIG. 27-5. Schematic for protein synthesis.

Eventually, a stop signal at the end of the gene is reached, the RNA polymerase is released from the DNA, and the new RNA chain is released. This new chain becomes messenger RNA (mRNA).

Once the information from a gene has been transcribed into an RNA molecule within the nucleus, the mRNA transports this information to cytosolic structures called ribosomes. mRNA attaches to the ribosome by a specific codon called the start codon. In humans, this codon is always an AUG codon and codes for the amino acid methionine.

Another form of RNA molecule called transfer RNA (tRNA) functions as an adaptor to translate the information on the mRNA into protein. Each amino acid is recognized by a special type of enzyme called aminoacyl-tRNA synthetase. These enzymes are responsible for linking the amino acids to their own specific type of tRNA. Each of the tRNA's has a three-nucleotide region called an anticodon. Thus, the amino acid at one end of each tRNA always corresponds to a specific set of three nucleotides in the anticodon region of the tRNA. As the tRNA molecules move amino acids floating free in the cell into position on ribosomes, the amino acids are linked together to form a protein chain (Fig. 27-5).

TECHNIQUES OF DNA AND RNA IDENTIFICATION

Making the diagnosis of a genetic or genetically related disease requires the isolation and characterization of specific small portions of what is an enormous human genome. To identify such small segments of DNA, the molecular biologist uses, among others, two very basic biochemical techniques.

Restriction Endonucleases

Restriction enzymes were first identified over a decade ago. These small biological molecules are actually de-

fenses of microscopic organisms such as fungi or bacteria against their only natural enemy: the virus. Because viruses are nothing more than naked "DNA" or RNA within a simple protein capsule, the only way for microorganisms to fight off these tiny predators is to be able to identify and specifically cut up their DNA, rendering them inactive. The discovery that these bacterial and fungal enzymes, called restriction endonucleases, could be useful in specifically cutting human and other forms of eukaryotic DNA represents one of the major advances in the field of medical molecular biology. The name of the restriction enzyme gives a clue as to what organism it is isolated or derived from. For example, *Eco*R1, one of the most commonly used restriction enzymes, is the first restriction enzyme isolated from *Escherichia coli*. Similarly, *Hin*fIII is the third restriction endonuclease from *Hemophilus influenza*. There are now hundreds of commercially available restriction endonucleases, each capable of dividing DNA strands in specific locations.

The restriction enzyme is capable of identifying a very specific pattern of four to six nucleotides within the DNA strand. This probably is a result of those differences in the distances of hydrogen bonding between the GC and AT pairs discussed earlier. This topographic recognition allows the enzyme to settle at or near its restriction site and to cleave the DNA in one of two specific patterns. *Blunt-ended patterns* are cleavages that are produced straight down the middle of a series of nucleotide pairs. This produces a blunt end where all nucleotides are paired with an existing complementary base on a second strand. *"Sticky"-ended* endonucleases cleave in a more complex fashion producing an irregular division between the strands. Thus, several unpaired nucleotides are exposed at the end of each strand following restriction enzyme digestion. The most significant aspect of this unbalanced division of the DNA strands is that these unpaired bases may subsequently reanneal with complementary bases on another strain. This allows easy annealing of the excised DNA with natural or artificially created DNA strands and is central to the concepts of cloning and gene therapy,

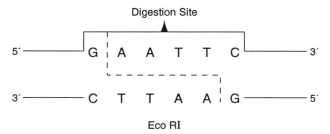

FIG. 27-6. Restriction endonucleases.

which will be discussed later. Restriction enzymes seem to work specifically at palindromic areas of DNA. For example, the identification site of the *Eco*R1 restriction enzyme is the nucleotides GAATTC, which if turned on themselves are complementary (Fig. 27-6).

Gel Electrophoresis

The second technique utilized by the molecular biologist is *gel electrophoresis*. Long utilized for the separation of proteins and other types of macromolecules, scientists in the last 15 years have begun to extensively utilize the technique for the separation of variously sized DNA and RNA molecules. Electrophoresis owes its specificity to differences in the size and charge of nucleic acid molecules. The DNA molecule may be divided into pieces of various sizes by restriction endonucleases. Restriction endonucleases, because of their almost absolute specificity for these palindromic sequences, will create precise and repeated consistent cuts in a DNA molecule, much like proteolytic enzymes, such as trypsin, create precise and consistent cuts in a protein. Thus, each time a particular strand of DNA is subjected to restriction enzyme digestion, the pieces of DNA that result from strand division will be identical in length and in sequence.

Gels consist of matrices of molecules, complex polymers, such as polyacrylamide, that form a sort of biological sieve allowing either rapid or slower passage of nucleic acids through the matrix. The most popular systems size DNA and RNA molecules by size alone because they utilize chemicals like sodium dodecyl sulfate (SDS), which are powerfully charged molecules that render the electrical charges on the DNA molecules identical. By passing an electric current through the gel matrix, the DNA molecules are drawn from a well in the negatively charged terminal toward the positively charged terminal at the opposite end of the gel. Based on the size (and sometimes the tertiary structure) of the DNA molecules, their progress through the gel may be rapid or slow. The smallest molecules tend to move through the gel most rapidly. If the time over which the electric current is passed through the gel is properly chosen, all of the DNA fragments resulting from a restriction enzyme digest will

be displayed on the gel and separated by size. These DNA fragments can then be identified either by the use of intercalating agents, such as ethidium bromide (Fig. 27-7), which identify all of the DNA fragments, or specifically by the use of molecular probes.

Each unique strand of DNA has its own special nucleotide sequence and thus will be cleaved in a slightly different fashion by restriction endonuclease digestion. Even minor differences (as few as one or two bases in length) can be differentiated on gel electrophoresis if proper gel composition and electrophoretic technique are utilized. These differences in the gel electrophoresis and restriction enzyme digestion patterns of DNA allow us to perform the "DNA fingerprinting" that is used for paternity testing and forensic identification purposes.

Blotting Techniques

After restriction enzyme digestion and gel electrophoresis, specific portions of the DNA molecule or other macromolecules, such as proteins, may be identified through a process known as blotting. Blotting techniques have become central to the task of the medical molecular biologist. There are three basic forms of evaluation, which have been given the names of Northern, Southern, and Western blotting. Although these procedures are often confusing to the clinician, blotting is actually a simple process and the differences between the three types of blots are easy to understand.

Blotting is a two-part procedure. The first involves the transfer and bonding of macromolecules to nylon or nylon-like filters. The second involves using a specific probe to identify the component part of the blot that is of interest. The differences in the three forms of blotting are summarized in Table 27-2. A Southern blot involves the bonding of DNA fragments to the filter and the use of complementary DNA molecules to identify the specific fragments of interest. This bonding occurs through the process of DNA/DNA hybridization—the specific annealing of complimentary nucleotides of a free-floating DNA molecule to a bonded DNA molecule on the filter. In the Northern blotting technique, RNA is bonded to the filter paper and is identified using hybridization of complimentary DNA to the specific segments of RNA on the filter. A third procedure, called a Western blot, involves the binding of protein to the nylon filter. Rather than complementary nucleic acid molecules, specific antibodies to the protein are then used for identification of the proteins of interest.

These three blotting techniques have in common the procedure of macromolecule transfer to nylon or other synthetic membranes. This stepwise procedure is demonstrated in Fig. 27-8. Initially, the macromolecules are separated by electrophoresis or chromatography techniques as described above. Next, the separated macromolecules

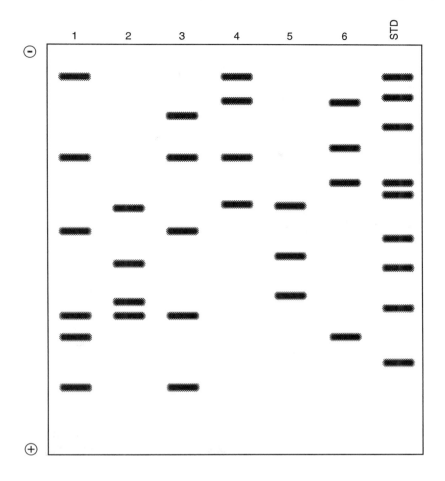

FIG. 27-7. Electrophoresis gel. Each lane represents DNA fragments resulting from digestion with different restriction endonucleases. The far right lane represents marker DNA fragments. Ethidium bromide was used to illuminate DNA fragments for photography with a Polaroid camera.

are transferred to a filter-like membrane by either osmotic or electrophoretic techniques. The macromolecule may then be fixed to the membrane either thermally or electrochemically. Finally, the membrane is bathed in a solution containing either radiolabeled or fluorescent-specific probe which will identify only the protein or nucleic acid of interest on the filter-like membrane. Autoradiography or fluorescence under ultraviolet light may then be used to identify the specific molecules.

In Situ Hybridization

Another form of identification used to demonstrate the presence or absence of either protein or nucleic acid in a specific tissue or at a specific time in the development of that tissue is called *in situ hybridization*. In this technique, small sections of the tissue are frozen and carefully mounted on slides without exposure to denaturing chemicals such as alcohol. These tissue sections become the equivalent of the membrane filters used for blotting. The sections are carefully bathed in droplets of a solution containing a specific DNA or antibody probe to identify the molecule of interest. Microscopic or electron micrographic evaluation of the tissue section will then demonstrate not only the presence but the specific tissue or intracellular location of the macromolecule. In situ hybridization may be utilized to answer questions, such as the presence of papilloma virus DNA in cells exhibiting invasive cervical cancer or cervical dysplasia and the presence and location of cells within the placenta that make human placental lactogen.

Cloning Techniques

Gene cloning was developed in the mid-1970s and has become a pivotal tool for the identification and characterization (sequencing) of specific DNA transcripts. A schematic representation of cloning is seen in Fig. 27-9. First, living cells are broken open either with mechanical forces or with a detergent. The next step is to remove ge-

TABLE 27-2. *Blots*

Type	Radiolabeled "probe"	Separated by gel electophoresis
Southern blot	DNA	DNA
Northern blot	DNA	RNA
Western blot	Antibody	Protein (antigen)

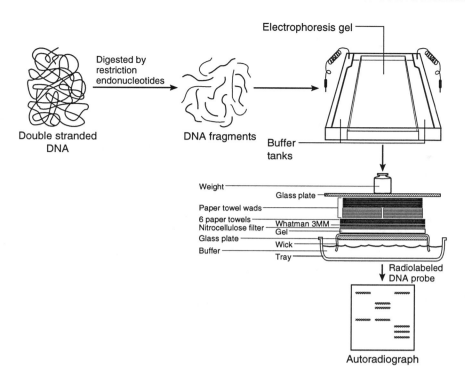

FIG. 27-8. Technique for Southern and Northern blots.

netic material from the cells and purify the DNA. One common method involves spooling DNA onto a glass rod. Next, DNA is cut using restriction endonucleases. These sections of DNA are then spliced into cloning vehicles that are able to carry the DNA sections into other living cells including bacterial cells. The spliced DNA molecule is also called a recombinant DNA molecule. Cells are allowed to multiply, forming a clone, having millions of identical cells with the recombinant DNA. The specific DNA splice is then translated to a protein product. Western blotting can then be used to detect colonies of cells that are producing the specific protein and thus contain the specific DNA of interest.

Polymerase Chain Reaction

Amplification of small fragments or sections of DNA into quantities large enough to be analyzed can be accomplished with the polymerase chain reaction (PCR). The specificity of PCR amplification is based on two oligonucleotide primers that flank the DNA section to be amplified. The oligonucleotide primers anneal to opposite strands and are usually composed of 15–25 nucleotides. There are three basic steps in the PCR technique: (1) denaturation of the double-stranded DNA sample by using elevated temperature; (2) annealing of the oligonucleotide primers to the DNA template at low temperatures (37–55°C); (3) extension of the primers using specific DNA polymerases. One set of the above steps is referred to as a cycle. Each successive cycle es-

sentially doubles the amount of DNA synthesized from the previous cycle. This results in exponential accumulation of the specific DNA fragment at approximately 2^N, where N represents the number of cycles (Fig. 27-10).

IDENTIFICATION OF GENETIC ERRORS AND DIFFERENCES

One of the major roles of the new molecular technologies is identification of the genetic differences and errors that characterize human disease. These errors can be the consequence of genetic errors as small as single nucleotide differences (such as that which creates sickle cell anemia) or result from huge additions or deletions to the human genome (Table 27-3).

Karyotyping

The largest defects in the human genome can be identified by procedures as gross as *karyotyping*. Major deletions or transpositions of chromosomal material and duplications such as trisomies and triploidies are easily identified by this technique. Such major anomalies, however, are relatively rare in the overall scope of human disease. The wide variety of other genetic diseases cannot be identified by such macroscopic techniques. Thus, other methods of identification are required for the identification of such defects at the genomic level, the intragenic level, or the level of single-protein codons or individual nucleotide bases. *Restriction length polymorphisms,*

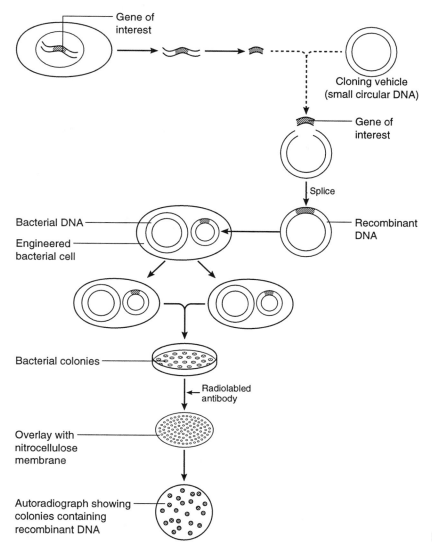

FIG. 27-9. Cloning.

Southern blot analysis, and *DNA sequencing* are examples of newly developed molecular biology technologies that are being utilized increasingly in the identification and management of genetically related diseases (Table 27-4).

Restriction Length Polymorphism

Restriction length polymorphisms (RFLPs) were among the first genetic differences to be associated with disease states. RFLPs are the result of genetic differences between individuals and do not necessarily occur within the abnormal gene of interest. It is customary, in fact, to find that the critical sequence differences in RFLPs are familial in nature and are found in areas that flank the gene to either side. Because genetic patterns are inherited within families, the presence of a signature RFLP for a genetic disorder in an individual is highly suggestive of the presence of the disease and, more particularly (in clinical use), the carrier state. Restriction length polymorphisms are identified when the human DNA is exposed to a predetermined group of restriction enzymes (endonucleases). Mutations within the specific segments of DNA either creating or eliminating unique restriction sites produce differences within the DNA strands in the pattern of restriction cleavage (Fig. 27-11).

RFLP technology is informative for genetic analysis only when two specific criteria are met. First, the restriction sites of the DNA region of interest must be different for individuals with normal and abnormal genes. Second, a large number of family members must be available for analysis not only of their DNA but for the presence or absence of the disease state in themselves, their ancestors, and their offspring. This family linkage analysis is often difficult to provide and as such RFLPs have gradually given way to other forms of evaluating

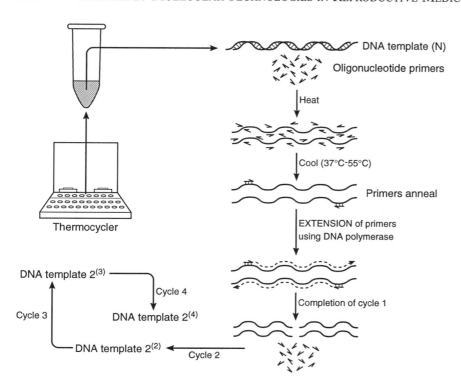

FIG. 27-10. Polymerase chain reaction.

the presence of the specific genes encoding proteins that cause genetic diseases.

Gene Error Identification

Because of tools like RFLP, linkage analysis, and "reverse genetics" (whereby abnormal proteins may be used as starting points to work backward toward identification of the genes from which they arise), we have, in recent years, increasingly been able to identify the specific genetic defects responsible for a variety of disease states. When these defects are reasonably large, ie, greater than three or four nucleotides in length, direct genetic analysis by Southern blot is an effective tool in differentiating individuals who carry abnormal genes from those who do not. Utilizing differences in probes for specific areas of DNA that can be as short as 20–30 bases (but more frequently are lengthier), it is usually possible to identify deletions or inserts in specific gene sequences. The ability of these sequences to anneal to complementary sequences is dependent on temperature, pH, and solute concentration of the hybridization solution.

TABLE 27-3. *Types of genetic abnormalities*

Numerical: Most commonly a result of nondysjunction
    Aneuploid
    Mosaic
    Polyploid
Structural: Rearrangements or translocations
Single-gene mutations: Follows Mendelian order of transmission
    with dominant or recessive pattern
    Autosomal
    X-linked

CURRENT APPLICATIONS OF MOLECULAR TECHNIQUES

As technologies in molecular biology advance, specific methodologies and techniques considered to be the state of the art change on a continuous basis. Molecular

TABLE 27-4. *Some disorders that can be detected with DNA-based techniques on research or diagnostic basis*

Albinism
α-Thalassemia
Antitryspin deficiency
Ataxia-telangiectasia
β-Thalassemia
Charcot–Marie–Tooth disease
Congenital adrenal hyperplasia (21-PH deficiency)
Cystic fibrosis
Fragile X syndrome
Gaucher's disease
Growth hormone deficiency (hereditary)
Huntington's disease
Kallman's syndrome
Lesch–Nyhan syndrome
Malignant hyperthermia
Muscular dystrophy, Duchenne–Becker type
Muscular dystrophy, Emery–Dreyfus type
Neurofibromatosis
Osteogenesis imperfecta
Phenylketonuria
Polycystic kidney disease, adult
Prader-Willi syndrome
Retinitis pigmentosa
Retinoblastoma
Sickle cell anemia
Tay-Sachs disease
Testicular feminization
von Willebrand's disease
Xeroderma pigmentosum

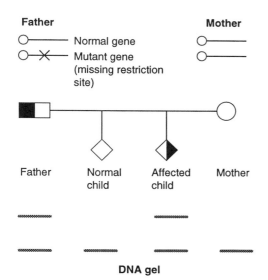

FIG. 27-11. Restriction fragment length polymorphism.

biology techniques clinical application that bridge the research and clinical disciplines of medicine. Exploitation of molecular technology vastly expands the capability of the reproductive biologist to diagnose and treat reproductive dysfunctions. Applications of these new techniques range from prenatal diagnoses to direct and indirect gene analyses for specific abnormal genes.

The power of the new DNA technology is its use as a tool for diagnosis. There are two types of molecular lesions that lead to disorders. The lesions, insertions, or rearrangements of genes compose the first type of molecular lesion. The second type of abnormality presents itself in the form of a single-nucleotide abnormality (point mutations) in critical regions of genes. By employing the older methods of chromosome analysis in the form of karyotyping and banding techniques, one will elicit gross abnormalities. The newer molecular biology techniques allow the discovery of more subtle abnormalities of the gene. Application of the previously described molecular biology technique may be in the form of direct or indirect gene analysis. Examples of these applications will be briefly discussed in the following paragraphs.

Prenatal Diagnosis

Genetically determined disease affects approximately 3% of newborn infants. The identification of pregnancies involves a search for risk factors. These increased risk factors include advanced maternal age, familial history of birth defects, and ethnic and racial factors. Fetal DNA can easily be isolated from cells obtained from amniocentesis or chorionic villus sampling. Ultrasound-guided amniocentesis is usually performed between 14 and 16 weeks. Viable cells are cultured for karyotyping or DNA extraction. Chorionic villus sampling is performed by aspirating tissue through a transcervical catheter or transabdominal needle, again with ultrasound guidance. This

procedure is usually performed between 10 and 12 weeks gestation. For gestations >18 weeks, percutaneous umbilical blood sampling or fetal biopsy may be used to obtain cells for DNA extraction. Although the list of cloned genes for prenatal diagnosis is impressive, there is not yet available a cloned gene for all genetic disorders.

Recurrent Pregnancy Loss

Progress in DNA technology has allowed the exploration of molecular mutation associated with embryonic loss. Many feel that lethal mutations occur in genes that are necessary for early embryologic and fetal development. These genetic defects, which lead to abortions in humans, appear to have a normal karyotype with past techniques. As an example, mouse models suggest that mutations in critical genes result in embryonic death. DNA insertions inactivate mouse type 1 collagen gene by blocking the initial transcription. Thus, blood vessels are affected leading to rupture and eventually death of the developing embryo. In addition, genes that direct cell differentiation in early morphologic development theoretically acquire mutations yielding severely deformed nonviable embryos or even massive embryonic disorganization that results in a blighted ovum.

Sexual Differentiation

Progression of sexual differentiation depends on molecular events. In the case of male sexual differentiation, gene sequences critical for sex determination (SRY) have been limited to a segment of the Y chromosome by elimination studies of certain intersex patients using Y-specific DNA probes. Once SRY is produced and testicular development initiated, the seminiferous tubals appear and surround the germ cells. Mullerian-inhibiting factor

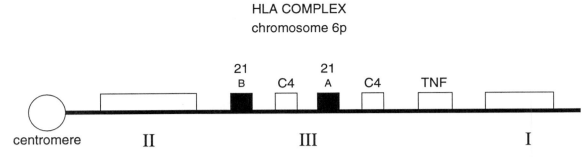

FIG. 27-12. 21B represents the active gene for 21-hydroxylase. 21A represents a pseudogene (nonsense gene). C, compliment; TNF, tumor necrosis factor.

(MIF) from the Sertoli cells is the next major molecular event evoked. The gene encoding for MIF has been isolated. This gene has five exons that encode a protein of 550 amino acids. The C-terminal domain of this peptide is highly conserved and demonstrates marked homology with human transforming growth factor–β and the β chain of porcine inhibin. Other DNA-mediated steps that are crucial for normal sexual development include the production of human chorionic gonadotropin and the enzymes responsible for steroidogenesis. Genes encoding for the development of receptors can result in potentially critical defects. In the case of androgen receptors, androgen insensitivity could result.

Female sexual differentiation is for the most part independent as compared with male differentiation. However, with newer DNA techniques, it is possible that gene expression during embryogenesis may uncover the basic drive for female sexual differentiation. The use of DNA probes will make diagnoses, such as uterine anomalies, possible in the future. As with early sexual differentiation in the embryo, a cascade of molecular events is necessary for pediatric and adolescent statural growth and pubertal development.

Genes necessary for encoding specific hormones, such as growth hormone, gonadotropin-releasing hormone (GnRH), insulin growth factors, cortical adrenal–stimulating hormone, the gonadotropins, somatostatin, and others, are all prerequisite. Critical molecular defects of any of these genes potentially alters growth and secondary sexual development. A classical example is growth hormone deficiency, which is the prototype for such defects. Although several syndromes for growth hormone deficiency have been described, one particular syndrome, type 1A, is a result of a deletion. Likewise, isolated deficiency of GnRH may provide an opportunity for identifying a specific gene defect. This syndrome has been associated in a variety of hereditary settings including autosomal recessive, autosomal dominant, X-linked recessive, and isolated forms. It is possible that different gene mutations might be responsible for this variety of forms.

Congenital Adrenal Hyperplasia

An autosomal recessive disorder in which a deficiency in an enzyme is important for adrenal steroidogenesis (most commonly 21-hydroxylase) results in a partial or complete block in cortisol biosynthesis. Classical genetic studies reveal that this autosomal recessive disorder is linked to the human leukocyte antigen (HLA) major histocompatibility locus on the short arm of chromosome 6 (Fig. 27-12). Recently, molecular analysis of this region has actually elucidated the structural gene for cytochrome P450-21-hydroxylase. Nonclassical cases of congenital adrenal hyperplasia (CAH) through RFLP analysis reveal ultrastructural defects in the form of deletions and point mutations responsible for the expression of "late-onset" CAH. Other instances of similar molecular analyses presently being explored include GnRH, gonadotropin-associated peptide (GAP), and the gonadotropins.

FUTURE DIRECTION OF THE MOLECULAR BIOLOGY

Human Genome Project

An international effort is currently underway with the goal of sequencing the entire human genome. There are approximately 3 billion base pairs of DNA encoding for the estimated 75,000–100,000 genes in the human genome. The human genome project is estimated to take 10–15 years to complete. The genomic sequence will provide a basis for advances in gene therapy and identification of specific biological disorders.

Genome Imprinting

The concept of genome imprinting continues to evolve. Investigators have been striving to identify the molecular nature of the genome imprint, which is a process that temporarily and erasably imprints or marks the genes passed on by females and males in different ways. Traits

TABLE 27-5. *Disorders that are clinically suspected of being associated with genonic imprinting*

Prader–Willi syndrome
Angelman's syndrome
Huntington's disease
Cystic fibrosis
Beckwith–Wiedemann syndrome
Diabetes (insulin-dependent, maturity-onset)
Myotonic dystrophy
Neurofibromatosis (II)
Fragile X mental retardation

associated with genome imprinting do not obey normal Mendelian observations. Parents may contribute exactly identical genes to their offspring but the genes may have different sex-specific imprints that influence normal development and alter expression of diseases. Table 27-5 lists disorders that are suspected to be influenced by genetic imprinting.

Recombinant Medication

In addition to diagnosis of gene abnormalities encoding for critical hormones and enzymes, recombinant DNA technology provides feasibility of commercially available medication in patients with these missing substances. Once genes are isolated and characterized, they can be transfected into prokarocytes (bacteria and yeast) or eukaryotic cells that are designed to produce large portions of a specific protein product. For example, recombinant medications include preparations of insulin, growth hormone, follicle-stimulating hormone, and luteinizing hormone. Many other products are in the process of development for the management of a wide range of disorders. These engineered synthetic medications provide increased purity and improved flexibility for individualized patient management.

Gene Therapy

Although there have been rapid advances in gene isolation for various diseases, the majority of inheritable diseases are without adequate treatment. Protocols are currently being investigated for gene transfer in therapy by the Recombinant DNA Advisory Committee. Two approaches for gene transfer are in vivo delivery and ex vivo delivery followed by autologous return of these cells to the patient. An example of the ex vivo approach is the transfer of a gene into bone marrow cells. Gene therapy is targeted to bone marrow stem cells and these cells are then returned to the patient. In contrast, in vivo gene delivery requires a vector for transfer of the gene. Both viral and nonviral methods are being investigated. Viral vectors include retroviruses, adenoviruses, adeno-associated viruses, and herpes simplex viruses. Nonviral methods include the transport of genes by macromolecules such as fusogenic lipid vesicles. The wide range of diseases that may be treated by gene therapy include liver disease, hematopoietic disease, cancer, respiratory disease, and muscular disease. The impact of the new genetic technology has already been considerable, but with the rapid advancement of knowledge and techniques seen over the past several years, this may only be the beginning of the way medicine is practiced in the future.

SUGGESTED READING

Collins F, Galas D. A new five-year plan for the U.S. human genome project. *Science* 1993;262:43.
Drlica K, ed. *Understanding DNA and Gene Cloning. A Guide for the Curious.* Toronto: John Wiley and Sons, 1984.
Morsy MA, Mitani K, Clemens P, Caskey CT. Progress toward human gene therapy. *JAMA* 1993;270:2338.
Sapienza C. Parental imprinting of genes. *Sci Am* 1990;263:52.
Sinden RR, ed. *DNA Structure and Function.* San Diego: Academic Press, 1994.

Clinical Reproductive Medicine,
Edited by Bryan D. Cowan and David B. Seifer
Lippincott-Raven Publishers, Philadelphia © 1997

APPENDIX

Resource List

Adoptive Families of America   *3333 Highway 100 North, Minneapolis, MN 55422, 1-800-372-3300*

American College of Obstetricians & Gynecologists Resource Center   *409 12th Street, SW, Washington D.C. 20024-2188, 202-638-5577*

American Society of Andrology   *P.O. Box 15171, Lenexa, KS 66285-5171, 913-541-9077*

The American Society for Reproductive Medicine   *1209 Montgomery Highway, Birmingham, AL 35216-2809, 205-978-5000*

American Urological Association, Inc.   *1120 North Charles Street, Baltimore, MD 21201-5559, 410-727-1100*

DES Action USA (East Coast Office)   *Long Island Jewish Medical Center, New Hyde Park, NY 11040, 516-775-3450*

DES Action USA (West Coast Office)   *1615 Broadway, Oakland, CA 94612, 510-465-4011*

The Endocrine Society   *9650 Rockville Pike, Bethesda, MD 20814, 301-941-0200*

Endometriosis Association   *8585 North 76th Place Milwaukee, WI 53223 1-800-992-3636 (in the United States) 1-800-426-2363 (in Canada)*

National Adoption Center   *1500 Walnut Street, Suite 701, Philadelphia, PA 19102, 1-800-TO-ADOPT or 215-735-9988*

National Adoption Information Clearinghouse   *11426 Rockville Pike, Suite 410, Rockville, MD 20852, 301-231-6512*

National Committee for Adoption   *1930 17th Street, NW, Washington D.C. 20009-6207, 202-328-1200*

National Society of Genetic Counselors   *233 Canterbury Drive, Wallingford, PA 19086, 610-872-7608*

North American Menopause Society   *University Hospital of Cleveland, 2074 Abington Road, Cleveland, OH 44106, 216-535-3334*

OURS, Inc.   *3333 Highway 100 North Minneapolis, MN 55422, 612-535-4829*

Resolve, Inc.   *1310 Broadway, Somerville, MA 02144-1731, 617-623-0744*

SHARE: Pregnancy and Infant Loss Support, Inc.   *Joseph Health Center, 300 First Capitol Drive, Saint Charles, MO 63301, 314-947-6164*

Turner's Syndrome Society of the United States   *Twelve Oaks Center, 15500 Wayzata Boulevard, Suite 811, Wayzata, MN 55391, 612-475-9944*

Subject Index

A

Abortion
  immunologic mechanisms of
    antiphospholipid antibodies, 261
    induction of trophoblast antigen
      expression, 261
    suppressor cell deficiency, 260–261
  spontaneous
    of human chorionic gonadotropin-
      stimulated conceptions, 237
Acromegaly
  clinical syndrome in, 122t, 127
  suppression tests for, 123t, 127
ACTH. See Adrenocorticotropin hormone
    (ACTH)
Activin
  gonadal secretion and, 27, 27f
Adenohypophysis. See Anterior pituitary
    (adenohypophysis)
Adenomas
  hepatocellular
    oral contraceptive-associated, 137
Adhesion molecules
  implantation and, 164–165
Adrenal glands
  androgen production by, 97, 97f
Adrenarche
  puberty and, 51–52
Adrenocorticotropin hormone (ACTH)
    stimulation test
    for ACTH deficiency, 121t, 126
    for congenital adrenal hyperplasia, 99f,
      99–100
Age
  effect on GIFT outcome, 216t, 217t
  effect on IVF outcome, 215, 216, 216t
  oocyte donation and, 222
  reproduction and, 173t, 173–174,
    174f
Agenesis
  Mullerian, 187–188
  uterine cervix, 188, 188f
Alcohol
  recurrent pregnancy loss from, 244
Aldosterone
  biosynthesis of, 15, 16f, 17
  structure of, 15f
Alloimmunity
  recurrent pregnancy loss and, 245
Amenorrhea
  postpill, 137
Amenorrhea/anovulation

chronic, 76–79
  classification of, 77t
  gonadotropin-ovarian interaction in,
    76–77, 77t
  polycystic ovarian syndrome and, 76,
    77, 78, 79, 79f
  sex hormone-binding globulin in,
    77–78, 78t
classification of, 76t
from CNS-hypothalamic-pituitary
    dysfunction, 79–81
diagnosis of, 81–82
  algorithm for, 81f
evaluation interpretation in, 82
exercise-induced, 80
from gonadal dysgenesis, 81
from hyperprolactinemia, 82–83
from hypothalamic-pituitary interactions
    faulty, 80–81
from Mullerian and outflow tract
    defects, 81
primary and secondary, 76
psychogenic, 80
treatment of, 173
Aminoacids, 268, 268t
Androgen insensitivity (testicular
    feminization)
complete, 42–43
partial, 43
Androgen receptor, 20, 20t
Androgens
  biosynthesis of, 15, 16f
  conversion to estrogens by peripheral
    aromatase, 76, 77f
  disorders of. See also Hirsuitism
  for endometriosis, 178
  excess production of. See
    Hyperandrogenism
  in hair growth, 96, 97t
  ovarian
    and adrenal biosynthesis of, 41f
    synthesis of, 8
  production of
    in women, 97, 97f
  in sexual development, 40, 40t
  in utero excess of
    female pseudohermaphroditism from,
      44, 44t
Androstenedione
  in androgen biosynthesis, 15, 16f
  production rates of, 16t
  synthesis of, 8

Androsterone
  in estrogen biosynthesis, 17, 17f
Anorexia nervosa
  amenorrhea/anovulation in, 79–80, 80t
  characteristics of, 80t
Anterior pituitary (adenohypophysis)
  anatomy of, 5f, 6, 7
  controlling factors in, 6t, 7t
  hormones of, 6t, 7t
Antibodies. See Immunoglobulin(s)
Antigens
  definition of, 249
  production of, 256
Antisperm antibodies (AsAb)
  etiology of
    in male reproductive tract, 262
    in uterus, 262
  evaluation of, 261
  prevalence of, 261
  testing for, 262
Antrum
  fluid in, 149
  follicular, 147f, 148, 149
Apoptosis
  in follicle atresia, 34
ART. See Assisted reproductive technology
    (ART)
Arteries
  hypophyseal, 4, 5f
Assisted embryo hatching
  definition of, 219
  selection criteria for, 219–220
  technique for, 220f
Assisted fertilization
  for sperm-related barriers, 218–219,
    219f
Assisted reproductive technology (ART)
  acronyms in, 214
  comparison of 1993 procedure
    outcomes, 215t
  definitions in, 214
  historical perspective on, 214
  success of
    age and, 215, 216, 216t
    male factor infertility and, 215,
      216t
  success rates with, 214–215
Atresia
  follicular, 34, 149, 149f
  vaginal, 187, 187f, 189
Autoimmunity
  recurrent pregnancy loss and, 245

B

Bacterial colonization
    recurrent pregnancy loss from, 243–244
Basal body temperature
    in infertility evaluation, 168
Bleeding
    abnormal vaginal. *See* Dysfunctional
        uterine bleeding (DUB)
    breakthrough
        oral contraceptive-associated, 139
    in ectopic pregnancy, 193
    during menopausal hormone therapy,
        113
Blotting technique(s)
    basic procedure in, 272–273, 273t
    Northern, 272, 274f
    Southern, 272, 274f
    Western, 272
Bromocriptine
    for hyperprolactinemia, 90
    pharmacokinetics of, 90, 91f
    routes of administration of, 90
    side effects of, 90
    suppression of
        in hyperprolactinemia, 123t, 127

C

CA-125
    in endometriosis diagnosis, 176
CAH. *See* Congenital adrenal hyperplasia
        (CAH)
Cancer risk
    with estrogen replacement therapy, 110
Cardiovascular disease
    complications of, 108
    oral contraceptive-associated, 135
    postmenopausal, 107–108
    premenopausal, 108
CBG. *See* Cortisol-binding globulin
        (CBG)
Celomic metaplasia theory
    of endometriosis, 176–177
Central nervous system-hypothalamic
        interaction
    faulty
        amenorrhea/anovulation from, 79–80
Cerebrovascular disease
    oral contraceptive-associated, 135
Cervix uteri incompetence
    recurrent pregnancy loss from, 242
Chlorpromazine stimulation test
    for prolactin deficiency, 117, 119t
Chocolate cysts, ovarian, 177
Cholesterol
    conversion to testosterone, 41, 41f
    from LDL cholesterol uptake, 13, 14f
    storage of, 13
    structure of, 13f
Cholesterol desmolase (P450scc)
        deficiency, 41–42 42f
Chromophobe adenoma
    hyperprolactinemia from, 87
Chromosomal anomalies
    in aborted pregnancies, 240–241
Clomiphene citrate
    adjunctive agents with, 233–234
    for anovulatory infertility, 173

complications with, 234, 234t
    contraindications to, 233
    dosing and response with, 233, 233t
        monitoring of, 234
    historical perspective, 232
    indications for, 233
    mechanism of action of, 232–233, 233t
    ovulation and pregnancy with, 235, 235t
    pharmacology of, 232
    physiology of, 232
    pregnancy rates with, 233, 234f
    toxicology of, 234–235
Clomiphene stimulation test
    for gonadotropin deficiency, 117, 119t
Cloning, 273–274, 275f
Congenital adrenal hyperplasia (CAH),
        44–45
    diagnosis of, 99f, 99–100
    late-onset, 98t, 98–99
        diagnosis of, 99f, 99–100
        steroidogenesis pathway and enzyme
            defects in, 99, 99f
    peripheral precocious puberty from, 57
    restriction length polymorphism
        identification of, 278, 278t
Congenital lipoid adrenal hyperplasia
        (CLAH). *See* Cholesterol
        desmolase (P450scc) deficiency
        (congenital lipoid adrenal
        hyperplasia [CLAH])
Constitutional delay
    in hypogonadotropic delayed puberty,
        54t, 55
Contraception
    anti-human chorionic gonadotropin
        vaccines for, 263t, 263–264
    current methods for, 263
    immunologic vaccines for
        advantages of, 263
        anti-sperm antigen vaccine for, 264
        anti-zona pellucida vaccine, 264
        limitations of, 264
    during menopause, 113–114
    postcoital, 139
Controlled ovarian hyperstimulation
    in ART, 216–217, 217t
Corpus luteum
    structure and function of, 64f, 66
Corticotropin (ACTH) deficiency, 120t,
        126
    corticotropin-releasing factor
        stimulation test for, 121t, 126
    glucagon stimulation test for, 121t, 126
    insulin-induced hypoglycemia
        stimulation test for, 121t, 126
    metyrapone stimulation test for, 121t,
        126
    synthetic corticotropin stimulation test
        for, 121t, 126
Corticotropin (ACTH) excess (Cushing's
        syndrome)
    clinical syndrome in, 124t, 127–28
    suppression testing for, 125t, 127–128
Corticotropin-releasing hormone (CRH)
        stimulation test
    for ACTH deficiency, 121t, 126
    ACTH response to

in Cushing's syndrome, 125t,
        127–128
Cortisol
    in Cushing's syndrome, 100
    function of, 15
    structure of, 15f
Cortisol-binding globulin (CBG)
    estrogen effect on, 136
C protein
    in gonadotropin action, 25, 26f
Craniopharyngioma
    amenorrhea/anovulation from, 80
Cumulative probability
    of pregnancy, 171
Cushing's syndrome
    in hirsutism, 100
    recurrent pregnancy loss from, 243
    screening for, 100
Cyproterone
    for endometriosis, 178
Cytochrome P450 enzymes
    in cholesterol biosynthesis, 14, 15t
Cytokine(s). *See also* named class, e.g.
        Interferon(s)
    characteristics and functions of, 252t
    colony stimulating factors, 252t
    interferons, 252t, 255–256
    interleukins, 252t, 252–255
Cytotrophoblast(s)
    in immunotolerance of pregnancy
        chorionic, 258
        extravillous, 259

D

Danocrine
    for endometriosis, 178
Decidual suppressor cells
    production of immunosuppressive
        factors by, 259f, 259–260
Dehydroepiandrosterone (DHEA)
    structure of, 15, 16f
    synthesis of, 8
Dehydroepiandrosterone-Sulfate
        (DHEAS), 15, 16f
Delayed puberty, 53–54
    differential diagnosis of, 54t, 54–55
    eugonadotropic conditions in, 54, 54t
    hypergonadotropic hypogonadism, 54t,
        54–55
    hypogonadotropic hypogonadism, 54t,
        55
    schematic evaluation of, 56f
Deoxyribonucleic acid (DNA). *See* DNA
        (deoxyribonucleic acid)
17:20-Desmolase deficiency, 42
Dexamethasone suppression tests
    for corticotropin excess, 125t, 127–128
    for hyperandrogenism, 125t, 128
DHEA. *See* Dehydroepiandrosterone
        (DHEA)
Diabetes mellitus
    estrogen replacement therapy and, 108
    recurrent pregnancy loss from, 243
DNA (deoxyribonucleic acid)
    double helix model of, 269, 269f
    function of, 268–270
    genes in, 270–271

genetic code and, 269t
identification techniques, 271–274
nucleotide bases in, 268, 268f
nucleotide linkage in, 269, 269f
packaging of, 270f
phosphate molecules in, 269
protein synthesis in, 271, 271f
RNA polymerase in, 270–271
structure of, 268t, 268–270
Dopamine
in prolactin secretion, 86
DUB. *See* Dysfunctional uterine bleeding
(DUB)
Dynamic testing. *See also* Stimulation
testing; Suppression testing
basic principles of, 116, 118t–1225t
difficulties with, 116
stimulation, 116
suppression, 116
value of, 116
Dysfunctional uterine bleeding (DUB)
breakthrough, 70
diagnosis of
algorithm for, 71t
medical history in, 70
menstrual calendar in, 70
pelvic examination in, 70
progestin withdrawal test in, 71
differential diagnosis of, 70, 70t
laboratory evaluation of, 71, 71f
medical management of, 71–73
medication-associated, 70, 70t
surgical therapies for, 73
treatment of
hospitalization for, 71–72
outpatient, 71
withdrawal, 70
Dyspareunia
menopausal, 106

E
Ectopic pregnancy
case-fatality rate for, 192
conservative treatment of
complications of, 196–197
diagnosis of, 193–194
algorithm for, 194, 196f
histopathology of, 192–193
implantation sites for, 192, 193f
incidence of, 192, 192t
nonsurgical treatment of, 197–198
operations for
in distal tubal, 195, 197f
historical perspective, 194–195
in proximal tubal, 195–196, 197f
reoperation second-look procedures for,
209, 211
risk factors for, 192, 192t, 208–209
salpingectomy for, 209, 209f
salpingostomy for
endoscopic linear, 209, 210f
spontaneous resolution of, 197–198
surgery for
reproduction following, 197
Embryo
biopsy of
for genetic diagnosis, 220f, 220–221

placenta from, 160
transfer in IVF, 218
trophoblast from, 160
Embryogenesis, 151–152, 152f
Empty sella syndrome
amenorrhea/anovulation from, 80–81
hyperprolactinemia in, 87–88
Endometrial cancer
oral contraceptive reduction of, 137
Endometriomas, 177
Endometriosis
adhesions in, 177
definition of, 176, 177
diagnosis of, 176, 204
epidemiology of, 176
etiology of, 176t
extrapelvic, 179
fertility and, 178–179
historical perspective on, 176
hysterectomy for, 178
incidence of, 176t
medical therapies for, 177t, 177–178
pain in, 177, 177t
pathogenesis of, 176–177
pathology of, 177
prevalence of, 176, 179
surgery for
aqua- or hydrodissection in, 205, 205f
laser ablation of implants, 205
surgical resection for, 179
pregnancy rates with, 179, 179f
symptoms of, 177, 177t
treatment of, 172–173
fecundity rate with, 172–173
Endometrium
ablation of
for dysfunctional uterine bleeding, 73
biopsy of
in infertility evaluation, 169
histologic changes during menstrual
cycle, 64f, 68
preparation for oocyte donation, 221f,
221–222
Endoscopic surgery
advantages versus disadvantages of,
203t
versus laparotomy, 202
Enzyme-linked assays for sperm
antibodies, 262
17β-Estradiol
in estrogen biosynthesis, 17, 17f
micronized, 111–112
Estrogen receptor, 19, 20t
Estrogen replacement therapy
schedules for, 105f
selected estrogens and starting doses,
105t
for vasomotor instability, 104
Estrogens
administration of
injectable, 110
transdermal, 110
vaginal, 110
biosynthesis of, 17
classes of, 110, 112t
conjugated, 112
derivation from androgens, 76, 77f

esterified, 112
in hair growth, 96–97, 97t
in oral contraceptives, 132, 132t
production of
gonadotropin-dependent, 76, 77f
peripheral gonadotropin-independent,
76, 77f
routes of administration of, 110
selected, 105t, 111–112
Estrone, 112
in estrogen biosynthesis, 17, 17f
Exercise
amenorrhea/anovulation from, 80
Exocytosis
process of, 7–8, 24

F
Fecundity
definition of, 171
with endometriosis treatment, 172t,
172–173
Female pseudohermaphroditism, 44t,
44–46
from congenital adrenal hyperplasia,
44–45
from gonadal development disorders,
45–46
from X0 monosomy, 45–46
Fertility
age-related decline in, 173t, 173–174,
174f
Fertilization, 151–151, 152f
intracytoplasmic sperm injection in,
219, 219f
Fetal alcohol syndrome, 244
Fibroids. *See* Myomas, uterine
Fimbrial expression
for unruptured ampullary gestation, 195
Flutamide
for hirsutism, 101
Folistatin
gonadal secretion and, 27, 27f
Follicles
atresia of, 34
classification of, 148
depletion of, 34
development of
FSH in, 152–153
hormonal control in, 152–153
fetal development of
gonadotropin-dependent, 34
gonadotropin-independent, 33–34
growth of, 148f, 148–149
maturation of, 147f, 148
number of
age-dependent, 149f
tertiary
meiosis in, 149–150, 150f, 151f
Follicle-stimulating hormone (FSH)
in amenorrhea evaluation, 82
effects of, 22
in follicular development, 152–153,
152–153
in follicular recruitment, 63, 63f
function of, 8–9
in late follicular phase of menstrual
cycle, 65–66

in puberty, 50, 50f, 51f
secretion of
gonadal protein hormones in, 26–27, 27f
in spermatogenesis, 156–157
surge of, 63f
synthesis, storage and release of, 24, 24f
Folliculogenesis, 145, 147, 147f. *See also* Follicles
Friberg agglutination test, for sperm antibodies, 262
FSH. *See* Follicle-stimulating hormone (FSH)

G

Galactorrhea
oral contraceptive-associated, 137
Gallstones
oral contraceptive-associated, 137
Gamete intrafallopian transfer (GIFT)
age-dependent outcome in women age 40 and older, 217t
definition of, 214
1993 outcome rates with, 215t
pregnancy rates in women over age 40, 216t
GAP. *See* Gonadotropin-associated protein (GAP)
Gastrointestinal tract endometriosis, 179
Gel electrophoresis, 272, 273f
Genes
base sequences in, 270, 270f
expression of, 270, 271
identification of errors and differences in, 274–275, 276r
prenatal diagnosis of, 277
mRNA molecule from, 271
signals and markers in, 270, 270f
transcription and translation by, 270
tRNA from, 271
types of abnormalities in, 276t
Gene therapy, 279
Genetic diagnosis
preimplantation
embryo biopsy for, 220f, 220–221
fluorescent in situ hybridization technique in, 221
polymerase chain reaction testing in, 220, 221
Genital duct embryology, 38, 39f, 182, 183f, 184f
Genitalia
ambiguous
differential diagnosis of, 46f, 47
evaluation of, 46f, 46–47
embryology of, 39–40, 40f
Genome imprinting
for genetic disorders, 278–279, 279t
Germ cells (oogonia)
migration of, 144
number of, 144, 146f
proliferation of, 144
Gestagens. *See* Progestins
Gestrinone
for endometriosis, 178
GH. *See* Growth hormone

GIFT. *See* Gamete intrafallopian transfer (GIFT)
Glucagon stimulation test
for ACTH deficiency, 121t, 126
Glucocorticoid receptor, 19–20, 20t
Glucocorticoids
adjunctive with clomiphene citrate, 233
Glucose
serum
estrogen effect on, 136
Glucose suppression test
for growth hormone excess, 123t, 127
GnRH. *See* Gonoadotropin-releasing hormone (GnRH)
GnRH-A. *See* Gonadotropin-releasing hormone analogs (GnRH-A)
Gonadotropin-associated protein (GAP)
in prolactin secretion, 86, 88t
Gonadotropin deficiency
clinical syndrome and etiologies of, 116–117, 118t
clomiphene stimulation test for, 117, 119t
GnRH stimulation test for, 116–117, 119t
Gonadotropin-ovarian interaction
in follicular maturation and steroidogenesis, 77f
Gonadotropin receptor system
components and action of, 25, 25f
Gonadotropin-releasing hormone analogs (GnRH-A)
for hirsutism, 101
Gonadotropin-releasing hormone (GnRH)
for dysfunctional uterine bleeding, 72–73
gonadotropin responses to, 227
historical perspective on, 226, 227
mechanism of action of, 24, 24f
native, 226
in puberty, 50, 50f, 51f
pulsatile secretion of, 8–9
receptor interaction with, 226, 227f
Gonadotropin-releasing hormone (GnRH) agonists, 227t, 227–228
adverse reactions to, 229, 229t
clinical applications of, 228–229, 229t
for endometriosis, 178
for ovarian hyperstimulation, 216, 217t
for precocious puberty, 58
Gonadotropin-releasing hormone (GnRH) antagonist
for ovarian hyperstimulation, 216–217, 217t
Gonadotropin-releasing hormone (GnRH) antagonists, 227t, 228
in clinical use, 228t
response to, 228, 228f
Gonadotropins
circulating
chemistry of, 22t
half-life of, 23t
mechanism of action of
stimulatory cascade, 25, 25f, 26f
inhibitory cascade, 25, 26f
sialic acid content of, 23t
Gonads

development of, 38, 38f
dysgenesis of
mixed, 43–44
XX, 46
XY, 43
failure of
amenorrhea/anovulation in, 81
peptides of, 25–27, 27f, 28f
glycosylation of, 22, 22t
in regulation of ovarian function, 28f
G protein
in gonadotropin action, 25, 26f
Granulosa cell
in folliculogenesis, 147f, 148
Growth factors
decidual
in pregnancy immunotolerance, 163t, 163–164
Growth hormone (GH)
deficiency of, 117, 118t, 126
insulin challenge test for, 119t
L-dopa stimulation test for, 119t
stimulation tests for, 119t
excess production of. *See* Acromegaly
in pubertal development, 50–51
Growth hormone-releasing hormone (GHRH) stimulation test
for gonadotropin deficiency, 117–118, 119t
for growth hormone deficiency, 119t

H

Hair disorders. *See* Hirsutism
from androgen excess
postmenopausal, 106
Hair follicle
growth and development of, 96, 96f
pilosebaceous unit of, 96, 96f
Hair growth
sex steroid effects on, 96–97
HCG. *See* Human chorionic gonadotropin (hCG)
Hematocolpos, 186, 186f
Hemorrhage
from dysfunctional uterine bleeding
treatment of, 72
Hermaphroditism. *See* Pseudohermaphroditism; True hermaphroditism
Hirsutism
diagnosis of, 97, 98t
differential diagnosis of, 98t, 98–100
evaluation in, 97–98
idiopathic, 98, 98t
laboratory assessment for, 97–98, 99t
pharmacotherapy for, 100–101
in pregnancy, 100
versus virilization, 96, 96t
Histocompatibility (MHC) antigen
expression of
trophoblast limitation of, 162
hMG. *See* Human menopausal gonadotropin (hMG)
HSG. *See* Hysterosalingography (HSG)
Human chorionic gonadotropin (hCG)
adjunctive with clomiphene citrate, 233–234

biosynthesis of, 23f, 23–24, 233t
apoprotein synthesis in, 23, 23f
assembly in, 24
glycosylation in, 23f, 23–24
steps in, 22f, 23t
cancer risk with, 237
effects of, 22, 22f
measurements for ectopic pregnancy, 193–194, 194f, 194t
ovulation induction with
complications of, 236–237
evaluation for, 235
results of therapy, 237–238, 238f
treatment protocol for, 235–236
Human chorionic gonadotropin (hCG) test
for hyperandrogenism, 125t, 128
Human genome project
molecular biology in, 278
Human menopausal gonadotropin (hMG)
for chronic anovulatory infertility, 173
for ovarian hyperstimulation, 216, 217t
11β-Hydroxylase deficiency, 45
17α-Hydroxylase deficiency, 41f, 42, 45, 54t, 55
21-Hydroxylase deficiency, 44–45
3β-Hydroxysteroid dehydrogenase deficiency, 41f, 42, 45
17β-Hydroxysteroid dehydrogenase deficiency, 42
Hyperandrogenism
clinical syndrome in, 124t
suppression tests for, 125t, 128–129
Hypergonadotropic hypogonadism, 54t, 54–55
Hyperprolactinemia
clinical presentation of, 89
clinical syndrome in, 122t, 127
idiopathic, 88
imaging studies of pituitary for, 90, 90t
laboratory evaluation of, 89t, 89–90
pathologic causes of, 86–88, 88t
pharmacotherapy for, 90–91, 91f
physiologic causes of, 88–89
during pregnancy, 92
radiotherapy for, 91–92
suppression tests for, 123t, 127
surgery for, 91, 91f
Hypertension
estrogen replacement therapy and, 108
oral contraceptive-associated, 136
Hyperthyroidism
clinical syndrome in, 122t, 127
suppression tests for, 122t
Hypogonadotropic delayed puberty, 54t, 55
Hypogonadotropic hypogonadism
amenorrhea/anovulation from, 80
tumor-induced, 83
Hypothalamic hypopituitarism
amenorrhea/anovulation from, 80
Hypothalamus
anatomy of, 4–6
developmental changes in, 51f
hormones of
delivery of, 5f
hypothalamohypophsial blood vessels and, 4, 5f

intrahypothalamic neural connections of, 4
nuclei of, 4, 5f
Hypothalamus-pituitary axis
circulation of, 5f, 8
function of, 8
menstrual cyclicity and, 8–9
Hypothalamus-pituitary-ovarian (HPO) axis, 4–9
hormone interrelationships in follicular recruitment, 63f, 64
Hypothalamus-pituitary unit, 4, 4f
Hypothyroidism. See Thyroid stimulating hormone (TSH) deficiency
Hysterectomy
for cornual ectopic pregnancy with hemorrhage, 196
for dysfunctional uterine bleeding, 73
for endometriosis, 178
Hysterosalpingography (HSG)
algorithm for use with infertile couples, 203f
comparison with surgical findings, 202, 202t
in diagnosis of pelvic disease, 202
in infertility evaluation, 169

I
ICSI. See Intracytoplasmic sperm injection (ICSI)
Immune response
antibodies in, 250–252
antigens in, 249, 256
cellular, 256–258, 257f
cytokines in, 252–256
effector cells and, 248t, 248–249
humoral, 256, 256f
major histocompatibility complex in, 249f, 249–250, 250f
Immunobead technique for sperm antibody testing, 262
Immunogens
hCG-specific, 263t, 263–264
sperm-specific, 264
zona pellucida-specific, 264
Immunoglobulin(s)
classification and properties of, 250, 251t
functions of, 250–251
IgA, 251, 251t
IgD, 251, 251t
IgE, 251–252
IgG, 250–251
IgM, 251
structure of, 250, 251f
Immunology of pregnancy. See Immunotolerance of pregnancy
Immunotolerance of pregnancy
immunosuppression by pregnancy-associated factors, 259–260
trophoblast regulation of, 162–164
Immuntolerance of pregnancy
antiphospholipid antibodies in, 261
immunosuppression by pregnancy-associated factors in, 259f, 259–260

induction of trophoblast antigen expression in, 261
selective antigen expression in, 258–259
theories for, 258
trophoblast resistance to immune effector cells in, 259
Imperforate hymen
surgery for, 184
Implantation
adhesion molecules and, 164–165
definition of, 160
placenta and, 160–162
Infertility
adjunctive, 170t
definition of, 168
endometriosis in, 178–179
surgery for, 179, 179f
etiology of, 168, 168t
immunologic
female, 262–263
male, 261–262
management algorithm for, 170f
prevalence of subfecundity and, 168
testing for
male factor in, 168
ovulation factor in, 168–169
strategy for, 170–171
timing of studies in, 169–170
tuboperitoneal evaluation in, 169
uterine factors in, 169
tests for
basic, 170t
treatment of
male factor, 171–172, 172t
measures of success and, 171, 172t
for ovulation defects, 173
in tubal disease, 172–173
for unexplained infertility, 173
treatment outcomes in, 171, 172t
uterine factors in, 169
Inhibin
and gonadal secretion, 26–27, 27f
Insemination
for male factor infertility
donor, 172
homologous, 171–172, 172t
In situ hydridization, 273
Insulin challenge test
for ACTH deficiency, 121t, 126
for growth hormone deficiency, 119t
Insulin growth factor (IGF-I)
in pubertal development, 51
Insulin-induced hypoglycemia
in suppression testing for prolactin excess, 123t, 127
Integrins
behaviors of, 164
in extracellular matrix binding, 164f
in reproduction, 164t, 164–165
Interception (postcoital contraception), 139
Interferons (IFNs)
action of, 255–256
characteristics and principal activity of, 252t
Interleukin(s)
characteristics and functions of, 252t
IL-1, 252–253

IL-2, 252t, 253
IL-3, 253
IL-4, 253
IL-5, 253–254
IL-6, 254
IL-7, 254
IL-8, 254
IL-9, 254
IL-10, 254–255
IL-11, 255
IL-12, 255
IL-13, 255
Intracytoplasmic sperm injection (ICSI)
   comparison with subzonal insemination,
      219
Intrauterine synechiae
   surgery for, 208
In vitro fertilization (IVF)
   definition of, 214
   embryo transfer in, 218
   fertilization in, 217
   incubation of inoculated oocytes,
      217–218, 218f
   medications for ovarian
      hyperstimulation in, 216–217, 217f
   oocyte retrieval in, 217, 217f, 218f
   1993 outcome rates with, 215t
   pre-embryo stage in, 217–218
   semen collection in, 217
   stimulation protocols in, 216–217
IVF. See In vitro fertilization (IVF)

K
Karyotyping, 274–275, 276t

L
Lactation
   hyperprolactinemia in, 88, 89f
   oral contraceptive effect on, 138
Laparoscopy
   in infertility evaluation, 169
Laser versus electrosurgery, 202–203
Late onset adrenal hyperplasia (LOAH)
   adrenal stimulation test for, 125t,
      128–129
L-dopa
   suppression of
      in hyperprolactinemia, 123t, 127
Leiomyoma
   surgery for
      indications for, 206
Leydig cell hypoplasia, 44
LH. See Luteinizing hormone (LH)
   in amenorrhea evaluation, 82
   in follicular recruitment, 63, 63f
   in late follicular phase of menstrual
      cycle, 65–66
   in puberty, 50, 50f, 51f
   in spermatogenesis, 156–157
   surge of, 63f, 65
   synthesis, storage and release of, 24, 24f
Lipoproteins
   cardiovascular risk and, 108
   structure of, 13, 14f
Liquor folliculi, 149
LOAH. See Late onset adrenal hyperplasia
      (LOAH)

Luteinizing hormone (LH)
   effects of, 22
   function of, 8–9
Luteoma of pregnancy
   hirsutism from, 100
Lymphatic/hematogenous transport theory
   of endometriosis, 177
Lymphocyte(s)
   B lymphocyte, 248, 248t
   classification of, 248t, 248–249
   natural killer cells, 248t, 248–249
   T lymphocyte, 248, 248t

M
Macrophages, 249
Major histocompatibility complex (MHC)
   class I and class I antigens in
      comparison of, 249t
   class II molecules
      structure of, 249f
   class I molecules in
      function of, 249–250, 250
      structure of, 249f
Male factor dysfunction
   evaluation of, 168, 168t
   incidence of, 168
Male factor infertility
   effect on IVF outcome, 215, 216t
Male hermaphroditism
   from androgen deficiency, 41f, 41–42
   from androgen insensitivity, 42–43
   from Mullerian inhibiting substance
      defects, 43
   from deficient testosterone conversion,
      43
   from gonadal formation errors, 43–44
McCune-Albright syndrome
   peripheral precocious puberty from, 57
Medications
   hyperprolactinemia from, 88
   recurrent pregnancy loss from, 244
Medroxyprogesterone acetate (MPA)
   for dysfunctional uterine bleeding, 72
   for precocious puberty, 59
Meiosis
   cellular division during, 144, 146f
   inhibitors of, 150, 151f
   phases in, 144, 146f
Menarche, 53
Menopause
   breast tenderness in, 113
   cardiovascular disease in, 107–108
   changes in, 104–108
   climacteric syndrome in, 104
   clinical tips for, 112–114
   contraception during, 113–114
   definition of, 104
   endocrinology of, 104
   hormone replacement therapy in,
      108–112
      compliance with, 109–110
      contraindications to, 109, 110t
      cost and benefit of, 114
      estrogen, 105t, 110, 111–112, 112t
      evaluation for, 109, 111t
      indications for, 108–109
      progestins, 107t, 110–111, 112, 112t

      treatment regimens for, 105f, 105t,
         111
   inappropriate uterine bleeding during,
      113
   osteoporosis in, 106–107
   psychological changes in, 105
   sexual function in, 106
   skin and hair disorders in, 106
   smoking cessation in, 113
   therapy for, 112–113
   urogenital atrophy in, 105–106
   vasomotor instability in, 104–105, 111f
Menotropins. See also Human chorionic
      gonadotropin (hCG)
   commercially available, 235
   historical perspective on, 235
Menstrual cycle
   endometrial changes in
      late proliferative, 67
      postmenstrual, 67
   follicular phases of
      follicle selection, 64, 64f
      late (gonadotropin surge and
         ovulation), 64f, 64–66, 65f
      recruitment, 63f, 63–64, 64f
   luteal phase of
      postovulatory, 66
      premenstrual, 66–67
   ovarian
      in fertility test timing, 169–170, 170f
   ovulation in, 64f, 65, 65f
   uterine changes in
      late luteal phase, 68
      luteal phase, 67–68
   uterine events in, 64f, 67
Menstruation
   cyclicity of
      hypothalamic-pituitary axis in, 8–9
   recurrence of
      with estrogen replacement therapy,
         109, 110
   reflux
      endometriosis and, 176
Mesonephric (Wolffian) ducts, 182, 183f,
      184f
Metabolism
   alterations in
      hyperprolactinemia from, 88
Methotrexate
   for unruptured ectopic pregnancy, 198
Metoclopramide stimulation test
   for prolactin deficiency, 117, 119t
Metroplasty
   hysteroscopic
      for uterine septum, 207–208
Metyrapone stimulation test
   for ACTH deficiency, 121t, 126
MFP. See Multifetal pregnancy (MFT)
MHC. See Major histocompatibility
      complex (MHC)
Mineralocorticoid biosynthesis, 15, 15f, 16
Mineralocorticoid receptor, 20, 20t
Miscarriage. See Recurrent pregnancy loss
Mitosis
   phases in, 144, 145f
Molecular technology(ies)
   applications of

current, 276t, 276–278
future, 278–279
DNA and RNA identification, 271–274
identification of genetic errors and
differences, 274–276
Monocytes, 249
Mosaicism, 45–46
Mullerian agenesis (Rokitansky-Kuster-
Hauser syndrome), 187
McIndoe vaginoplasty for, 187–188
nonoperative vaginal construction in, 187
presentation of, 187
Mullerian anomalies
amenorrhea from, 81
in infertility evaluation, 169
Mullerian ductal system
congenital anomalies of, 182–188
associated heritable disorders in, 185t
classification of, 182, 185f
imperforate hymen, 184
incidence of, 182
obstetric consequences of, 188–189,
189t
obstructive, 182, 184, 185t
surgery for, 189
uterine cervix, 188
vaginal, 184–188
embryology of, 182, 183f, 184
obstructive fusion defect of, 188
Mullerian inhibiting substance (MIS), 38f,
40–43
Multifetal pregnancy (MFP)
following human chorionic
gonadotropin-stimulated ovulation,
237
Myomas
uterine
recurrent pregnancy loss from, 242,
242t
Myomectomy
indications for, 206
techniques in, 206

N
Naloxone
effect on GnRH release, 9
Natural killer (NK) cells
in cell-mediated immunity, 257–258,
258f
functions of, 248t, 248–249
Neoplasm(s)
adrenal and ovarian
precocious puberty from, 57, 57f
oral contraceptive-associated, 137
pituitary
hyperprolactinemia from, 86–88
Neosalpingostomy
for distal tubal occlusion, 204, 205f
Neurohypophysis. See Posterior pituitary
(neurohypophysis)
Neuropeptides
in psychological changes of menopause,
105
NK. See Natural killer (NK) cells
Nomifensine
nonsuppression with prolactinomas,
123t, 127

Nonsteroidal antiinflammatory drugs
(NSAIDs)
for dysfunctional uterine bleeding, 72
Norgesterone
for dysfunctional uterine bleeding, 72

O
OHS. See Ovarian hyperstimulation
syndrome (OHS)
Oocyte
meiosis of, 31–33, 32f
regulators of, 33f
Oocyte donation
age and, 222
uterine preparation for, 221f, 221–222
Oocyte maturation inhibitor (OMI), 32–33,
33f, 150, 151f
Oogenesis. See also Folliculogenesis
meiosis in, 144, 146f
mitosis in, 144, 145f
Oogonia. See Germ cells (oogonia)
Oral contraceptives
components of, 132t, 132–133
contraindications to, 138t
drug interaction with and pregnancy,
138–139
for dysfunctional uterine bleeding, 72
effects of
cardiovascular, 135–136
endocrine, 136
galactorrhea, 137
gastrointestinal, 136–137
metabolic, 135
postpill amenorrhea, 137
for endometriosis, 177t, 178
formulations currently available, 133,
134t
for hirsutism, 100
historical perspective and, 132
initiation of, 138–139
for interception (postcoital
contraception), 139
mechanism of action of, 133–135
missed dose of, 138, 138t
neoplasia and, 137
noncontraceptive benefits of, 137t,
137–138
progestin-only pill for, 140
response to
in hyperandrogenism, 125t, 128
risk factors with, 138t
selection of, 132
side effects of, 139
Osteoporosis
postmenopausal
calcium and exercise for, 107
drugs for, 107
hip fracture from, 106
risk for, 107–108, 109t
tamoxifen for, 107
risk factors for, 109t
Outflow tract defects
amenorrhea from, 81
Ovarian hyperstimulation syndrome
(OHS)
classification of, 236–237, 237t
etiology of, 236, 237f

human chorionic gonadotropin-induced,
236
Ovary(ies)
anatomy and function of, 8
androgen production by, 97, 97f
androgen-secreting tumors of
hirsutism from, 100
coelemic epithelial cells of, 30
embryogenesis of, 30f, 30–31
embryology of, 38, 38f
historical perspective on, 30
mesenchymal cells of, 30
premature failure of
causes of, 81, 81t
primordial germ cells of
migrational path of, 30f, 30–31
time line of, 31f
Ovulation, 64f, 65, 65f
clomiphene citrate-induced
rates of, 235, 235t
dysfunctional
evaluation of, 168–169
human chorionic gonadotropin-induced,
236, 236f
induction of
clomiphene citrate for, 232–235
menotropins for, 235–238
patient selection for, 232
induction rates for
with menotropin therapy, 237
WHO classification of, 231, 232
Oxytocin
secretion and release of, 5f, 7, 7f

P
Pain
in endometriosis, 177
Paramesonephric (Mullerian) ducts, 182,
183f, 184f. See also Mullerian
ductal system
PCOS. See Polycystic ovary syndrome
(PCOS)
Pelvic adhesions
infertility and
treatment of, 172
lysis of, 203–204, 204f
prevention of, 203
surgical adjuvants for, 203, 204f
surgery for, 203–204, 204f
Pelvic disease. See also Reproductive
surgery
diagnosis of, 202
hysterosalpingography for, 202, 202t,
203f
Pergolide
for hyperprolactinemia, 91
Persistent ectopic pregnancy, 196–197
after conservative surgery, 209
Pituitary. See Anterior pituitary; Posterior
pituitary
developmental changes in, 51f
imaging studies of
in hyperprolactinemia, 90, 90t
secretion of LH and FSH by, 8–9
tumors of
amenorrhea/anovulation from, 80
Placenta

comparative development of, 160–161
functions of, 160
genesis of, 160
Grossner classification of, 161, 162t
human hemomonochorial villous
    structure, 162, 162f, 163f
regulatory factors in, 163t, 163–164
Polycystic ovary syndrome (PCOS)
androgens in, 76
anovulation in, 76
differential diagnosis of, 79
genesis of, 78–79, 79f
hirsutism in, 98, 98t
SHBG metabolism in, 78
Polymerase chain reaction, 274, 276f
Porcine follicular fluid (pFF)
in vitro inhibition of FSH, 26, 26f
Posterior pituitary (neurohypophysis), 5f,
    6, 6t
anatomy of, 5f, 7, 7f
hormones of, 7, 7f
Precocious puberty
central (gonadotropin-dependent),
    55–56
combined, 57
differential diagnosis of, 57t
evaluation of, 57, 58f
peripheral (gonadotropin-independent),
    57
treatment of, 58–59
Pregnancy
molecular techniques, 277
prenatal diagnosis of genetic disorders,
    277
Pregnancy loss
chromosomal anomalies and, 240–241,
    241t
genetic component of, 240–241,
    241t
incidence of, 240
recurrent
    from acquired uterine defects, 242,
        242t
    age-associated, 244
    causes and incidences of, 241t
    from chromosomal rearrangements,
        242–243
    counseling and follow-up in, 245
    from environmental toxins, 244
    evaluation in, 244–245, 245t
    from immunologic infertility, 244
    from infection, 243–244
    from pharmacologic toxins, 244
    from progesterone deficiency, 243
    from systemic disease, 243
    therapies for, 245, 245t
    from uterine anomalies, 241–242,
        242t
Premature ovarian failure, 54t, 55
Prenancy. See also Recurrent pregnancy
    loss
criteria for, 240
cumulative probability of, 171
hirsutism in, 100
hyperprolactinemia in, 92
immunotolerance of. See
    Immunotolerance of pregnancy

oral contraceptive inhibitory mechanism
    and, 134
rates of
    clomiphene citrate-induced, 235, 235t
    with menotropin therapy, 237–238
Progestagens. See Progestins
Progesterone
biosynthesis of, 15, 16f
deficiency of
    recurrent pregnancy loss from, 243
monitoring of
    for ectopic pregnancy, 194, 195f
serum measurements of
    in infertility evaluation, 169
synthesis of, 8
Progesterone receptor, 19, 20t
Progestins
adverse effects of, 133
in hair growth, 97, 97t
menopausal replacement, 110–111
    natural progesterone, 111, 112t
    selected and dosages of, 107t, 112,
        112t
    synthetic, 111, 112t
in oral contraceptives, 132t, 132–133
pharmacokinetics of, 133
Progestin withdrawal test
in amenorrhea evaluation, 82
estrogen-stimulated
    in amenorrhea evaluation, 82
Prolactin
in amenorrhea evaluation, 82
deficiency of, 117, 118t
    chlorpromazine stimulation test for,
        119t
    insulin-induced hypoglycemia test for,
        119t
    metoclopramide stimulation test for,
        119t
    stimulation tests for, 119t
    thyrotropin-releasing hormone
        stimulation test for, 117, 119t
excess of
    tumor-induced, 82–83
excess production of. See
    Hyperprolactinemia
secretion of
    circadian, 86, 86f, 88
    dimeric and polymeric, 86, 87f
    regulators of, 86, 88t
    stimulation of, 86
Prolactinomas
surgery for, 91, 91f
Prostaglandin
local injection of
    for unruptured ectopic pregnancy, 198
Protestogens. See Progestins
Proximal tubal occlusion
cannulation and balloon tuboplasty for,
    207
resection in, 206
tubal anastomosis of, 206–207, 207t
Pseudocyesis
amenorrhea/anovulation in, 79
Pseudohermaphroditism. See also Female
    hermaphroditism; Male
    hermaphroditism

female, 44t, 44–46
male, 41t, 41–44
Pseudomenopause
for endometriosis, 178
Pseudovaginal perineoscrotal hypospadias.
    See 5α-Reductase deficiency
    syndrome
Pubarche, 53
Puberty
breast development in, 52, 52f–53
delayed, 53–55. See also Delayed
    puberty
linear growth in, 50–51
onset of, 50
    anatomic components of, 50f
precocious. See Precocious puberty
pubic hair development in, 53
Pulmonary endometriosis, 179
Purines, 268, 268f
Pyrimidines, 268, 268f

Q
Quinagolide
for hyperprolactinemia, 91

R
Radioimmunoassays for sperm antibodies,
    262
Recombinant medication, 279
Recurrent pregnancy loss
documentation of, 240
genetic component of, 240–241
molecular techniques and, 277
incidence of, 240
5α-Reductase deficiency syndrome, 43
Reproduction
age impact on, 173t, 173–174, 174f
Reproductive surgery
adhesion prevention in, 203, 204t
for distal tubal occlusion, 204
for ectopic pregnancy, 208–209
for endometriosis, 204–205
endoscopic versus laparotomy, 202,
    203t
indications for, 202
for intrauterine synechiae, 208
laser versus electrosurgery, 202–203
for leiomyoma, 206
for pelvic adhesion, 203–204
principles of, 202–203
for proximal tubal occlusion, 206–207,
    207t
reoperation versus second-look
    procedures, 209-211
for salpingitis isthmica nodosa, 206,
    206f
for sterilization reversal, 207
for uterine septum, 207–208
Resection
for proximal tubal pregnancy, 195–196
Restriction endonucleases
in genetic diagnosis, 271–272, 272f
Restriction length polymorphism,
    275–276, 277f
Ribonucleic acid. See RNA (ribonucleic
    acid)
RNA (ribonucleic acid), 271

identification. *See* DNA (deoxyribonucleic acid)
Rokitansky-Kuster-Hauser syndrome. *See* Mullerian agenesis (Rokitansky-Kuster-Hauser syndrome)

S
Salpingectomy, 194–195
  partial, 197f
Salpingitis isthmica nodosa
  hysterosalingogram of, 206f
  surgery for, 206
Salpingostomy
  for unruptured ampullary gestation, 195, 197f
Semen
  specimens
    for IVF, 217
Semen analysis
  for male infertility, 168, 168t
Septae
  uterine, 189, 189f, 207–208
    recurrent pregnancy loss from, 242
  vaginal, 186f, 186–187, 189
Sex differentiation
  male and female, 38, 38f, 39f, 40f
Sex hormone-binding globulin (SHBG)
  characteristics of, 78t
  function of, 77–78
  production of, 78
  testosterone binding by, 97
Sexual development. *See also* Pseudohermaphroditism
  disorders of
    ambiguous genitalia, 46–47
    causes of, 40, 40t
    pseudohermaphroditism, 41–45
  normal, 38–40
Sexual differentiation
  DNA diagnostic techniques and, 277–278
Sexual function
  CNS-releasing hormones in, 109t
SHBG. *See* Sex hormone-binding globulin (SHBG)
Skin disorders
  from postmenopausal androgen excess, 106
Smoking
  cessation in menopause, 113
  miscarriage from, 244
Sperm
  antibodies to. *See* Antisperm antibodies (AsAb)
  autoimmunity of, 262
Spermatid
  in spermiogenesis, 154f, 155, 156
Spermatocytes, 154, 154f
Spermatocytogenesis
  spermatocyte divisions in, 154f, 154–155
  spermatogonia in
    differentiation of, 154, 154f, 155f
Spermatogenesis, 153f
  definition of, 153
  fetal and postnatal, 153
  gonocytes in, 153, 153f

phases of, 153
  prespermatogonia in, 153, 153f
  process of, 154f, 154–155
  spermatocytogenesis in, 154f, 154–155, 155f
  spermatogonia in, 154, 154f, 155f
  spermiogenesis in, 154f, 155, 155f, 156f
Spermatogonia
  differentiation of, 154, 155f
  formation and division of, 154, 154f
Spermiation, 155
Spermiogenesis, 154f, 155f, 155–156, 156f
  hormonal control of, 156–156
  transformation of spermatid to spermatozoon, 155–156, 156f
Spironolactone
  for hirsutism, 100–101
Spontaneous abortion
  clinical, 240
  incidence of, 240
  unrecognized, 240
Steroid receptors
  characterization of, 19–20, 20t
Steroids
  biosynthesis of, 12, 13f
    cholesterol and, 13–15
  carbon content of, 12, 12t
  catecholestrogen metabolism in, 18f
  conjugation of, 17t
  cyclopentanophenanthrane ring and, 12, 12f
  elimination of, 17–18
    metabolic alternatives in, 17t
  glucocorticoid pathyway of, 12, 13f
  hormones of
    mechanisms of action of, 18–20
  mineralocorticoid pathway and, 12, 13f
  nomenclature for, 12–13
  numerical schema for, 12, 12f
  in regulation of ovarian function, 28f
  synthesis of
    cholesterol uptake and utilization in, 13–15
Steroid-steroid receptor interactions, 18–19, 19f
Stimulation tests, 116–117, 119t, 121t, 126, 128–129
  definition of, 116
  difficulties with, 116
  value of, 116
Stromal hyperthecosis
  hirsutism in, 98, 98t
Subzonal insemination (SUZI), 218
  comparison with intracytoplasmic sperm injection, 219
Suppression tests, 123t, 125t, 127–129
  definition of, 116
  difficulties with, 116
  value of, 116
SUZI. *See* Subzonal insemination (SUZI)
Swyer's syndrome (46,XY karyotype)
  diagnosis of, 54
  hormone replacement for, 54–55
Synctiotrophoblast
  in immunotolerance of pregnancy, 259

T
TBG. *See* Thyroid-binding globulin (TBG)
Testis(es)
  embryology of, 38, 38f
Testolactone
  for precocious puberty, 59
Testosterone, 15, 16f
  after bilateral ovariectomy, 113
  biosynthesis from cholesterol, 41, 41f
  for endometriosis, 178
  free and protein-bound, 97, 98f
  origin in normal women, 76, 78f
  production of, 97, 97f
  production rates of, 16t
TET. *See* Tubal embryo transfer (TET)
Tetraploidy
  in aborted pregnancies, 241
Theca
  in folliculogenesis, 147f, 148
Thoracic cage endometriosis, 179
Thromboembolism
  venous
    oral contraceptive-associated, 135–136
Thrombosis
  estrogen replacement therapy and, 108
Thymine, 268, 268f
Thyroid-binding globulin (TBG)
  estrogen effect on, 136
Thyroid function
  in amenorrhea evaluation, 82
Thyroid hormone
  excess production of. *See* Hyperthyroidism
Thyroid-stimulating hormone (TSH)
  deficiency, 117, 118t
  clinical syndrome in, 117, 118t
  thyrotropin-releasing hormone stimulation test for, 117, 119t
Thyrotropin-releasing hormone (TRH)
  for growth hormone excess, 123t, 127
  in prolactin secretion, 86
Thyrotropin-releasing hormone (TRH) stimulation test
  for prolactin deficiency, 117, 119t
  response in hyperthyroidism, 123t, 127
  for thyroid deficiency, 117, 119t
TPET. *See* Tubal pre-embryo transfer (TPET)
Translocation
  chromosomal
    recurrent pregnancy loss from, 243
TRH. *See* Thyrotropin-releasing hormone (TRH)
Triiodothyronine (T_3) suppression test
  for hyperthyroidism, 123t
Trisomy
  in aborted pregnancies, 241
  recurrent pregnancy loss from, 243
Trophoblast
  attachment to endometrium, 160, 160t, 161f
  in immunotolerance of pregnancy, 162–164, 163t
  enhanced function of, 260, 260f
  induction of antigen expression by, 261

resistance to immune effector cells, 259
secretion of immunoregulatory macromolecules by, 260
resistance to maternal effector cells, 162–163
Trophoblast HLA-G
in immunotolerance of pregnancy, 258–259
True hermaphroditism, 44
Tubal anastomosis
for proximal tubal occlusion, 206
for sterilization reversal, 207
technique for, 207, 208f
for tubal disease, 173
Tubal embryo transfer (TET), 214
Tubal pre-embryo transfer (TPET), 214
Tuboperitoneal disease
in infertility evaluation, 169
Turner's syndrome (XO monosomy), 45–46
in aborted pregnancies, 241
clinical features of, 45
diagnosis of, 45, 54
hormone replacement for, 54–55

U

Ultrasonography
transvaginal
for ectopic pregnancy diagnosis, 194, 194f
Unicoruate uterus, 185f
Ureterovaginal anomalies
obstetric consequences of, 188–189, 189t
Urethral syndrome, 106
Urinary incontinence, 106
Urinary tract endometriosis, 179
Uterine bleeding

dysfunctional. *See* Dysfunctional uterine bleeding (DUB)
during menopausal hormone therapy, 113
Uterine didelphys, 186f, 188
Uterus
acquired defects of
recurrent pregnancy loss from, 242, 242t
congenital anomalies of
classification of, 185f
diethylstilbestrol-induced, 242
obstetric outcome in, 189
recurrent pregnancy loss from, 242t, 242–242
curettage of, 73
dysfunctional bleeding from. *See* Dysfunctional uterine bleeding (DUB)
in infertility evaluation, 169
in menstruation, 67
postovulation changes in, 67–68
in prolactin production, 86
septum of
hysteroscopic metroplasty for, 207–208
transcervical hysteroscopic diversion for, 189, 189f
surrogate, 222
Uterus didelphys, 186f

V

Vagina
atresia of, 187, 187f
surgical outcome in, 189
atrophy of
menopausal, 105–106
longitudinal septum of, 186f, 186–187
transverse septum of, 184–186, 186f

associated hematocolpos in, 186, 186f
surgical outcome in, 189
surgical technique for, 185–186
symptoms of, 184
Vasoactive intestinal peptide (VIP)
in prolactin secretion, 86
Vasomotor disturbance
menopausal, 104–105
hormone replacement for, 104–105
LH elevation and, 111f
pharmacotherapy for, 105
Vasopressin
secretion and release of, 5f, 7, 7f
VIP. *See* Vasoactive intestinal peptide (VIP)
Virilization
hirsutism versus, 96, 96t

W

Weight gain
oral contraceptive-associated, 136
Wolffian ducts. *See* Mesonephric (Wolffian) ducts

X

XO monosomy. *See* Turner's syndrome (XO monosomy)

Z

ZIFT. *See* Zygote intrafallopian transfer (ZIFT)
Zona drilling
for fertilization, 218
Zona pellucida
in folliculogenesis, 147f, 148
Zygote intrafallopian transfer (ZIFT)
definition of, 214
1993 outcome rates with, 215t

ISBN 0-397-51186-8

9 780397 511860